Essentials *of* Neuroanatomy *for* Rehabilitation

Leah Dvorak
Concordia University Wisconsin

Paul Jackson Mansfield
Milwaukee Area Technical College

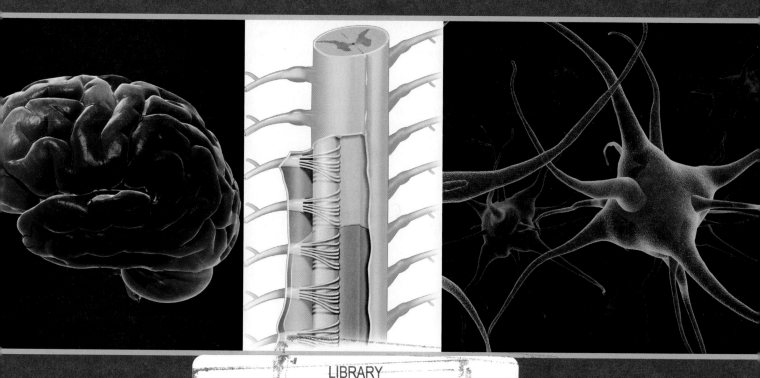

PEARSON

Boston Columbus Indianapolis New York San Francisco Upper Saddle River
Amsterdam Cape Town Dubai London Madrid Milan Munich Paris Montreal Toronto
Delhi Mexico City Sao Paulo Sydney Hong Kong Seoul Singapore Taipei Tokyo

Publisher: Julie Levin Alexander
Publisher's Assistant: Regina Bruno
Editor in Chief: Mark Cohen
Executive Editor: John Goucher
Editorial Project Manager: Melissa Kerian
Editorial Assistant: Erica Viviani
Development Editor: Marion Waldman, iD8 Triple SSS Press
Director of Marketing: David Gesell
Executive Marketing Manager: Katrin Beacom
Marketing Specialist: Michael Sirinides
Senior Managing Editor: Patrick Walsh
Project Manager: Patricia Gutierrez
Senior Operations Supervisor: Ilene Sanford

Operations Specialist: Lisa McDowell
Design Director: Andrea Nix
Art Director: Maria Guglielmo
Text and Cover Designer: Ilze Lemesis
Cover Art: Lateral view of the brain-3D4Medical/ Photo Researchers, Inc., Human brain neurons-CLIPAREA/Shutterstock Images
Media Editor: Amy Peltier
Lead Media Project Manager: Lorena Cerisano
Full-Service Project Management: Patty Donovan
Composition: Laserwords
Printer/Binder: R.R. Donnelley/Roanoke
Cover Printer: Lehigh-Phoenix Color/Hagerstown
Text Font: 10/12 Times Ten

Credits and acknowledgments for content borrowed from other sources and reproduced, with permission, in this textbook appear on appropriate page within text.

Library of Congress Cataloging-in-Publication Data
Dvorak, Leah.
  Essentials of neuroanatomy for rehabilitation / Leah Dvorak, Paul Jackson
Mansfield.—1st ed.
     p. ; cm.
  Includes bibliographical references and index.
  ISBN-13: 978-0-13-502388-4
  ISBN-10: 0-13-502388-2
 I. Mansfield, Paul Jackson.   II. Title.
  [DNLM: 1. Nervous System—anatomy & histology.   2. Nervous System Diseases—rehabilitation.
3. Nervous System Physiological Phenomena. WL 101]
  LC Classification not assigned
  612.8—dc23
                                                              2011045177

10 9 8 7 6 5 4 3 2 1

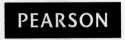

ISBN 10: 0-13-502388-2
ISBN 13: 978-0-13-502388-4

Dedication

This book is dedicated to my father, Earl A. Dvorak, for always encouraging and supporting my education.

—Leah

To Anne and Madilynn, you have shown a level of courage and perseverance that is unrivaled by anyone I know. And to my parents, I love you.

—Paul

Preface

Essentials of Neuroanatomy for Rehabilitation is intended to provide students with a solid foundation in the structure and function of the human nervous system. Our goal in writing this book was to make the incredibly complex and beautiful human nervous system as clear, transparent, and easy to understand as possible. We intend this text to be a prerequisite or corequisite for students in health care professions who are preparing to treat patients with neurological challenges. Hallmarks of this book include clear, lucid writing illuminated by simple, vivid artwork, along with clinical notes and patient case studies.

Why We Wrote *Essentials of Neuroanatomy for Rehabilitation*

Students in health care professions must digest a tremendous amount of information within a short time—typically only two or three years. The volume of information that is known about the nervous system is continually expanding. Mastering this large and complex body of knowledge is a daunting task for many students. Neuroanatomy is a necessary prerequisite for more advanced coursework in neurological assessment, evaluation, and treatment. Knowledge of the structure and function of the brain, spinal cord, and peripheral nervous system is both fundamental and vital to becoming a top-notch clinician. Furthermore, health care professionals are frequently called on to be patient educators; the ability to explain neurological signs and symptoms in a clear and accurate manner is critical for success in any clinical setting. To that end, we have written this text with three primary goals:

1. Clear, vivid, lucid writing that eliminates unnecessary detail and presents the most essential information
2. Clear, simple illustrations that make the material concrete and understandable
3. Clinical relevance, so that readers can apply the book's content to real patients and bring it to life

About This Book

This book uses the organizational scheme used by the authors over many years of effective teaching in neuroanatomy. Chapter 1 provides the book's context and describes the overall function of the nervous system, setting the stage for the rest of the text. Chapter 2 gives the reader an overview of basic brain and spinal cord structures. After completing this chapter, students will be able to identify the most important regions of the nervous system, as well as their supporting structures (skull and spine, meninges, and vascular supply). Chapters 3 and 4 contain relevant information about neurons and glial cells. Without excessive detail, these chapters allow students to grasp the basics of action potentials, synapses, and neurotransmitters. Chapters 5 through 9 provide the reader with the structure and function of the major structural nervous system subdivisions: cerebral cortex, diencephalon, brainstem, and spinal cord, as well as the peripheral nervous system. The autonomic nervous system follows in chapter 10, and chapters 11 through 14 address the major functional systems: general sensation, special sensation, movement (including the cerebellum and the basal ganglia), and cognition/emotion/behavior. Chapter 15 discusses how the nervous system develops, along with changes that occur with aging. Finally, chapter 16 is a summative chapter describing neuroplasticity. This chapter ties the text together and provides the biological context for changes that occur in the nervous system due to experience, and that form the basis of learning, healing, and growth.

Although this text is not intended to be a treatment book, clinically relevant examples are woven throughout the text in order to allow readers to connect the various brain regions and structures to real-life examples. Each chapter contains clinical boxes that discuss clinical pathologies relevant to chapter content, followed by challenge questions that ask students to apply their learning immediately. Chapters also contain neuroscience notes boxes that provide interesting pathological examples that illustrate the chapter content and stimulate interest in the chapter material. Summary tables called Review Concepts are sprinkled throughout, as needed, in order to effectively and efficiently organize complex material. Every chapter ends with patient scenarios. These simple patient cases are drawn from real-life situations and serve to bring the content to life. Each patient scenario concludes with several questions designed to allow students to apply chapter material to that patient. Each chapter also contains a list of key terms with definitions, and a series of review questions that instructors can use to stimulate class discussions or as brief homework assignments. The review questions also serve as a tool for students to check their learning; they should be able to answer the review questions if they have truly mastered the chapter material.

Distinctive Features of This Book

- *Outstanding artwork:* The art in this text is designed to be large, clear, and revealing. All relevant structures are included, yet no extraneous details clutter the images.
- *Clinical boxes with challenge questions:* These boxes apply important concepts to clinical situations, and ask the students to solve a question related to the topic.
- *Patient scenarios:* Real-world examples provide students with the opportunity to apply what they've learned.
- *Neuroscience notes:* Interesting clinical examples relevant to the study of neuroscience are featured.
- *Combined authorship:* The expertise of the two authors gained from over 30 combined years of teaching experience in neuroanatomy and neurology along with many related fields provides a rich blend of knowledge that informs this text.
- *Clear writing style:* This text strives for clarity of expression and understanding that is appropriate for students at all levels. Reviewers consistently commented on the outstanding writing style in the book.

Ancillary Materials for This Book

- PowerPoint presentations for each chapter, including all images (images are also available separately for instructors who wish to create their own PowerPoints)
- Question banks with short-answer, multiple-choice, and true/false questions for each chapter (making the preparation of quizzes or exams very simple)
- Student review questions in the same formats so that students can prepare for the real quiz or exam (this resource is found at www.myhealthprofessionskit.com)

Conclusion

This text is a valuable resource for instructors in a variety of health professions and academic settings who need a clearly written, engaging text that presents all relevant information related to neuroanatomy, yet does not overburden students with extraneous details. When neuroanatomy is presented in a clear and relevant format, students' mastery of this complex topic is enhanced. Ultimately, our goal is to promote the development of excellent clinicians across the health professions who are both competent practitioners and outstanding communicators.

About the Authors

The authors are both experienced educators who have taught a diverse population of health care students at all levels, from the associate (two-year) degree to the doctoral level.

Leah Dvorak holds a Ph.D. in anatomy and has taught neuroanatomy to students in physical therapy, occupational therapy, and physical therapy assistant programs for 17 years. She also teaches human gross anatomy, physiology, pathology, and pharmacology to physical therapy, occupational therapy, nursing, athletic training, pharmacy and physician assistant students. She has a strong grasp of the educational needs and challenges that face health care students. Dvorak is also a sought-after speaker for clinicians seeking continuing education in neuroanatomy; she combines clarity with humor and clinical relevance in her presentations.

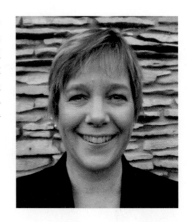

Paul Jackson Mansfield has practiced physical therapy for over 15 years, and is director of the Physical Therapy Assistant Program at Milwaukee Area Technical College. He teaches neurology to physical therapist assistant students, as well as numerous other courses, including musculoskeletal anatomy, kinesiology, orthopedics, and advanced therapeutic exercise. Mansfield continues to practice physical therapy and is engaged in the application of real-world clinical content to the courses he teaches. He has also coauthored a textbook for PTA students focused on anatomical kinesiology.

Together, the authors possess many years of teaching experience with the students who are the intended readers of this text. Their combined knowledge and experience represent a rich blend of classroom, laboratory, and clinical practice expertise, along with an in-depth understanding of the many challenges that health care students face when learning neuroanatomy. Both authors are themselves outstanding classroom teachers who value and exemplify teaching excellence and who use their knowledge of brain-based learning and neuroplasticity to inform and enhance their teaching.

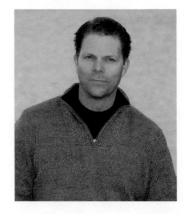

Acknowledgments

Thank you to my friends and colleagues, Dr. Terry Steffen and Dr. Kathryn Zalewski—both of whom made me believe I could teach neuroanatomy and write a book about it—for their many years of support and good advice. Mr. Alan Becker, M.S., P.T., provided many of the clinical patient scenarios used in this book, and was a constant source of encouragement; his dedication to life-long learning is an inspiration. Thanks are also due to the University of Wisconsin–Milwaukee and Concordia University Wisconsin for allowing me time to work on this project, and to my many friends and colleagues at both places. It is a pleasure to work with all of you! I am deeply grateful to Paul Jackson Mansfield who was an outstanding co-author and provided constant support and encouragement; I could not have completed this project without his valuable contributions. I give special thanks for their love and support to my family: Earl, Joy, Andy, Steph, and Michael, and to my husband Brad Condie, whose love never wavers. Finally, I thank all the many students I have taught: You are the reason I wrote this book. Never stop learning!

—Leah Dvorak

One of the primary components of being an excellent educator is the ability to break down complex subjects into easy-to-understand "nuggets" that not only interest and engage students but also excite them enough to want to push forward on their own. I am grateful to have the opportunity to thank the primary author of this text, Dr. Leah Dvorak, for bringing this brilliance to our book. Leah, thank you for your perseverance and friendship over the course of this project; I have learned so many things from you during this time. For that, I will always be grateful.

I also thank my family for their unending support. To my beautiful wife Heather—thank you for your continued inspiration and encouragement. I couldn't have done this without you. To my children, Rachael, Daniel, Megan, Hannah, and Beckett, thank you for the ongoing flow of hugs, smiles, and laughter that you bring into my life. One of the reasons I continue to do these types of projects is that I hope the profound love and respect I have for education—and learning in general—is somehow expressed by my commitment to teaching, learning, and sharing what I know.

—Paul Jackson Mansfield

Reviewers

Chris Barrett, PT, M.Ed.
Lake Area Technical Institute
Watertown, South Dakota

Marja P. Beaufait, MA, PT
St. Petersburg College
St. Petersburg, Florida

Linda Biggers, PT, MHS, CLT
University of Indianapolis
Indianapolis, Indiana

Peggy Block, PT, MHS
West Kentucky Community and Technical College
Paducah, Kentucky

Carey Bumgarner, PT, DPT
Jefferson College of Health Sciences
Community Hospital of Roanoke Valley
Roanoke, Virginia

Tammie L. Clark, PT, DPT
Nash Community College
Rocky Mount, North Carolina

Laurie Clute, PT, MS
New Hampshire Community Technical Community College
Claremont, New Hampshire

James Duley, MSPT, NCS
Delta College
University Center, Michigan

Susan Edelstein, PT, M.Ed
Broward College
Coconut Creek, Florida

Patricia A Erickson, PT, DPT
Colby Community College
Colby, Kansas

Mayra P. Eschbach, PT
Seminole State College
Altamonte Springs, Florida

Ruth Freeman, PT, M.Ed.
Concorde Career Institute
Jacksonville, Florida

Carla Gleaton, PT, M.Ed.
Kilgore College
Kilgore, Texas

Cosette Hardwick, PT, DPT, ACCE
Western Missouri State University
Joseph, Missouri

Patricia Harris, PT, MS
Sacramento City College
Sacramento, California

Joanne Howell, PT, M.Ed., DPT
Delaware Technical & Community College
Georgetown, Delaware

Kristen M. Johnson, PT, MS, NCS
San Diego Mesa College
San Diego, California

Becky Keith, PT, MSHS
Arkansas State University
State University, Arkansas

Allison Kellish, PT, MPA, DPT
Union County College
Plainfield, New Jersey

Malorie Kosht, PT, DPT
University of Pittsburgh at Titusville
Titusville, Pensylvania

Ken Mailly, PT
Essex County College
Newark, New Jersey

Paula Provence, PT, Med
Arapahoe Community College
Littleton, Colorado

Kathy Robert, CPTA, BS
Colby Community College
Colby, Kansas

Mary Ann Sharkey, Ph.D., MS, PT
Spokane Falls Community College
Spokane, Washington

Laurie Shimko, MPT
Concorde Career Institute
Jacksonville, Florida

Table of Contents

Essentials *of* Neuroanatomy *for* Rehabilitation

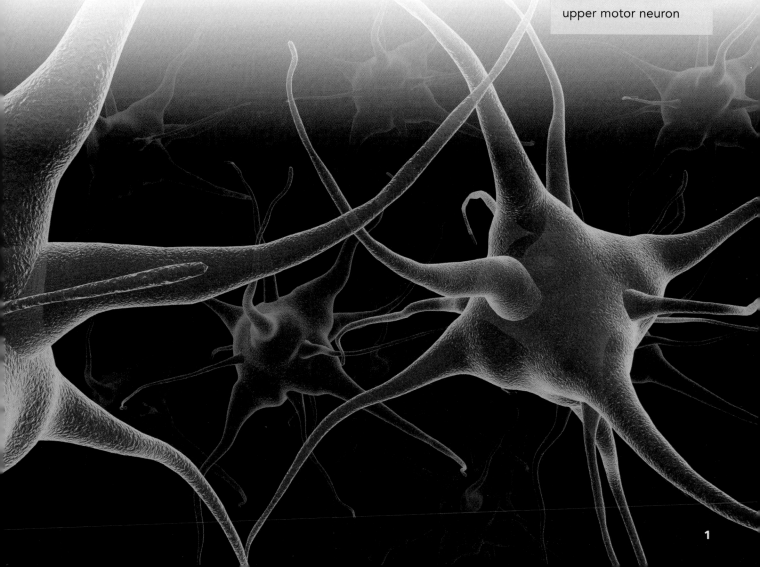

1

Introduction to Neuroanatomy

CHAPTER OBJECTIVES

After completing this chapter, the reader will be able to:

1. Discuss some key functions of the brain.

2. Explain why the brain is different from other organs in the human body (why it is unique to each person).

3. Describe the location of the spinal cord, indicate its functions, and discuss the major effects of spinal cord injury.

4. Identify the location of the peripheral nerves, and describe their general functions.

5. Define the term *neuroplasticity*.

KEY TERMS

autonomic neuron

central nervous system (CNS)

lower motor neuron

neuropathy

neuroplasticity

paralysis

paresis

peripheral nerve

peripheral nervous system (PNS)

proprioception

reflex

upper motor neuron

Essential Facts···

The nervous system is formed by the brain, the spinal cord, and the peripheral nerves.

▶ Thought, language, emotion, and sensation are processed in the brain.

▶ The brain controls the movement of the body.

▶ The brain is flexible and can modify its connections based on experience.

▶ The spinal cord connects the brain with the body.

▶ Peripheral nerves connect the body to the spinal cord and brain.

The brain is the body's most complex and amazing organ. It weighs about 3 pounds and contains over 10^{12} (1,000,000,000,000) nerve cells and even more supporting cells, all of which fit neatly inside the skull. The brain communicates with the body via the spinal cord and peripheral nerves. Together, they form the human nervous system. This system is essential for normal functioning of the human body. If you work in health care or rehabilitation, many of your patients will have diseases and disorders of the nervous system.

This book has been written to provide a simple, clear understanding of the structure and function of the nervous system. To become an effective clinician, you must have a solid understanding of the science behind the treatments you provide. In addition, the ability to explain the "why" of treatments to clients will improve your ability to communicate with and educate your patients. Often, the therapist, therapist assistant, or nurse is the person with whom patients and their families communicate most often concerning their diagnosis and prognosis.

The nervous system can be subdivided into the central nervous system and the peripheral nervous system (**Figure 1-1**). The **central nervous system (CNS)** consists of the brain and the spinal cord. The **peripheral nervous system (PNS)** is formed by cranial nerves (from the brain) and spinal nerves (from the spinal cord). Together, the CNS and PNS control body movement, regulate basic functions such as heart rate, respiration, and blood pressure, and detect sensation. The brain is also responsible for functions such as thought, emotion, and language: the so-called higher functions that are unique to human beings.

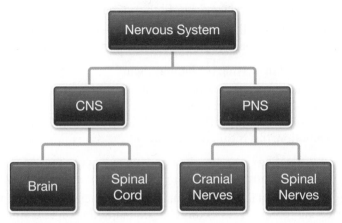

FIGURE 1-1 Divisions of the nervous system: central (CNS) and peripheral (PNS).

Overview: The Brain

The brain has many essential functions (see Figure 1-2). These functions will be described in detail later in this book, but for now, let's consider some of the specific functions of the brain:

- Perceiving and interpreting (understanding) sensations
  - We are only aware of pain, touch, taste, and so on, when these sensations reach the brain.
  - The brain permits us to understand and make sense of what we are experiencing.

- Generating movements that are functional and coordinated
  - The brain allows us to move when we choose to; this is called *voluntary* or *volitional movement.*
  - The brain is responsible for our ability to move efficiently and smoothly; damage or injury to the brain often results in uncoordinated movement.

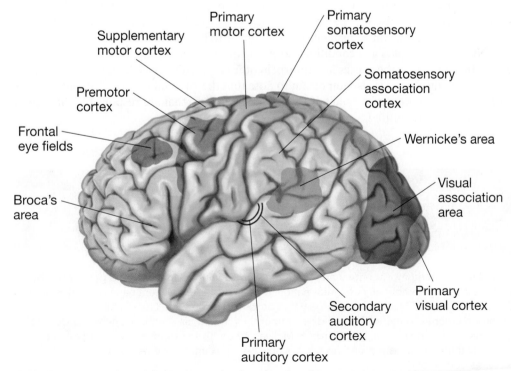

FIGURE 1-2 Overview of the brain's major functional regions.

- Understanding and producing language, both spoken and written
  - We are born with the ability to learn any language, but this ability lessens with age.
  - Sign languages and oral languages are learned using the same brain regions.

- Feeling emotions and displaying (or hiding) them
  - We often refer to our feelings as being located in our hearts, but that is because the brain affects the speed and strength of the heartbeat when we are "emotional."
  - People with disease or injury affecting the brain's emotional regions may feel little or no emotion; this is called *loss of affect.*

- Understanding ("reading") the emotions and behaviors of other people, and communicating with others nonverbally (using facial expressions and body language)
  - Brain regions involved in emotions connect to our facial muscles, so we can display our feelings on our faces; actors are good at faking these emotions!
  - The ability to understand other people's emotions and intentions is a very important component of social behavior.

- Thinking, planning, organizing, and problem solving
  - These abilities are often called the *executive functions,* and they are needed for independent adult life.
  - These functions are some of the last to develop when the brain matures.

- Controlling basic body functions like heart rate, blood pressure, digestion, respiration (breathing), sweating, shivering, urination, and defecation
  - These functions are partially automatic (such as control of blood pressure) and partly voluntary (such as urination)

- Creating, storing, and accessing memories, including facts and figures, our own life stories, and patterns of movements and behaviors
  - The ability to remember is central to your self-identity: Diseases such as Alzheimer's disease can profoundly affect memory, drastically changing "who" that person is.

The brain is the center of the self; it is the organ that makes each person unique. You can receive a new kidney, a new heart, or even have a face transplant and still be yourself, but if you received a brain transplant you would "become" the person whose brain you received. This is because that person's memories, personality, and mind are all centered in the brain. (Luckily, brain transplants do not appear to be on the horizon.)

Numerous diseases and conditions affect the brain, some of which are described in this book. In some cases, the causes are known; in other cases, scientists do not understand the cause of the disease. It is also important to note that the "mental illnesses" are all diseases of the brain. In some cases, specific regions and chemicals that are responsible for mental illnesses can be identified.

Neuroscience Notes Box 1-1:
Anterograde Amnesia

If the brain's memory centers are damaged due to injury or disease, the patient will be unable to remember any new information. In a classic case, a patient named Henry Molaison (known as H.M.) had brain surgery that produced a complete lack of ability to form any new memories. Although he could remember things from his childhood, he was unable to remember anything new afterwards. H.M. lived to be 82 years old. He was studied extensively throughout his life, and his brain is now being examined for clues about the cellular basis of memory.

Treatment of brain illnesses is not yet at the level of treatment of other body illnesses. The brain is a challenging organ for scientists and doctors to study, because so many of its functions are unique to human beings, and because its functions are so complex and interconnected. However, progress has been made in the development of new medications and other treatments for certain diseases. Medical researchers now know more about how movement and exercise can affect the brain. This knowledge can allow clinicians to develop more effective and functional treatments for patients who have diseases affecting the nervous system.

At one time it was believed that the brain was "fixed": after you became an adult, your brain's wiring was basically unchangeable. However, scientists now know that the human brain is actually quite flexible and adaptable; the brain's ability to reorganize is referred to as **neuroplasticity.** It means that the brain's wiring can change and modify itself based on life experiences. The ability to learn something new, and to "unlearn" something old, is based on neuroplasticity. In most cases, nerve cells in the brain (and spinal cord) cannot regrow (regenerate) if they are injured. However, the nervous system can find other ways to re-establish function after it is damaged. This is good news for clinicians who must design treatments to help patients. It means that well-designed therapies can help "rewire" the brain, allowing people to learn new ways of moving after brain injury or disease.

Overview: Spinal Cord

The spinal cord is a long cylindrical structure that runs from the top of the neck to the upper lumbar part of the spine (see **Figure 1-3**). At its thickest point it is about as wide as a thumb. The spinal cord contains long nerve fibers that interconnect the body's **peripheral nerves** with the brain. Peripheral nerves communicate with muscles, skin and subcutaneous tissue, and include both cranial nerves arising from the brain and spinal nerves arising from the spinal cord. Thus, the brain and body communicate via the spinal cord. Within the cord, neurons that connect the brain's movement centers to the peripheral nerves are known as **upper motor neurons.** Upper motor neurons control the activity of peripheral motor nerves (lower motor neurons; see below), and thereby control skeletal muscle and movement. Some nerve cells in the spinal cord are interconnected to form **reflexes,** which allow for very rapid, involuntary responses to sensations.

Injury to the spinal cord may cause two major problems:

1. Loss of feeling (sensory loss), because sensations such as touch or pain cannot travel from the body to the brain
2. Loss of movement **(paralysis),** because the brain cannot tell skeletal muscles when to move

Many spinal cord injuries are traumatic and result from accidents. Tumors and diseases of the spine can also injure the cord. Because the spinal cord is part of the central nervous system, it does not regenerate (re-grow) if it is damaged.

Overview: Peripheral Nerves

Peripheral nerves are located throughout the body and the head (see **Figure 1-4**). They send signals to and from the skin and subcutaneous (beneath the skin) tissue, the bones, joints and skeletal muscles, glands, and the internal organs. Peripheral nerves contain three

Neuroscience Notes Box 1-2:
Spinal Cord Injury

People who have suffered a spinal cord injury lose feeling and movement. As a result, they become vulnerable to developing decubitus ulcers (bedsores). These are caused by lack of mobility, which puts pressure on body parts where bones come into close contact with skin. Muscle atrophy (wasting) due to lack of movement makes the problem worse, as does the fact that patients may not be able to feel these sores. In some cases, they can be fatal; the actor Christopher Reeve died from complications of an infection caused by a bedsore.

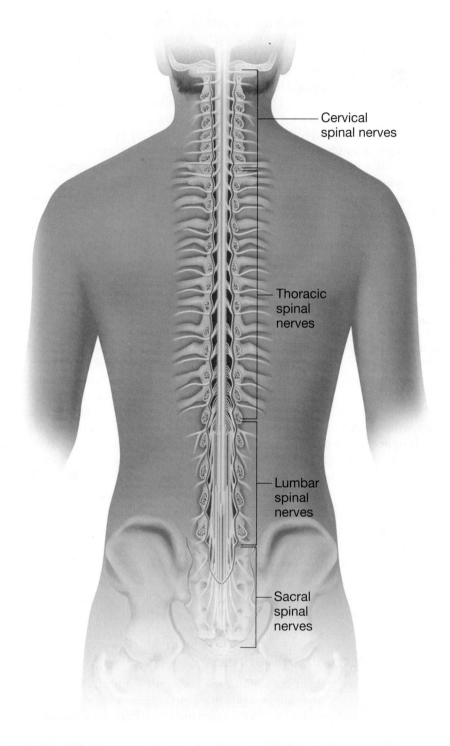

FIGURE 1-3 The spinal cord is located within the spinal column, and gives rise to the peripheral nerves.

kinds of nerve cells (neurons): (1) sensory nerve cells, (2) motor nerve cells, and (3) autonomic nerve cells. Peripheral nerves usually regenerate (re-grow) if they are damaged.

An important function of peripheral nerves is to detect and transmit sensations. They do this via sensory nerve cells (neurons). Some sensations originate outside the body, including:

- Smell (odor)
- Taste
- Sound
- Sight (vision)
- Touch (including pain, touch, pressure, temperature)

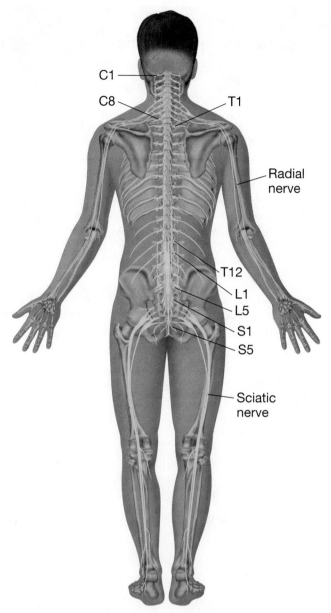

FIGURE 1-4 A posterior view of the spinal cord, spinal nerves, and some representative peripheral nerves.

These functions are essential for survival. For example, we must be able to recognize potential threats and dangers and determine what foods are good to eat and which are not.

Other sensations come from inside the body, including the following:

- Hunger, nausea, thirst
- Pain (from internal organs, bones, and joints)
- **Proprioception** (the body's position sense; your position and location in space)

Some of these sensations are conscious (we are aware of them—for example, hunger or thirst), whereas others are subconscious (such as proprioception). The sensory nerve cells transform all of these into nerve impulses that are sent to the spinal cord and brain for processing.

The peripheral nerves also control contraction of skeletal muscles via motor nerve cells (neurons). This control is necessary for normal movement. Injury to a peripheral nerve can impair the ability to move, causing paralysis or **paresis,** also known as muscle weakness. The motor neurons located in peripheral nerves are known as **lower motor neurons.** The brain controls the activity of lower motor neurons, and thus allows us to move voluntarily.

Some peripheral nerves regulate internal functions such as heart rate, blood pressure, and breathing rate; they also control digestion, elimination (defecation), urination, and sexual function. Peripheral nerves do this by sending signals from the brain and spinal

Neuroscience Notes Box 1-3: Diabetic Neuropathy

In people with diabetes, the high levels of blood glucose (blood sugar) produce chemicals that damage peripheral nerve fibers. This condition is called diabetic peripheral **neuropathy.** Peripheral neuropathy is felt first in the most distal (distant) body parts (the feet and the hands). In the early stages, people typically feel a constant, painful "pins and needles" feeling, most often in their feet. As the disease progresses, the painful sensations are replaced by numbness (a lack of feeling). This condition is dangerous because people may not realize that they have a foot injury (a blister or sore). Sores often fail to heal in people with diabetes, so neuropathy combined with poor wound healing may cause long-lasting sores as well as infections, and sometimes make amputation of a limb necessary. About half of all people with diabetes will develop peripheral neuropathy.

cord to internal organs, adjusting the contraction of smooth and cardiac (heart) muscle. The nerve cells that perform these functions are called **autonomic neurons.**

Peripheral nerves can be injured when:

- There is trauma to a body part (e.g., a crushing injury).
- They are compressed somewhere in the body (e.g., carpal tunnel syndrome in the wrist).
- They are damaged by disease (e.g., diabetes mellitus).

Review Questions

1. Which part of the nervous system is responsible for emotion, language, memory, and thought?

2. What kinds of nerve signals travel in the spinal cord? How would an injury to the spinal cord affect the ability to feel pain and to move muscles?

3. What are the primary functions of the peripheral nerves?

4. What is meant by the term *neuroplasticity*?

Further Reading

1. Damasio, A. (2010). *Self comes to mind.* New York: Pantheon Books.

2. Gazzaniga, M. S. (2008, June/July). Spheres of influence. *Scientific American Mind*, pp. 33–39.

3. Pinker, S. (2007). *The stuff of thought: Language as a window into human nature.* New York: Viking Penguin.

4. Rempel-Clower, N. L., Zola, S. M., Squire, L. R., & Amarai, D. G. (1996). Three cases of enduring memory impairment after bilateral damage limited to the hippocampal formation. *J. Neuroscience* 16(16): 5233–5255.

5. Scoville, W. B., & Milner, B. (1957). Loss of recent memory after bilateral hippocampal lesions. *J. Neurology, Neurosurgery and Psychiatry, 20,* 11–21.

2

Regional Anatomy

CHAPTER OBJECTIVES

After completing this chapter, the reader will be able to:

1. Identify each major anatomical region of the brain, and explain its general function.

2. Locate major anatomical regions of the spinal cord, and discuss the concept of a spinal cord segment.

3. Identify the meninges surrounding the brain and spinal cord, as well as the spaces between them.

4. Locate the four ventricles of the brain, and describe the function of cerebrospinal fluid.

5. Describe the major arteries supplying the brain and spinal cord, and the major venous sinuses that drain them.

6. Explain the functions of the blood-brain barrier and blood-nerve barrier.

KEY TERMS

basal ganglia
blood-brain barrier
brainstem
calvaria
cerebellum
cerebral cortex
cerebrospinal fluid
cerebrum
cranial base
diencephalon
grey matter
hypophysis (pituitary gland)
hypothalamus
infarct
meninges
spinal cord
thalamus
ventricles
white matter

Essential Facts ··

The brain and spinal cord are protected by bone, connective tissue (meninges) and cerebrospinal fluid.

▶ The brain has four major regions:
   1. The cerebrum is responsible for thought, emotion, and language.
   2. The diencephalon connects other brain areas to the cerebrum and controls physiological responses.
   3. The brainstem controls basic life functions.
   4. The cerebellum is responsible for coordination and balance.

▶ The spinal cord has four major regions: cervical, thoracic, lumbar and sacral.

▶ The brain uses 20% of the blood pumped by the heart.

▶ The brain and spinal cord are separated from the blood by a blood-brain barrier.

The central nervous system is composed of the brain and the spinal cord. This chapter provides an overview of the anatomy of the brain and its surrounding structures, and the spinal cord and its surrounding structures. In addition, it describes the extensive network of blood vessels that supports the nervous system. Specific details about the function of each brain and spinal cord region will be discussed in subsequent chapters. A number of pathologies affecting the central nervous system are presented because damage to the brain, to the spinal cord, or to the surrounding anatomical structures such as the skull, spine. and intervertebral discs, can have serious consequences for function. Clinicians need a thorough knowledge of brain and spinal cord anatomy in order to be most effective in treating patients.

Anatomy of the Brain and Spinal Cord

As discussed in chapter 1, the brain and spinal cord form the central nervous system. Each consists of many nerve cells (neurons), surrounded by supporting (glial) cells. The structure and function of the cells are discussed further in chapter 3.

Gross Anatomy of the Brain

The human brain weighs about 3 pounds and consists of approximately 10^{12} individual nerve cells (neurons). It also contains about 500^{12} glial (supporting) cells that surround the neurons. Although the brain's size varies among individuals, brain size is not related to intelligence. However, the parts of the brain responsible for thought, language, emotion, and other uniquely human characteristics are much larger in people than in other animals.

The brain can be divided into four major anatomical regions: the cerebrum, the diencephalon, the brainstem, and the cerebellum (see **Figure 2-1**).

The **cerebrum** is the largest part of the brain. It is divided into two cerebral hemispheres that are connected by a large band of nerve fibers (axons) called the corpus callosum (see **Figure 2-2**). The corpus callosum connects the right and left cerebral hemispheres

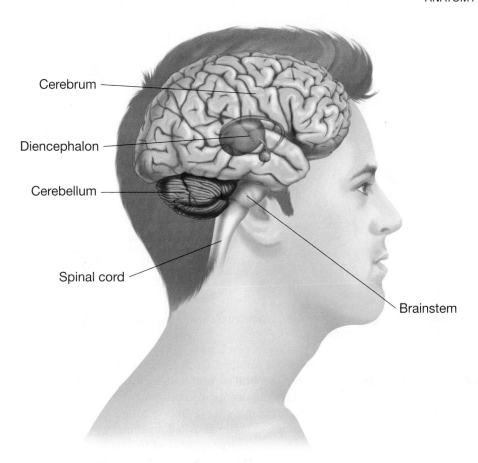

Cerebrum

Diencephalon

Cerebellum

Spinal cord

Brainstem

FIGURE 2-1 Subdivisions of the brain (lateral view).

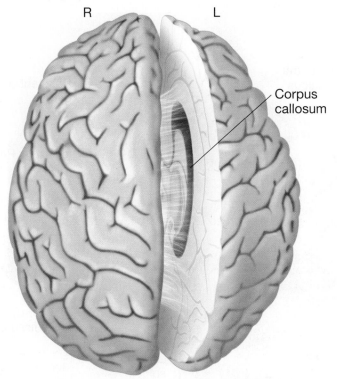

R   L

Corpus callosum

FIGURE 2-2 The cerebrum is divided into right and left hemispheres connected by a bundle of axons called the corpus callosum (superior view).

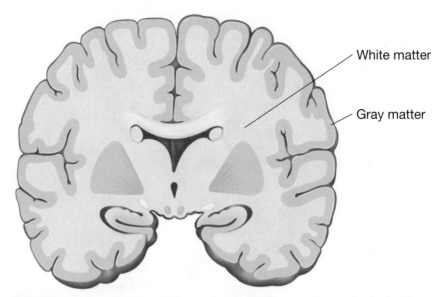

FIGURE 2-3 Frontal section of the cerebrum showing grey matter (neuron cell bodies) and white matter (axons).

so that they can communicate with one another. Each cerebral hemisphere is composed of an outer layer of **grey matter** (the **cerebral cortex**) that encloses an inner core of **white matter** (see Figure 2-3). Grey matter contains neuron cell bodies and dendrites, whereas white matter is formed by neuron processes (nerve fibers) called axons. Many of these axons are covered with a white, insulating material called myelin.

The cerebrum is tightly folded so that a large amount of tissue can fit inside the skull. Each fold or ridge is called a gyrus. Each gyrus is separated from the next one by a groove known as a sulcus. Some especially deep grooves are called fissures (see Figure 2-4).

Each cerebral hemisphere can be subdivided into four regions (lobes) that are named for adjacent skull bones. Most functions of the cortex involve the activity of several regions and lobes.

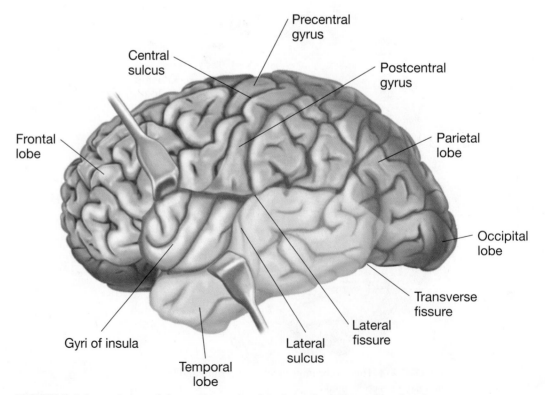

FIGURE 2-4 Lateral view of the cerebrum showing the major lobes and landmarks.

Neuroscience Notes Box 2-1:
Split-Brain Studies

The corpus callosum connects the left hemisphere to the right hemisphere, allowing each side of the brain to communicate with the other. At one time it was relatively common to cut the corpus callosum of people who suffered from severe seizures (epilepsy). This procedure was sometimes effective in limiting the number and severity of seizures. The inability of the two cerebral hemispheres to communicate also produced some interesting deficits. Studies of these "split-brained" people have helped to describe some of the functions and specializations of the left and right hemispheres. For example, language is usually centered in the left hemisphere, and nonverbal communication is located on the right.

The *frontal lobe* is located beneath the frontal bone. It is separated from the parietal lobe by the central sulcus, and from the temporal lobe by the lateral fissures. The inferior surface of the frontal lobe lies just above the eye sockets (orbits), so this part of the lobe is called the orbital surface. The *parietal lobe* lies just posterior to the frontal lobe, behind the central sulcus. It is separated from the occipital lobe by the small parieto-occipital sulcus, and from the temporal lobe by the lateral fissure. The *occipital lobe* is found at the back of the brain, under the occipital bone. It is the smallest cortical lobe. And finally, the *temporal lobe* is located inferior to the parietal lobe, and anterior to the occipital lobe. This lobe lies beneath the temporal bone.

All four cortical lobes are visible on a mid-sagittal section of the brain (see Figure 2-5). Some neuroscientists also describe a fifth "limbic lobe" that lies entirely in the center of the brain, not visible from the outside. The limbic lobe is a region of the cerebrum that contains portions of the four anatomical lobes, and is part of the limbic system (responsible for memory and emotion). Another region of the cerebrum that is not usually considered part of any anatomical lobe is the insula. The insula is hidden beneath parts of the frontal, parietal,

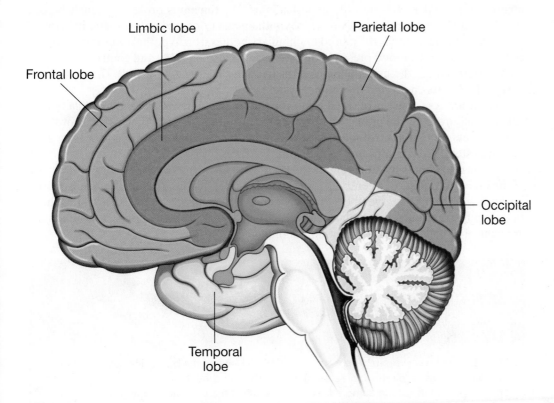

FIGURE 2-5 Mid-sagittal section of the brain showing the major lobes and regions.

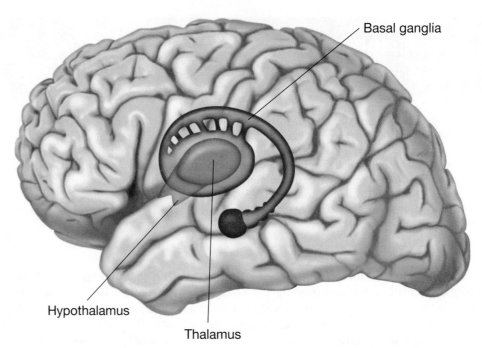

FIGURE 2-6 The basal ganglia and the diencephalon (thalamus and hypothalamus) (lateral view).

and temporal lobes, and can be seen by looking into the lateral fissure. It is connected to the limbic system, and is involved in awareness of sensation and emotion.

Deep inside the white matter of each cerebral hemisphere is a group of large subcortical structures made of grey matter known as the **basal ganglia** (basal nuclei) (see **Figure 2-6**). The basal ganglia include the caudate nucleus, the putamen, and the globus pallidus. These structures are involved in generating movement, thought, and emotion.

The **diencephalon** is located inferior to the cerebrum, and is visible only in a sectioned (sliced) brain. It is much smaller than the cerebrum. The diencephalon consists of two major parts: the thalamus and the hypothalamus. The **thalamus** processes signals before they are sent to the cerebral cortex. The **hypothalamus** is located anterior and inferior to the thalamus, and includes the paired mammillary bodies. The hypothalamus is involved in control of heart rate, blood pressure, digestion, and water balance, and controls the endocrine system. Under the hypothalamus is the **hypophysis** (pituitary gland). The pituitary is part of the body's endocrine (hormone) system.

The **brainstem** consists of three parts: the midbrain, the pons, and the medulla oblongata (see **Figure 2-7**). The brainstem connects the rest of the brain with the spinal cord, and contains centers that control many basic life functions such as breathing and heart rate. The brainstem also contains most of the cranial nerves.

The **cerebellum** is located behind the pons and below the occipital lobes at the back of the brain. It consists of a central vermis and two (right and left) cerebellar hemispheres. Three large bundles of nerve fibers (axons) connect the brainstem to the cerebellum. These fiber bundles are called cerebellar peduncles. The cerebellum's most important functions are control of balance and coordination of movement.

Neuroscience Notes Box 2-2:
Brainstem injury

The brainstem is extremely important for survival. Many of the body's life-sustaining functions such as respiration (breathing), swallowing, and heart rate are regulated by the brainstem. For this reason, tumors or strokes that affect the brainstem region are often fatal.

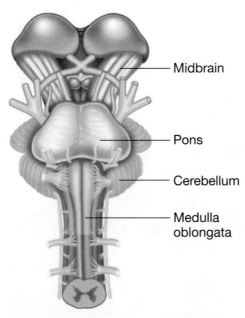

FIGURE 2-7 The brainstem and cerebellum: the brainstem consists of the midbrain, pons, and medulla oblongata (ventral view).

Review Concepts 2-1: Brain Anatomy

- The two cerebral hemispheres are connected by the corpus callosum.

- The four lobes of of the cerebral cortex are frontal, parietal, temporal, and occipital.

- Basal ganglia are located deep inside the cerebrum.

- The diencephalon consists of the thalamus and the hypothalamus.

- The brainstem is formed by the midbrain, the pons, and the medulla oblongata.

- The cerebellum is connected to the brainstem.

Gross Anatomy of the Spinal Cord

The **spinal cord** connects the brain with peripheral nerves in the body (see **Figure 2-8**). The cord conveys sensory information from the body to the brain, and also conveys signals from the brain to the body for control of skeletal muscles and organs. Damage to the cord has serious consequences for function, because spinal cord injury impairs transmission of essential information between the brain and the body.

The spinal cord extends from the base of the skull to vertebral level L_1. At its inferior end, the cord tapers to a point (the conus medullaris). It is anchored to the sacrum by a fiber of connective tissue called the filum terminale (terminal fiber). The cord is about 1.5 cm or about 0.6 inches in diameter at its widest point.

Like the spinal column, the spinal cord is composed of segments. Each spinal cord segment is a separate functional unit, and the segments generally correspond to the vertebrae that form the spine. There are 31 spinal cord segments. In the cervical region, there are 8 spinal cord segments (but only 7 cervical vertebrae). The thoracic region has 12 spinal cord segments, and the lumbar and sacral regions each have 5 segments. (There is also one coccygeal segment that has no functional significance.)

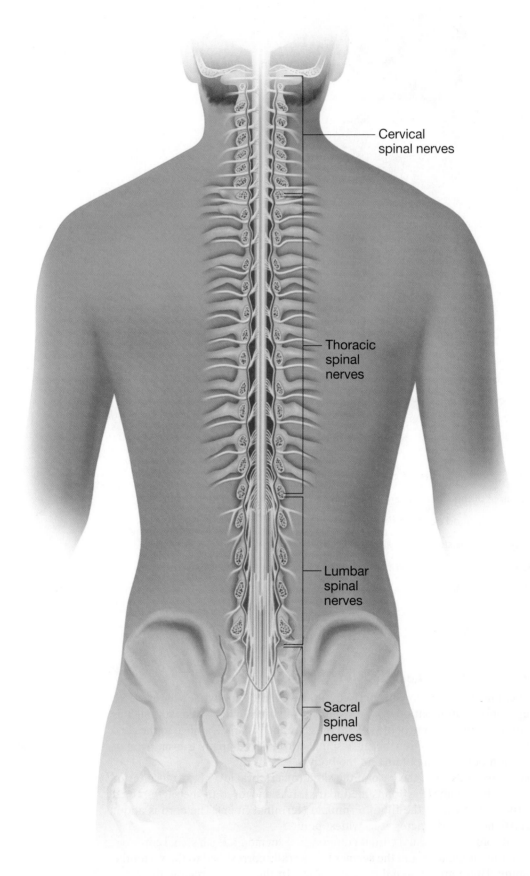

FIGURE 2-8 The spinal cord is located within the vertebral canal, and gives rise to the spinal nerves.

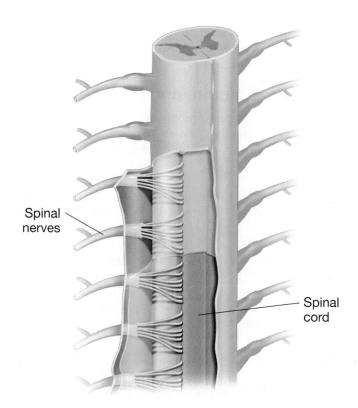

FIGURE 2-9 Spinal cord segment close-up with spinal nerves.

Each spinal cord segment gives rise to a pair of spinal nerves (right and left) (see **Figure 2-9**). These nerves contain motor, sensory, and autonomic axons (nerve fibers) that leave the spinal cord and form the peripheral nerves. The spinal nerves emerge from the vertebral column through holes called intervertebral foraminae. Each pair of spinal nerves leaves the spine adjacent to its corresponding numbered vertebra (except C8, which exits between vertebrae C7 and T1). Because the spinal cord ends at vertebral level L1 and is much shorter than the vertebral column, spinal nerve fibers from the lumbar and sacral portions of the cord must run inferiorly within the spinal column before exiting through the intervertebral foramen. These peripheral nerve fibers resemble a horse's tail, and are collectively referred to as the cauda equina.

A cross-section through the spinal cord reveals a central, butterfly-shaped core of grey matter surrounded by white matter (see **Figure 2-10**). The grey matter (made of neuron cell bodies and dendrites) is divided into regions known as horns. The three grey matter horns are the dorsal (posterior) horn, the lateral horn, and the ventral (anterior) horn. Motor

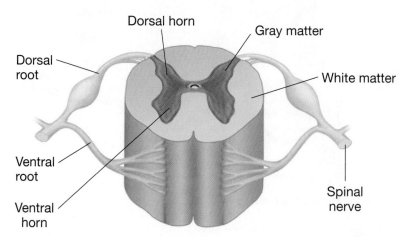

FIGURE 2-10 Cross-section of the spinal cord with peripheral white matter and central grey matter: grey matter is divided into dorsal and ventral horns that give rise to dorsal and ventral roots.

neuron cell bodies are located in the ventral horn, and autonomic neuron cell bodies are found in the lateral horn. The white matter consists of myelinated axons (nerve fibers) and it is organized into regions called columns.

The Skull, Vertebral Column, and Meninges

The central nervous system (brain and spinal cord) is surrounded by bones (skull and vertebral column) as well as three layers of connective tissue **(meninges).** Along with cerebrospinal fluid, these structures protect the delicate nerve tissue.

Anatomy of the Skull

The skull surrounds and protects the brain. The brain rests on the cranial base, and is surrounded by the skull cap (calvaria) (see **Figure 2-11**). The **calvaria** is formed from the frontal, parietal, occipital, and temporal bones. These bones are joined by fibrous joints called sutures, which are fused in adults but can expand in very young children to accommodate brain growth. Calvarial bones usually fuse by age 2.

The **cranial base** is formed by several bones and contains holes (foraminae) for nerves and blood vessels to pass to and from the brain (see **Figure 2-12**). The cranial base is subdivided into three regions called cranial fossae. The largest hole in the cranial base is the foramen magnum; the spinal cord passes through this opening to enter the vertebral column.

Clinical Box 2-1: Chiari Malformation

A Chiari malformation describes a condition in which the base of the brain (usually the brainstem and/or the cerebellum) "drops" through the foramen magnum. This compresses the brain and kills nerve cells. Chiari malformation is a dangerous condition and can result in death if left untreated.

Challenge question: If the cerebellum were compressed due to Chiari malformation, what functions would be affected?

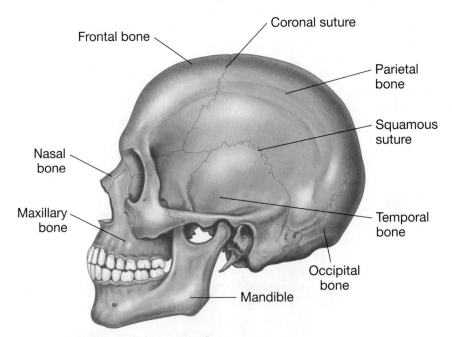

FIGURE 2-11 The skull (lateral view).

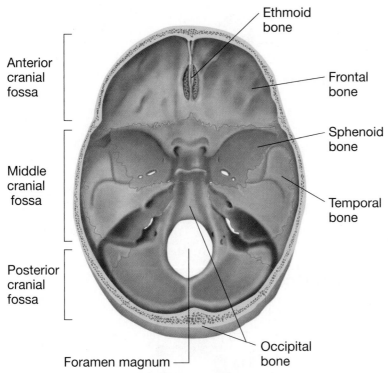

FIGURE 2-12 The skull: superior view of the cranial base.

Anatomy of the Vertebral Column

The spinal cord is surrounded by the spinal (vertebral) column that consists of 33 bones (vertebrae) (see Figure 2-13). The vertebral column can be subdivided into five regions: cervical (7 vertebrae), thoracic (12 vertebrae), lumbar (5 vertebrae), sacral (5 vertebrae, fused to form the sacrum), and coccygeal (3 to 5 small vertebrae).

The vertebrae in each region of the spinal column have a distinct structure (see Figure 2-14). All except the first cervical vertebra (C1) have a vertebral body that is round or oval in shape, and a vertebral arch composed of two laminae and two pedicles. Right and left transverse processes and a posterior spinous process serve as attachment points for muscles and ligaments. The vertebral foramen is the hole created by the vertebral body and the surrounding vertebral arch. When the vertebrae are stacked on top of one another, these foraminae create a long vertebral canal that surrounds the spinal cord.

The lateral side of each vertebra also has two spaces called notches. The notches of adjacent vertebrae combine to form a hole called the intervertebral foramen. This means that the spinal column has a row of intervertebral foraminae on both sides, between each pair of vertebrae. The spinal nerves that connect the spinal cord to the muscles, skin, and other structures leave the spinal canal via these intervertebral foraminae.

Individual vertebrae in the spinal column are separated by intervertebral discs (see Figure 2-15). The intervertebral discs consist of an outer shell of tough fibrocartilage (annulus fibrosus) that surrounds a gelatinous inner core (nucleus pulposus). Intervertebral discs allow for movement between the vertebrae, and also serve as shock absorbers. Each nucleus pulposus contains water that is squeezed out when the vertebral column bears weight (during standing and walking). This means that the discs are a bit smaller at the end of the day, and that one's height will be a bit less in the evening than in the morning. If excessive force is placed on the discs, they may bulge and put pressure on nearby structures, causing pain. A disc that is subjected to extreme force may rupture, allowing the nucleus pulposus to ooze out. This causes swelling, pain, and loss of function.

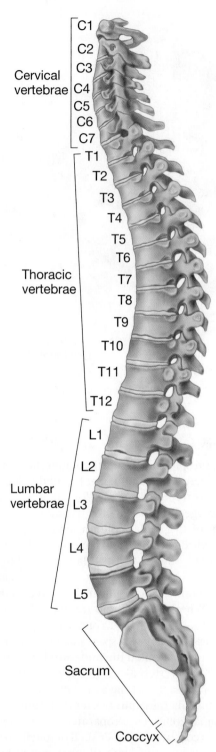

FIGURE 2-13 The vertebral column is divided into regions (lateral view).

The Meninges

Three layers of connective tissue are found inside the skull and the vertebral canal, surrounding the brain and spinal cord. Together they are called the **meninges** (see Figure 2-16). The meninges protect the central nervous system from infection and physical trauma.

The innermost meningeal layer is the pia mater. It is very thin and delicate, and attaches closely to the surface of the brain and spinal cord. The next layer is the arachnoid, which is thicker than the pia but still nearly transparent, and is named for its resemblance to a spider's web. Small fibers of arachnoid connect it to the pia; these are known as arachnoid

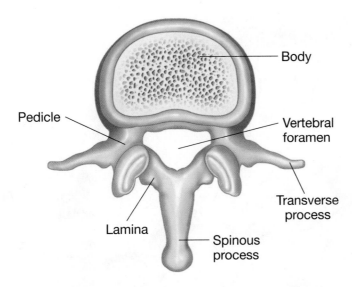

FIGURE 2-14 A representative vertebra.

trabeculae. Between the arachnoid and pia mater is a space (the subarachnoid space) that contains cerebrospinal (spinal) fluid (CSF). **Cerebrospinal fluid** is a watery fluid that helps to protect the brain and spinal cord. The average person has about 140 ml of this fluid.

The outermost layer of meninges is the dura mater. Dura mater is very thick and tough, and forms a strong covering around the CNS, the pia mater, and the arachnoid. It extends laterally along the spinal nerves as they exit the vertebral column, blending with connective tissue covering the spinal nerves. The dura mater has many sensory nerve endings, so it is very sensitive to pain.

Inside the skull, the dura mater has two sublayers: an outer periosteal dura and an inner meningeal dura. In most places the two layers of dura are tightly connected. However, they are separated in a few specific locations, creating a space between the layers that is called a dural sinus. Venous blood from the brain drains into the dural sinuses. Cerebrospinal fluid from the subarachnoid space also drains into the sinuses; thus the sinuses contain a mixture of blood and CSF. The sinuses drain into the jugular veins in the neck, and return blood and CSF back to the venous system.

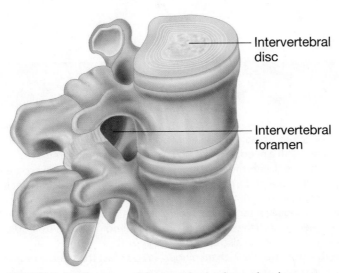

FIGURE 2-15 Segment of the vertebral column showing the intervertebral discs and intervertebral foramen.

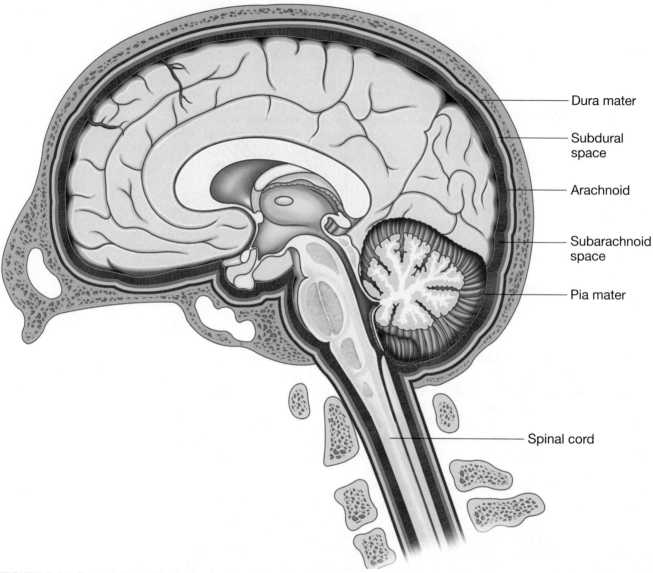

FIGURE 2-16 Sagittal view of the brain showing the meninges (dura mater, arachnoid, and pia mater); cerebrospinal fluid fills the subarachnoid space between the arachnoid and pia.

Labels:
- Dura mater
- Subdural space
- Arachnoid
- Subarachnoid space
- Pia mater
- Spinal cord

Clinical Box 2-2: Spinal Tap

In a lumbar puncture (spinal tap), a sample of cerebrospinal fluid is drawn out of the subarachnoid space with a needle. This is done in the lower lumbar region of the spine to avoid hitting the spinal cord with the needle. (Remember that the spinal cord ends at vertebral level L_1). Spinal taps are performed to diagnose a variety of conditions, including infections of the brain or spinal cord. A cloudy sample (full of white blood cells) may contain bacteria and indicate meningitis, a serious bacterial infection of the meninges. Blood in the sample can indicate bleeding into the **ventricles** or subarachnoid space. Antibodies to HIV (human immunodeficiency virus) can also be detected in CSF.

Challenge question: Which meningeal layers must the needle pass through to reach the subarachnoid space?

Clinical Box 2-3: Epidural and Spinal Anesthetics

Injection of an anesthetic into the epidural space causes temporary loss of sensation, without puncturing the dura mater and risking infection. Epidural anesthetics are used during childbirth and for some surgeries involving the lower extremities. In contrast to an epidural, a spinal anesthetic is administered directly into the cerebrospinal fluid in the subarachnoid space. This involves a greater risk to the patient because it requires piercing the dura mater. It can also cause a painful spinal headache, caused by a small leakage of CSF.

Challenge question: What structures are located in the epidural space that convey sensation and would be affected by an injection of anesthetic into this space?

Neuroscience Notes Box 2-3: Meningitis

Infection of the meninges is called meningitis, and can be a serious condition because the swelling and tissue damage that accompany infection can cause damage to the CNS. Meningitis is diagnosed by obtaining a sample of CSF, which is normally clear but looks cloudy when infection is present. Meningitis causes an intense headache because the dura mater contains many pain receptors. Other common signs include a high fever and a stiff neck.

In the spine (vertebral column), there is some space outside of the dura mater (epidural space), since the dura is not fused to the vertebrae. The epidural space contains the spinal nerve roots.

Vascular System, Ventricular System, and Cerebrospinal Fluid

The brain and spinal cord receive blood from several major arteries, each of which supplies a specific region of nerve tissue. In addition, the central nervous system contains hollow spaces (ventricles) that are filled with fluid. This fluid also surrounds the outside of the central nervous system, providing protection and nourishment for the nerve tissue.

The Vascular System

The human nervous system has a high metabolic rate and requires a large and consistent supply of oxygenated blood. About 20% of the blood pumped by the heart goes to the brain, even though the brain weighs only about 3 pounds (or about 2% of body weight). Nerve cells can live from 3 to 5 minutes without oxygen. An interruption in the supply of blood to brain and spinal cord tissue can cause irreversible loss of neurons and is a major cause of disability and death.

Four major arteries supply blood to the brain: two internal carotid arteries and two vertebral arteries (see **Figure 2-17**). The internal carotid arteries branch from the common carotid arteries in the neck. (This branching point is a common place for arteriosclerotic plaque to build up, impairing the flow of blood to the brain.) The vertebral arteries run alongside the medulla oblongata and give off small branches that form the spinal arteries (discussed below). Each vertebral artery also has a branch (the posterior inferior cerebellar artery) that supplies blood to the cerebellum. Near the brainstem, the two vertebral arteries merge to form the basilar artery that supplies blood to the pons and the cerebellum (via the superior cerebellar arteries and the anterior inferior cerebellar arteries).

The Circle of Willis (circulus arteriosus) is a ring of blood vessels that sits at the base of the brain (see **Figure 2-18**). It receives blood from both internal carotid arteries as well

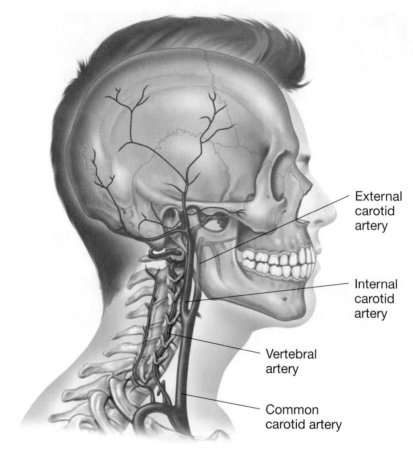

FIGURE 2-17 The arterial supply to the brain is derived from the vertebral arteries and the internal carotid arteries.

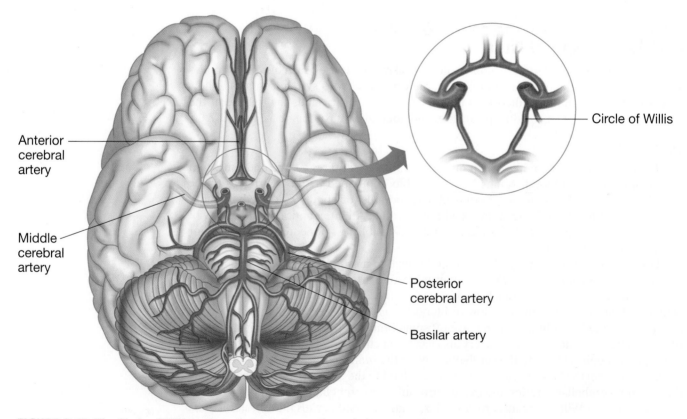

FIGURE 2-18 The Circle of Willis and cerebral arteries are the major sources of blood to the cerebrum (inferior view).

Neuroscience Notes Box 2-4:
Different Strokes

In the brain, each region receives blood from a single artery. This means that blockage of, or damage to, an artery will produce an area of dead nerve tissue called an **infarct.** Any disruption of blood flow to the brain is referred to as a *cerebrovascular accident* (*CVA* or stroke). Most strokes result from occlusion (blockage) of one artery; others occur when an artery ruptures, causing bleeding in the brain. The specific symptoms of a stroke are determined by which artery is affected, and according to which area of the brain is affected by the lack of oxygenated blood. Because every infarct is a bit different, each stroke will present with different signs and symptoms (see **Figure 2-19**).

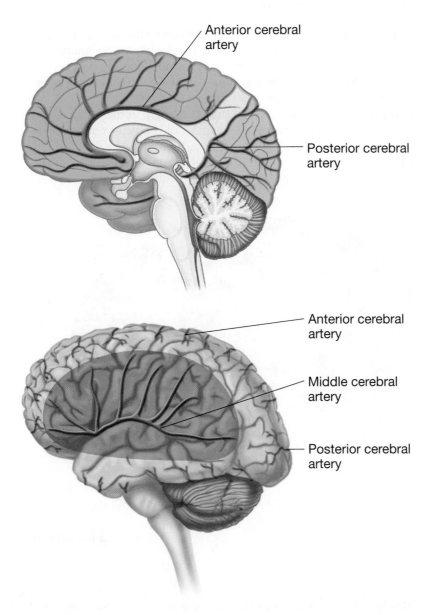

FIGURE 2-19 Primary regions of the brain supplied by the middle cerebral artery (purple), posterior cerebral artery (blue), and anterior cerebral artery (green). If an artery is occluded, the brain will likely suffer damage in the specified region.

as from the basilar artery. The Circle of Willis gives off three pairs of arteries: the anterior cerebral, the middle cerebral, and the posterior cerebral arteries. Together, these supply most of the brain with blood.

The anterior cerebral arteries run anteriorly between the frontal lobes in the central sulcus. They supply the anterior and inferior part of the frontal lobes and part of the parietal lobes. A small anterior communicating artery connects them and forms part of the Circle of Willis.

Two middle cerebral arteries also branch from the Circle of Willis. They run laterally between the frontal and temporal lobes. These arteries are the largest branches from the Circle of Willis and supply the largest region of the brain. Blood travels through the middle cerebral arteries to the lateral cerebrum, and to the diencephalon.

The posterior cerebral arteries branch from the Circle of Willis near the basilar artery. These vessels supply blood to the occipital lobe and have branches to the thalamus and midbrain.

Venous drainage of the brain occurs via small veins that drain blood into three large cerebral veins. The cerebral veins drain blood into the dural sinuses, spaces formed between two layers of dura mater. The dural sinuses empty into the internal jugular veins that leave the skull through the jugular foramen, and that return the blood to the heart (see **Figure 2-20**).

The spinal cord receives blood from three small spinal arteries that run the length of the cord (see **Figure 2-21**). One anterior spinal artery supplies the anterior two-thirds of the cord, and two smaller posterior spinal arteries provide blood to the posterior third. There are also small segmental arteries that supply individual spinal cord segments. An injury involving any of these vessels can cause a spinal cord infarct.

Two large central veins drain blood from the length of the spinal cord, supplemented by small segmental veins at each cord level. All of the veins empty into a large venous network (the epidural plexus) located in the epidural space. From the epidural plexus, the blood is drained into intervertebral veins that are found next to the segmental arteries, and then the blood moves into larger veins that eventually empty into the vena cavae.

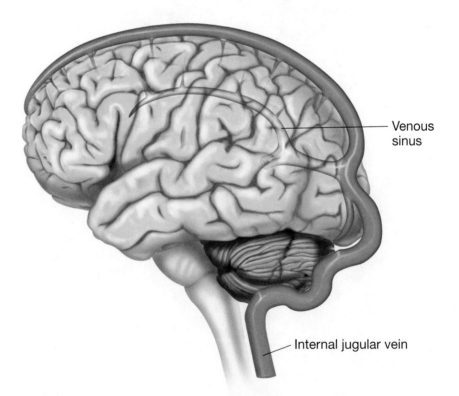

Venous sinus

Internal jugular vein

FIGURE 2-20 Venous drainage of the brain occurs via the venous sinuses; blood then drains into the internal jugular vein and returns to the heart.

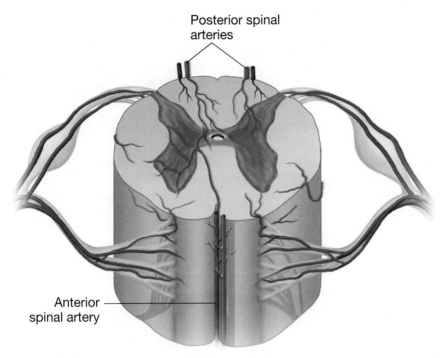

Posterior spinal
arteries

Anterior
spinal artery

FIGURE 2-21 The spinal cord is supplied with blood via the anterior spinal artery and the posterior spinal arteries.

Review Concepts 2-2: Blood Supply

- The anterior cerebral arteries supply the anterior part of the frontal lobes.

- The middle cerebral arteries supply the lateral portion of each cerebral hemisphere as well as the thalamus and hypothalamus.

- The posterior cerebral arteries supply the occipital lobes, the thalamus, and the midbrain.

- The basilar artery supplies the pons and part of the cerebellum.

- The vertebral arteries supply the medulla oblongata and part of the cerebellum.

- The anterior and posterior spinal arteries supply the spinal cord.

The central nervous system is protected from potentially harmful substances in the blood by a **blood-brain barrier** (see **Figure 2-22**). The blood-brain barrier is formed by tight connections (junctions) between cells in the capillaries that deliver blood to the brain and spinal cord. Glial cells called astrocytes secrete chemicals to stimulate formation of the tight junctions. The blood-brain barrier controls the passage of substances from the blood to the fluid that surrounds neurons. Substances that neurons need (oxygen, water, glucose, and amino acids) can cross the barrier, whereas many larger molecules cannot cross.

The blood-brain barrier forms during the midpoint of fetal development (about the 20th week). Before the barrier has developed, any chemicals a pregnant woman ingests can diffuse to the fetus's developing nervous system. This means that pregnant women must be careful to avoid exposure to toxic substances, including alcohol and drugs.

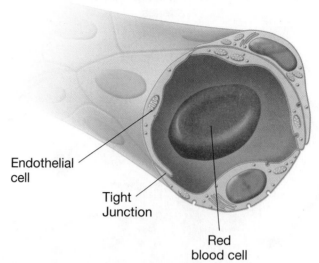

Endothelial cell

Tight Junction

Red blood cell

FIGURE 2-22 The blood-brain barrier is formed by tight junctions between capillary endothelial cells, and protects the brain from potentially harmful substances in the blood.

In the peripheral nervous system, a blood-nerve barrier protects peripheral neurons from substances found in the blood. The blood-nerve barrier is formed by cells that line the capillaries. In some places (for example, the neuromuscular junction where motor neurons contact skeletal muscle cells) the blood-nerve barrier is absent. This allows some viruses to avoid the blood-nerve barrier and to invade the nervous system. Viruses, including rabies and herpes zoster (chicken pox), use this method to infect the nervous system.

The Ventricular System and Cerebrospinal Fluid

The ventricles are four interconnected cavities that are found in the center of the brain (see Figure 2-23). All four ventricles contain cerebrospinal fluid (CSF), which also circulates in the subarachnoid space outside the brain and spinal cord.

Each cerebral hemisphere contains one lateral ventricle. The lateral ventricle is a roughly C-shaped space that has four defined regions called horns, each of which is located within one of the four cerebral lobes. Each lateral ventricle has a small hole (the interventricular foramen) that connects it to the third ventricle.

The third ventricle is located in the midline of the brain. From the third ventricle, a small tube called the cerebral aqueduct connects to the fourth ventricle. The fourth ventricle is a diamond-shaped space located between the pons and the cerebellum. From the fourth ventricle, cerebrospinal fluid can flow into the tiny central canal of the spinal cord, or into the subarachnoid space through small openings.

Cerebrospinal fluid is produced in all four ventricles, although most of it is formed in the right and left lateral ventricles. Each ventricle contains a choroid plexus, consisting of a network of capillaries surrounded by ependymal cells and some connective tissue. The ependymal cells filter blood plasma from the capillaries into the ventricle, creating CSF and assisting in its circulation.

The total volume of cerebrospinal fluid is about 140 ml, of which about 25 ml is found inside the ventricles and about 115 ml is in the subarachnoid space. CSF is produced continuously and is completely turned over about 3 times daily. It is reabsorbed from the subarachnoid space into the dural sinuses where it mixes with venous blood. Small arachnoid villi connect the subarachnoid space with dural sinuses, acting like tiny one-way valves.

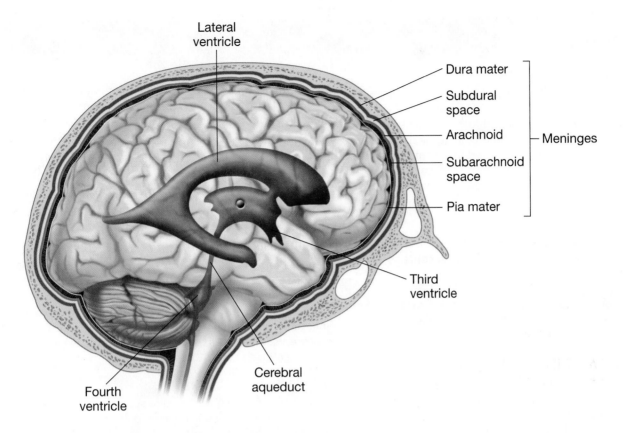

FIGURE 2-23 The ventricles of the brain: lateral ventricle, third ventricle, cerebral aqueduct, and the fourth ventricle. The subarachnoid space, which is also important for the transport of CSF, is pictured within the meninges.

Cerebrospinal fluid has several essential functions. First, it transports ions, nutrients, and hormones to neurons and removes wastes. Second, CSF regulates the composition of extracellular fluids that surround neurons and glial cells. In addition, CSF serves as a watery, protective cushion around the brain and spinal cord. The fluid can provide some shock absorption and keeps the brain from being compressed against the skull bones.

Neuroscience Notes Box 2-5:
Hydrocephalus

Normally there is a precise balance between the amount of CSF produced and the amount that is reabsorbed into the blood. If reabsorption is blocked, CSF will build up within the ventricles, causing hydrocephaly (hydrocephalus). In young children whose skull bones have not fused, hydrocephaly results in tremendous enlargement of the ventricles, the brain, and the skull. If the skull bones have fused, the ventricles enlarge and compress the brain against the skull from the inside. Nearby blood vessels and brain tissue may also be compressed, resulting in ischemia and brain damage.

Hydrocephalus can be caused by malformation of the ventricular system, by tumors that block CSF drainage, or by infections in which pus blocks drainage. Treatment involves implanting a shunt to bypass the obstruction and drain fluid out of the skull. Usually, the shunt is placed in one lateral ventricle.

PATIENT SCENARIOS

Patient Case 2-1 (Ryan)

Ryan is a 20-year-old college student. He woke up one morning with a high fever, sore throat, severe headache, and stiff neck. Ryan went to the college health center, where the doctor examined him and then sent him to the hospital for a spinal tap. The diagnosis was bacterial meningitis, and Ryan was admitted to the hospital for intravenous antibiotics.

Questions

a) Name the meninges surrounding the CNS and the spaces in between them. Which space contains cerebrospinal fluid?

b) Why does Ryan have such a painful headache?

c) Why would a spinal tap be a good way to diagnose meningitis? Which meningeal layers would be punctured to obtain the CSF sample?

Patient Case 2-2 (Florence)

While talking with a friend on the phone one afternoon, Florence, age 77, suddenly became confused and disoriented. She was unable to continue the conversation because she couldn't speak. In addition, the right side of her body felt numb, and she couldn't hold the phone in her right hand. Florence was taken to the hospital and diagnosed with a stroke (CVA) affecting her middle cerebral artery.

Questions

a) What regions of the brain could be affected by a CVA in the middle cerebral artery?

b) How long can nerve cells in the brain live if they are deprived of blood by a stroke?

Patient Case 2-3 (Maria)

Maria is 8 months old. She was born with part of her spinal cord and spinal meninges exposed (myelomeningeocele, a form of spina bifida). This was surgically repaired soon after her birth. Now, Maria's head circumference is unusually large for her age. She has been diagnosed with hydrocephalus, and will have a shunt implanted in her right lateral ventricle.

Questions

a) Describe the brain's ventricular system and the spaces through which cerebrospinal fluid flows.

b) Why is Maria's head enlarged?

c) What purpose will the shunt serve?

Review Questions

1. Name each major anatomical region of the brain, and locate each region on a diagram. State the general function of each.

2. Define the term *spinal cord segment*. How many spinal cord segments are found in each of the four anatomical regions of the spinal cord?

3. Name the three layers of meninges and identify them on a diagram. Describe the function of meninges. Also name the spaces located adjacent to the meninges and discuss the contents of each space.

4. Name each major artery that supplies blood to the brain and spinal cord. Explain the function of the dural sinuses.

5. Describe the function of the blood-brain and blood-nerve barriers. Name several substances that can cross the barrier.

Further Reading

1. Felten, D. L., & Shetty, A. (2009). *Netter's atlas of neuroscience* (2nd ed.). Philadelphia: Saunders.

2. Haines, D. E. (2011). *Neuroanatomy: An atlas of structures, sections and systems* (8th ed.). Philadelphia: Lippincott, Williams and Wilkins.

3. Kandel, E. R., Schwartz, J. H., & Jessel, T. M. (2000). *Principles of neural science* (4th ed.). Norwalk, CT: Appleton and Lange.

4. Moore, J. C. (1993). *Brain atlas and functional systems.* Rockville, MD: American Occupational Therapy Association.

5. Schuenke, M., Schulte, E., Schumacher, U., & Ross, L. (2010). *Head and neuroanatomy (THIEME atlas of anatomy).* Stuttgart, Germany: Thieme.

Neurons and Glial Cells

CHAPTER OBJECTIVES

After completing this chapter, the reader will be able to:

1. Describe the structure of a neuron, including the cell body, the dendrites and dendritic spines, and the axon and axon terminals.

2. Discuss the structure of the neuron cell membrane and explain how the resting membrane potential is maintained.

3. Explain how action potentials are generated and propagated in both unmyelinated and myelinated axons.

4. Define the refractory period and discuss its consequences for nerve cell function.

5. List the five types of glial cells found in the nervous system and state the function of each type.

6. Describe how injury affects nerve cells in the peripheral nervous system and in the central nervous system.

KEY TERMS

action potential (nerve impulse)

astrocyte

axon

axon terminal (synaptic terminal, synaptic knob)

dendrite

depolarization

ependymal cells

glial cell (neuroglial cell)

ion

ion channel

local potential

membrane pump

microglial cell

myelin

necrosis

neuron

neurotransmitter

oligodendrocyte

refractory period

resting membrane potential

safety factor

saltatory conduction

Schwann cell

Essential Facts···

▶ Neurons transmit information in the nervous system, supported by the glial cells.

▶ Neurons transmit signals in the form of action potentials, which travel along nerve fibers (axons).

▶ Myelin insulates axons and increases the speed of action potential transmission.

▶ Neurons in the central nervous system do not regenerate if injured, but neurons in the peripheral nervous system can regenerate.

This chapter explains how cells in the brain, spinal cord, and peripheral nervous system function. Nerve cells (neurons) are the primary cells that transmit information, and glial cells sustain and support the neurons. This chapter also describes how nerve cells respond to injury, and how and when healing takes place. Although neurons do not normally divide after birth, there are other mechanisms by which function can be regained after injury. Therapy and rehabilitation focus on activating neurons across the nervous system in order to promote and regain normal function.

Neurons

The nervous system contains two types of cells: neurons (nerve cells) and glial cells. **Neurons** generate and transmit information to control body functions, and allow for thoughts, emotions, and memories. **Glial cells (neuroglial cells)** surround and support the neurons, and some speed nerve transmission by insulating axons with myelin. The human brain contains about 10^{12} neurons, and about 50 times as many glial cells. Damage to neurons located in the brain and spinal cord results in their death, whereas neurons in the peripheral nervous system are capable of regeneration and healing.

Neuron Structure

Neurons come in many shapes and sizes. However, they have certain characteristics in common. All neurons have a cell body (soma) that contains the cell's nucleus (see **Figure 3-1**). Usually, the nucleus is in the middle of the cell body. It contains the cell's DNA.

In addition to the nucleus, the cell body contains ribosomes. Many of these are attached to membranes and form a structure called rough endoplasmic reticulum (RER); other ribosomes are not attached to anything and are called free ribosomes. All ribosomes produce proteins that are essential to the normal structure and function of the neuron. The cell body also contains the Golgi body, which is important for processing and exporting proteins. If its cell body is damaged, the neuron will die.

Most neurons have processes that are outgrowths of the cell body. These are known as **dendrites.** The size, shape, and structure of dendrites vary among different kinds of neurons. Many dendrites have branches, and some have small outgrowths on their branches called dendritic spines. Spines are usually where nerve cells receive input from other neurons. Some neurons have as many as 100,000 dendritic spines.

Neurons have a single long process that extends from the cell body and makes connections with other cells; this process is called an **axon.** Axons are also known as nerve fibers. Although neurons can have many dendrites, they have only one axon. Axons sometimes

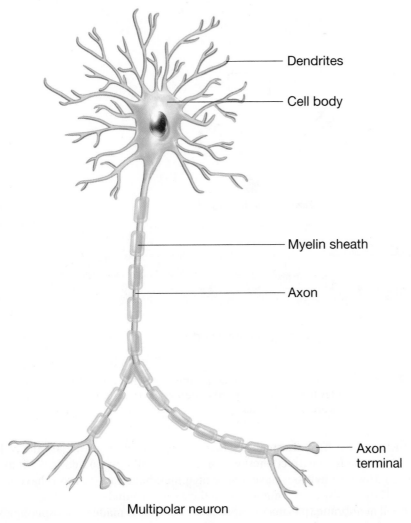

Dendrites

Cell body

Myelin sheath

Axon

Axon terminal

Multipolar neuron

FIGURE 3-1 A typical neuron with a cell body, numerous branched dendrites, and a single axon with many axon terminals.

have branches called axon collaterals. Each branch ends in a structure called an **axon terminal** (also called **synaptic terminal** or **synaptic knob**). Axon terminals make contact with other neurons, with muscle cells, or with glands. Some axons are short (a few millimeters), and others are quite long (up to 3 meters in some people).

Small intracellular "motors" called microtubules move substances around inside the neuron. Microtubules move molecules in both directions: toward the axon terminal (anterograde or orthograde transport) and away from the axon terminal (retrograde transport) (see Figure 3-2).

Neuroscience Notes Box 3-1: Dendritic Spines and Learning

Newborn babies have very few dendritic spines on their neurons. The number and density of spines increases as children grow and learn. In baby animals, learning is accompanied by an increase in the number of dendritic spines in the brain. These spines are most likely to be maintained if the animal (or human) practices the new skill or knowledge, and gets physical exercise. Recent evidence indicates that being physically active is correlated with learning and with retaining new knowledge and skills in people of all ages.

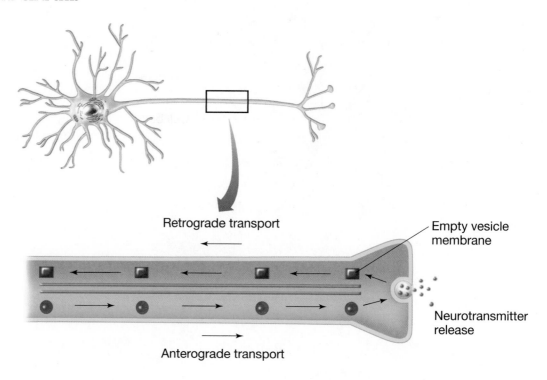

Retrograde transport

Empty vesicle
membrane

Neurotransmitter
release

Anterograde transport

FIGURE 3-2   Transport inside neurons (axoplasmic transport). Microtubules transport vesicles containing neurotransmitter to the axon terminal (anterograde transport). After neurotransmitter release, the empty vesicles are brought back toward the cell body (retrograde transport).

Mitochondria, which are small organelles found inside neurons, are the cell's powerhouses. Their role is to extract energy from glucose and oxygen and make it available to the neuron. Because neurons have a very high metabolic rate, neurons have many mitochondria. They are especially numerous in the axon terminals.

The cell membrane (plasma membrane) of neurons is made of phospholipids. The cell membrane forms a barrier between the fluid surrounding the neuron and the cell's internal cytoplasm. Small molecules such as oxygen (O_2), carbon dioxide (CO_2), nitrogen (N_2), and lipid-soluble molecules (e.g., ethanol) can diffuse across the membrane. Other molecules must move in or out of the neuron through membrane channels, or be moved across by specific carrier proteins. (For example, glucose enters nerve cells by a carrier protein.)

Many of the molecules that must cross the nerve cell membrane are **ions.** Ions are small, charged particles. Some ions that are important for neuron function include sodium (Na^+) and potassium (K^+). These ions are dissolved in the intracellular fluid (the cytosol), and in the fluid outside the cell (the interstitial fluid). Charged ions cannot diffuse through the cell membrane. They must pass through tiny channels in the membrane that are known as **ion channels** (see Figure 3-3). Channels are specific for certain kinds of ions. For example, a Na^+ channel is constructed so that it allows only Na^+ ions to pass through. Some channels allow more than one type of ion to pass: Na^+ –K^+ channels let both Na^+ and K^+ move through the channel. This specificity is called selective permeability.

MOVEMENT OF IONS   When ions diffuse across a membrane, they follow rules that guide the movement of all particles. First, ions move down their concentration gradient. This means that ions will move from a region of high concentration to a region of low concentration. The greater the concentration difference (gradient) on either side of the membrane, the faster the ions will move. Second, ions diffuse according to their charges: Positively charged ions are attracted to negative charges, and vice versa. Thus, ions will diffuse across cell membranes as a result of both concentration differences and charge differences. No energy (ATP) is required in either case. The movement of charged ions is called electrical current.

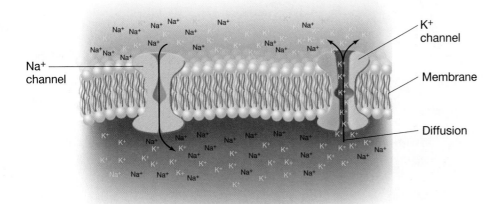

FIGURE 3-3   Each ion can only pass through its specific channel in the neuron cell membrane when the channel is open; in this example, the Na⁺ channel is closed and the K⁺ channel is open.

Sometimes it is necessary to move ions across the nerve cell membrane against a concentration gradient (i.e., from low to high). This requires a **membrane pump.** Membrane pumps are proteins embedded in cell membranes that use ATP to transfer ions across the membrane *against* their concentration gradient. A large percentage of the energy that nerve cells use is needed to keep these membrane pumps functioning. In the neuron cell membrane, there is an important membrane pump called the Na⁺ –K⁺ pump (see **Figure 3-4**). The Na⁺ –K⁺ pump is always on, whether the neuron is resting or is active. The pump moves K⁺ ions into the cell, and transfers Na⁺ ions out of the cell, using ATP for energy.

ION CHANNELS   Several kinds of ion channels are found in the neuron cell membrane. They can be classified into two groups: (1) nongated ("leak") channels and (2) gated channels. Nongated (leak) ion channels are always open. Ions flow through leak channels based on their charges and their concentration gradient. Gated ion channels have small molecular "gates" that can be closed (preventing the flow of ions) or open (allowing ions to flow). The gates open in response to a stimulus. Once the stimulus is removed, or after a set period of time in the open position, the channel gate closes again (see **Figure 3.5**).

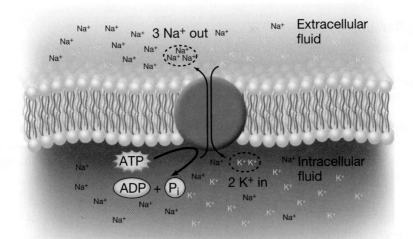

FIGURE 3-4   The Na⁺–K⁺ pump membrane pump. This pump pushes Na⁺ ions out of the cell, and pumps K⁺ ions into the cell. The pump requires energy in the form of ATP in order to function.

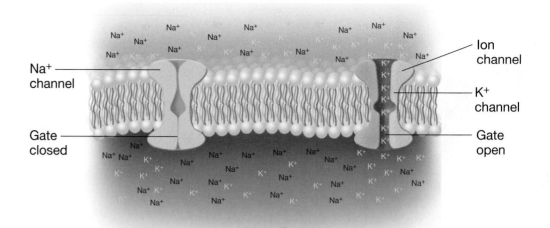

FIGURE 3-5   Two representative gated ion channels are shown. The sodium channel (green) is closed, preventing any Na⁺ ions from entering or exiting the cell. The potassium channel is pictured as open, allowing K⁺ ions to flow into or out of the cell.

Three kinds of gated channels are found in neurons: (1) modality-gated channels, (2) ligand-gated channels, and (3) voltage-gated channels. Each opens its gate in response to a different type of stimulus.

Modality-gated (sometimes called *pressure-gated*) ion channels open their gates in response to a physical (mechanical) stimulus. For example, a touch that causes deformation of tissue will cause this kind of channel to open. Other kinds of stimuli that open modality-gated channels include changes in temperature, sound waves, and various kinds of touch (pressure and vibration).

Ligand-gated (sometimes called *transmitter-gated*) channels open in response to the binding of a chemical to the ion channel protein. For example, if a stimulus causes damage to tissue so that cells break apart, the cells release chemicals that can bind to ligand-gated channels (resulting in pain). Some ligand-gated ion channels open in response to the binding of a chemical called a **neurotransmitter;** see chapter 4 for more about these important chemicals.

Voltage-gated ion channels open their gates when there are changes to the electrical charges found on each side of the cell membrane. There are many different kinds of voltage-gated ion channels. For example, some channels open slowly, while others open rapidly. Some are permeable to Na⁺, some to Ca⁺² , and some to K⁺ ions.

Resting Membrane Potential

When a neuron is "at rest," it is not transmitting information. At rest, the inside of the neuron (cytosol) has a net negative charge. This is because the fluid inside the cell contains proteins and amino acids that have negative charges. At the same time, the Na⁺–K⁺ pump in the cell membrane is on (as it always is), so K⁺ ions are being pumped into the cell, while Na⁺ ions are pumped out. The leak (nongated) ion channels in the cell membrane are open (as they always are, since they have no gates that can be closed). The leak channels are very permeable to K⁺, and slightly permeable to Na⁺. This means that most of the K⁺ ions being pumped into the neuron can diffuse right out again. However, most of the Na⁺ being pumped out must remain outside of the cell.

Taken together, all of this activity in the resting neurons means that:

• The inside of the cell membrane has a negative charge.
• The outside of the cell membrane has a positive charge.

Thus, the combination of the Na⁺–K⁺ pump, the leak channels and the negatively charged cytosol creates a charge difference (differential) across the cell membrane. This differential is called the **resting membrane potential** (see **Figure 3-6**). If measured with

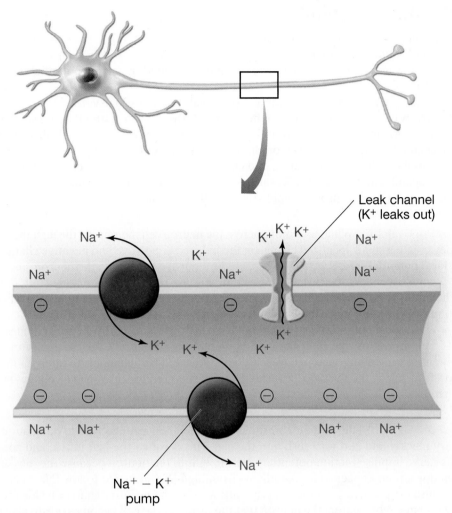

FIGURE 3-6 Resting membrane potential. Na$^+$ is pumped out of the cell by the Na$^+$–K$^+$ pump, and K$^+$ is pumped in but diffuses out through the leak channels. This causes positive ions to build up outside the cell and creates a resting membrane potential.

a tiny electrode, the resting membrane potential has a voltage of about –70 mV. (This is an average; the resting membrane potential can vary among neurons.) Because the interior of the cell has a negative charge, the resting membrane potential is defined as being negative.

Review Concepts 3-1: Neuron Function

- Neurons have a cell membrane that separates the cell's interior from the fluid outside the cell.

- Oxygen and carbon dioxide can diffuse through cell membranes.

- Ions are charged particles that pass through the neuron cell membrane using tiny ion channels embedded in the membrane.

- Ions move in or out of cells down their concentration gradient (from high to low), and according to their charges (opposite charges attract).

- At rest, the neuron cell membrane has more negative charges on the inside, and more positive charges on the outside.

- The resting membrane potential averages –70 mV.

The Action Potential

The function of neurons is to transmit information. This takes place by a flow of ions across the neuron cell membrane. The movement of ions sweeps like a wave along the cell membrane, and creates the electrical signal that is called the **action potential** or the **nerve impulse.**

A resting neuron has a membrane potential of about –70 mV. The inside of the cell is negatively charged with respect to the outside. If the neuron is stimulated, a small number of ion channels in the cell membrane will open in response to that stimulus. The type of ion channel that opens depends on the kind of stimulus. (For example, a physical/mechanical stimulus will cause pressure-gated channels to open, whereas a chemical stimulus will open ligand-gated channels.) Regardless of the type of stimulus, when some of the gated ion channels open, ions will be able to move through them.

LOCAL POTENTIAL When ions move across the neuron cell membrane through the channels, they create a small, localized change in the balance of positive and negative charges called a **local potential** (see **Figure 3-7**). It extends about 1–2 mm along the neuron, and lasts for a few milliseconds, after which the cell membrane returns to its resting state (–70 mV). The intensity of the stimulus determines the size of the local potential because a stronger stimulus will cause more ion channels to open.

If the local potential is strong enough so that the membrane potential reaches –55mV (15 mV more positive than the resting membrane potential), the change in membrane potential will be large enough to cause voltage-gated Na^+ channels to open. In most neurons, –55 mV is the average "threshold value" required for opening of voltage-gated Na^+ channels.

DEPOLARIZATION Once their threshold is reached, the voltage-gated Na^+ channels open very quickly and Na^+ ions rush into the cell. This is called the Na^+ influx, and constitutes the nerve impulse (action potential). Na^+ flows into the neuron because the ions are moving down their concentration gradient (from high $[Na^+]$ outside to low $[Na^+]$ inside), and because the positively charged ions are attracted to the negative charges inside the cell. In fact, so much Na^+ enters the neuron that the inside of the cell becomes positively charged. Thus, the action potential has a positive charge; at its peak, the inside of the neuron reaches a voltage of about +35 mV. Now, the neuron is **depolarized.**

The fast-opening Na^+ channels remain open for about 1 msec. As soon as they close, Na^+ ions are pumped out by the Na^+ –K^+ pump in the cell membrane. The voltage-gated Na^+ channels cannot be opened again until the membrane potential has regained its resting value (–70 mV). This means that the neuron cannot fire (generate another action potential) again for several milliseconds. The interval of time between action potentials is known as the **refractory period.**

When the neuron cell membrane reaches its threshold (–55 mV), slow-opening K^+ channels open. They allow K^+ ions to exit the cell at the same time that Na^+ ions are being pumped out. Together, the exodus of Na^+ and K^+ from the neuron re-establishes the resting membrane potential. Now the neuron is repolarized. In fact, so many positively charged ions exit the cell that there is a slight dip in membrane potential below the resting level. This is known as the after-hyperpolarization.

All action potentials are the same for each neuron: If the neuron's membrane potential reaches its threshold, there will always be an action potential. However, if the membrane potential fails to reach the threshold, there will be no action potential. It is impossible to have a partial action potential; for this reason, action potentials are referred to as being "all or none."

Action potentials always travel toward the axon terminal. As each section of cell membrane depolarizes, it causes voltage-gated channels in the section ahead of it to open (the "leading edge" of the action potential) (see **Figure 3-8**). In this way, each section of membrane depolarizes the next section. Thus, there is a wave of membrane depolarization that moves along the neuron. This wave always moves in the direction of the axon terminal. It cannot move backwards because of the after-hyperpolarization that occurs after each nerve impulse.

Local potential

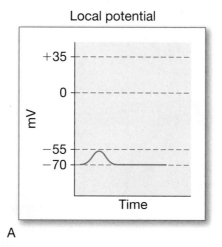

A

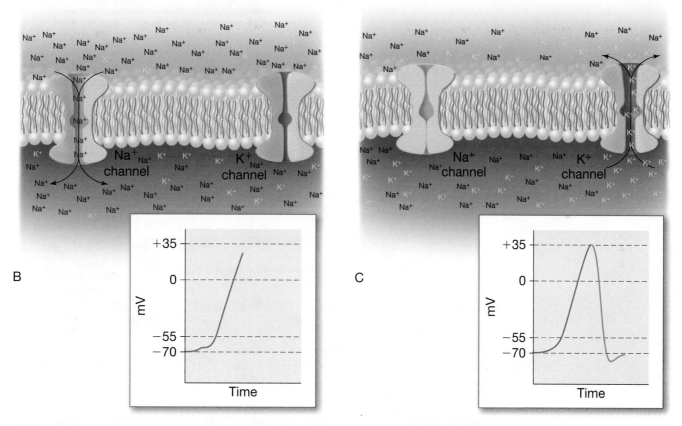

B   C

FIGURE 3-7 Excitation of the neuron cell membrane: local potential, depolarization (action potential), and repolarization. During depolarization, voltage-gated Na⁺ channels open and many Na⁺ ions flow into the neuron. During repolarization, the K⁺ channels open so K⁺ ions exit the neuron and restore the resting membrane potential.

Clinical Box 3-1: Topical Anesthetics

A topical anesthetic is applied to the skin to decrease pain from a surface wound. These drugs work by blocking Na⁺ channels, so that Na⁺ ions cannot enter the neuron and generate an action potential. Without an action potential, you do not feel the pain from an injury. Topical anesthetics include Lidocaine, Benzocaine, and Pramocaine. They are found in creams and gels used to treat minor cuts and scrapes, and also in gels used to numb teething pain and toothaches.

Challenge question: If a topical anesthetic blocked Na⁺ channels in motor axons as well as in sensory axons, what would happen?

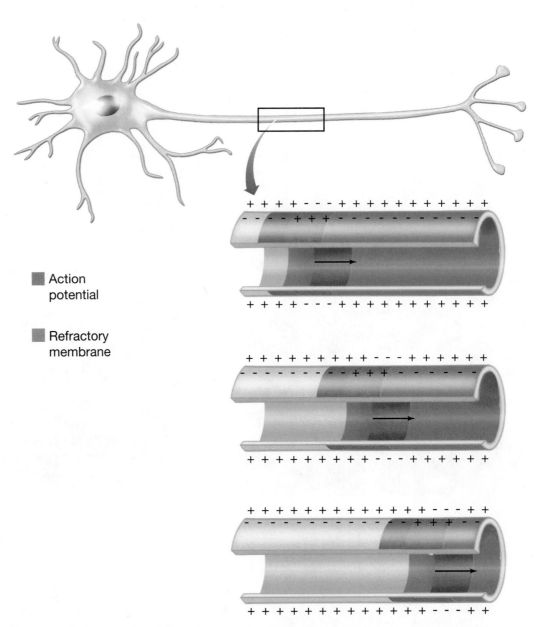

FIGURE 3-8 Propagation of the action potential. The action potential always moves toward the axon terminal. As each section of neuron cell membrane is depolarized, the Na⁺ influx depolarizes the next section of membrane.

Action potentials move along bare neuron cell membrane at a speed ranging between 0.6 m/sec and 2.3 m/sec, with an average speed of about 1 m/sec. Large diameter axons transmit signals faster than small axons. To further speed up signal transmission, many axons are insulated with **myelin.** Myelin is a fatty substance formed by glial cells. The glial cell membrane forms a sheath that wraps around each axon multiple times, similar to the way paper towels wrap around a cardboard tube. Each glial cell is separated from the others by a small gap, the node of Ranvier. Nodes are located about 1 mm apart along the myelin sheath. In myelinated axons, most of the voltage-gated ion channels are located at the nodes, with only a few channels found underneath the myelin. This allows the ions to flow inside the cell from one node to the next, depolarizing the channels at the next node. Action potentials therefore "skip" along the myelinated axon from node to node, a process called **saltatory conduction** (see **Figure 3-9**). This increases the speed of the action potential 10 to 100 times, averaging about 100 m/sec.

Conduction of action potentials is very reliable. This reliability is described as the **safety factor** of the neuron. The safety factor is the ratio between the amount of current

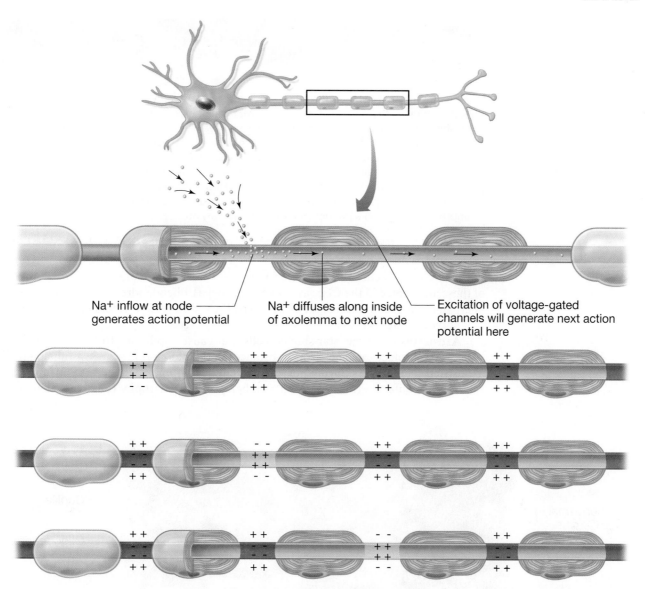

FIGURE 3-9 Saltatory conduction in a myelinated axon. As each node of Ranvier is depolarized, ions flow inside the axon to depolarize the next section of unmyelinated cell membrane. Saltatory conduction allows the action potential to move along the axon very rapidly. The action potential can "skip" from one node of Ranvier to the next.

(ion flow) that is available to stimulate an action potential, compared to the amount of current that is needed to stimulate it. In a healthy myelinated axon, the safety factor is usually between 5 and 6. This means that there is about 5 times as much current available as the neuron really needs. If the safety factor falls below 1, action potentials cannot be transmitted; this is called a conduction block.

Glial Cells

Glial cells (neuroglia) are the supporting cells of the nervous system. There are about 50 times as many glial cells as neurons. (Unlike most neurons, glial cells can divide throughout life, so most brain tumors are actually glial cell tumors.) Neuroglia have many different functions, including maintaining the fluid surrounding neurons, removing debris from the nervous system, and forming the myelin sheath that insulates axons. In addition, some glial cells can communicate with neurons to influence their functions (Fields & Stevens-Graham, 2002).

Clinical Box 3-2: Multiple Sclerosis

Conditions that damage the myelin sheath are called demyelinating diseases. The most common of these is multiple sclerosis (MS). Multiple sclerosis is an autoimmune disease in which the immune system attacks and injures myelin in the brain and spinal cord. People with MS cannot transmit action potentials effectively. Symptoms vary depending on the specific places in the CNS where myelin is damaged. Common symptoms include sensory loss and spastic paralysis. High temperatures make the symptoms of MS worse, so therapists must be careful to avoid overheating when working with people who have MS.

Challenge question: Would a medication that decreases immune system function improve sensation in a patient with MS? Why or why not?

Five kinds of neuroglial cells are found in the nervous system (see **Figure 3-10**). Four of these are located in the CNS: astrocytes (astroglia), oligodendrocytes (oligodendroglia), microglia, and ependymal cells. The fifth type (Schwann cells) is found only in the peripheral nervous system (PNS).

Astrocytes are large, star-shaped cells that cause capillaries to form a blood-brain barrier that protects neurons from substances in the blood. Astrocytes also help growing axons find their targets during nervous system development. If the CNS is injured, the astrocytes proliferate (increase their numbers) and hypertrophy (enlarge). They form a

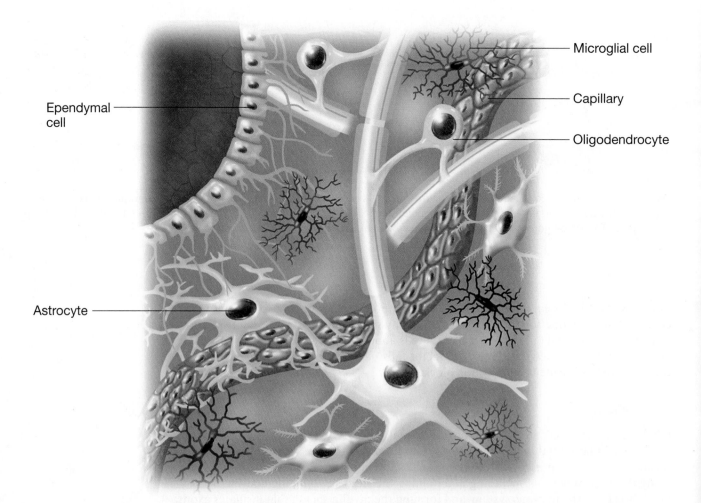

FIGURE 3-10 Glial cells in the central nervous system include the astrocytes (stimulate creation of the blood-brain barrier), oligodendrocytes (form myelin sheath), microglia (phagocytosis), and ependymal cells (secrete cerebrospinal fluid).

kind of meshwork around injured areas that isolates the affected area from the rest of the nervous system.

Oligodendroglial cells **(oligodendrocytes)** are also found in the CNS. They form the myelin sheath that insulates axons in the brain and spinal cord. Each oligodendrocyte can contribute to the myelination of between 7 and 70 axons. Oligodendrocytes are targets of the immune system in people with multiple sclerosis, causing de-myelination and impairing transmission of action potentials.

Microglia are small cells found in the CNS. Microglia are activated if there is an injury or illness. When activated, microglia migrate to the site of injury to surround damaged neurons. They act like phagocytes, removing and degrading dead or damaged cells from the nervous system (Fetler & Amigorena, 2005). Microglia have cell-surface receptors for the virus that causes AIDS (HIV), and thus can act as a hiding place for the virus within the nervous system.

Ependymal cells line the ventricles of the brain, and the central canal of the spinal cord. Some ependymal cells inside the ventricles produce cerebrospinal fluid, and assist in its circulation.

Schwann cells (also called neurilemmal cells) are located in the peripheral nervous system. Schwann cells surround and protect peripheral nerve fibers (axons), and their cell membranes form the myelin sheath that insulates peripheral axons. In addition, Schwann cells assist in axon regeneration by forming small tunnels that guide regrowth, and by secreting chemicals (growth factors) that stimulate axon growth after injury.

Neuron Injury and Repair

Neurons can be injured by disease, trauma, and lack of oxygen (anoxia). Diseases that kill neurons include Parkinson disease, Alzheimer disease, polio, and amyotrophic lateral sclerosis (Lou Gehrig disease). Trauma can result from head injury, nerve compression, and ischemia (lack of blood supply). This can damage neurons directly, and can also disrupt blood flow to the region surrounding the traumatic injury. Lack of oxygen often results from an interruption in blood flow to the nervous system, due to a stroke or heart attack.

When neuron cell bodies are damaged, the entire nerve cell dies. Cell death caused by injury or illness is called **necrosis.** When neurons die, they release chemicals that can be toxic to nearby cells. This means that necrosis can spread from an area of initial damage to nearby regions.

If axons (instead of cell bodies) are damaged, the axon will degenerate as a result (see **Figure 3-11**). In the CNS, this kills the entire neuron. Apparently, CNS neurons cannot regenerate their axons. This probably occurs because the CNS lacks chemicals that

Clinical Box 3-3: Guillain-Barre Syndrome

Guillain-Barre Syndrome (GBS) is the most common cause of acute (nontraumatic) paralysis. The syndrome is caused by an autoimmune reaction that destroys the myelin surrounding peripheral nerve fibers. Symptoms include flaccid paralysis, sensory loss or sensory hypersensitivity, blood pressure fluctuations, dysarthria (difficulty speaking), and dysphagia (difficulty swallowing). The peripheral nerves that innervate the diaphragm (phrenic nerves) may be compromised. If this occurs, the patient will require mechanical ventilation to assist with breathing. Typically, within a few weeks of the original de-myelination, the Schwann cells begin to regenerate and nerve transmission begins to be restored. Therapy for patients with GBS initially focuses on preventing pressure sores and maintaining range-of-motion as the patient progresses toward the most acute phase. As nerve function (action potential transmission) returns, patients begin to recover, and clinicians focus treatment on regaining strength, balance, and gait training.

Challenge question: What do MS and GBS have in common? How are they different?

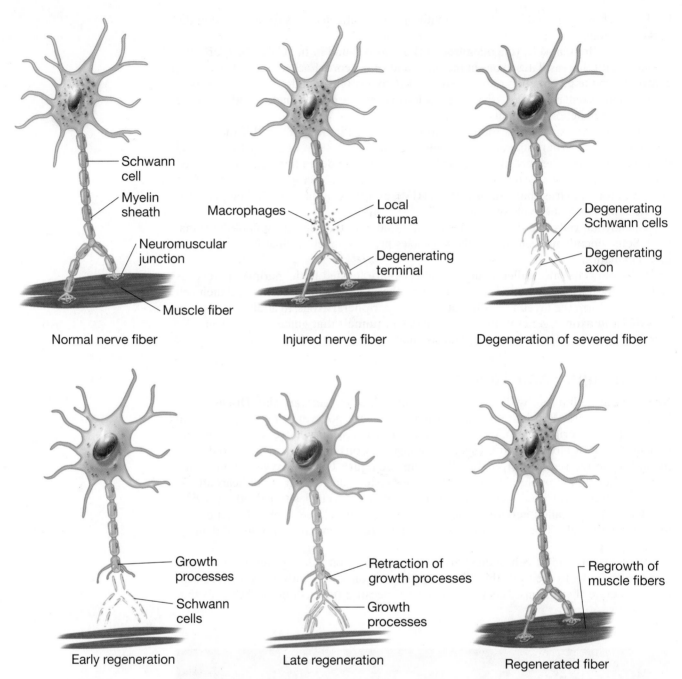

FIGURE 3-11 Regeneration of an injured neuron. When an axon in the peripheral nervous system is damaged, it degenerates, and then regrows. This growth is guided by Schwann cells. If the regenerating axons find a target and form synapses, they are retained and function can be restored.

facilitate axon regeneration, and contains chemicals that inhibit regrowth. Thus, injury to an axon in the brain or spinal cord almost always causes the entire nerve cell to die.

In the peripheral nervous system, damage to an axon usually does not cause the neuron to die. After injury, the axon degenerates within a few weeks. After that, a new axon sprouts from the cell body. The new axon grows until it reaches a target cell (another neuron, or a muscle cell), where it forms a new synapse. In part, this occurs because the Schwann cells produce chemical growth (trophic) factors that stimulate axon growth (Kablar & Belliveau, 2005), and form tunnels that guide the regenerating axons toward their targets. The new axons must form connections with other cells in order to survive. If they fail to do this, they will die and be removed from the nervous system (this is called "pruning"). Axons in the PNS can regenerate at a rate of about 1 mm per day. Thus, it may take several years for a long axon to regenerate completely.

When neurons die, they are not usually replaced. In adults, neurons can reproduce in only a few selected locations (the hippocampus and the olfactory bulb). This means that loss of neurons can cause death or permanent disability. When people regain function after nervous system injury, the improvement is due to new connections among existing neurons (rewiring).

Review Concepts 3-2: Neuron Regeneration

- When neuron cell bodies are injured, the neurons die and are not replaced.
- Central nervous system axons cannot regenerate, so the entire neuron dies.
- Peripheral nervous system axons can regenerate, aided by Schwann cells that stimulate growth.

PATIENT SCENARIOS

Patient Case 3-1 (Wayne)

Wayne is 55 years old. He began to experience blurred vision, fatigue, numbness, and difficulty walking. These signs and symptoms worsened until he needed a wheelchair for mobility. MRI scans revealed a number of sclerotic plaques in Wayne's brain and spinal cord. He was diagnosed with multiple sclerosis (MS).

Questions
a) How does MS affect transmission of nerve impulses?
b) Does MS affect the CNS or the PNS?
c) Which glial cell is the target of the damage in MS?

Patient Case 3-2 (Alison)

About a week after recovering from the flu, Allison, age 23, began to feel weakness and numbness in both of her legs. This began in her feet and moved up, and over the next few days it began to affect her arms as well. Allison was diagnosed with Guillain-Barre Syndrome.

Questions
a) How does GBS affect transmission of nerve impulses?
b) Does GBS affect the CNS or the PNS?
c) Which glial cell is the target of the damage in GBS?

Review Questions

1. Identify all parts of a neuron, including the cell body, dendrites, axon, and axon terminals.

2. Explain how modality (pressure)-gated, ligand (transmitter)-gated and voltage-gated ion channels work. What types of stimuli cause each channel to open its gate?

3. Describe the neuron when it is at rest (not transmitting information). What factors contribute to the resting membrane potential? What is the average voltage of the resting potential?

4. Discuss how an action potential is generated. Include the role of voltage-gated Na^+ and K^+ channels in depolarization and repolarization.

5. Why do myelinated axons transmit nerve signals faster than unmyelinated axons? Define the term *saltatory conduction.*

6. Describe the functions of glial cells (astrocytes, oligodendroglial cells, microglia, ependymal cells, and Schwann cells). In which part of the nervous system is each type of glial cell located?

7. Describe what happens when a neuron is injured. Distinguish the process in the peripheral nervous system from what happens in the central nervous system.

References

1. Fetler, L., & Amigorena, S. (2005). Brain under surveillance: The microglia patrol. *Science, 309,* 392–393.

2. Fields, R. D., & Stevens-Graham, B. (2002). New insights into neuron-glial communication. *Science, 298,* 556–562.

3. Kablar, B., & Belliveau, A. C. (2005). Presence of neurotrophic factors in skeletal muscle correlates with survival of spinal cord motor neurons. *Developmental Dynamics, 234,* 659–669.

4. Oh, S., Huang, X., & Chiang, C. (2005). Specific requirement of sonic hedgehog signaling during oligodendrocyte development. *Developmental Dynamics, 234,* 489–496.

Further Reading

1. Long, S. B., Campbell, E. B., & MacKinnon, R. (2005). Voltage sensor of Kv1.2: Structural basis of electromechanical coupling. *Science, 309,* 903–908.

2. Pascual, O., et al. (2005). Astrocytic purinergic signaling coordinates synaptic networks. *Science, 310,* 113–116.

3. Yang, Y. et al. (2004). Mutations in SCN9A encoding a sodium channel alpha subunit in patients with primary erythermalgia. *J. Med. Genetics, 41*(3), 171–174.

PEARSON
myhealthprofessionskit™

Use this address to access the Companion Website created for this textbook. Simply select "Physical Therapy" from the choice of disciplines. Find this book and log in using your username and password to access self-assessment questions, a glossary, and more.

Synapses

KEY TERMS

denervation
excitatory postsynaptic potential (EPSP)
exocytosis
gene expression
inhibitory postsynaptic potential (IPSP)
neural plasticity
neuromuscular junction
neurotransmitter
postsynaptic neuron
presynaptic neuron
synapse
synaptic cleft
synaptic pruning
synaptic receptors
synaptic vesicles
synaptogenesis

Essential Facts···

▶ A synapse is a connection between two neurons.

▶ At synapses, chemicals called neurotransmitters move from one neuron to another.

▶ Neurotransmitters bind to receptors and modify neuron function.

▶ Many diseases and conditions of the nervous system involve changes in the structure and function of synapses.

▶ Changes in synapse function are associated with learning and memory.

The human nervous system contains about 10^{12} individual neurons (nerve cells). Each of these is connected to many other nerve cells at structures called **Synapses**. Synapses are the structures that give the nervous system its rich complexity. Synapses are continually created, modified, and removed ("pruned"). This flexibility in the networks of nerve connections is called synaptic plasticity, and it is the basis of learning. Physical, occupational, and speech therapy take advantage of plasticity to allow patients to recover from damage or disease involving the nervous system. Clinicians design rehabilitation sessions and protocols to maximize the nervous system's ability to rewire and reorganize in order to regain functional ability.

Synapse Structure and Function

A synapse is the place where neurons communicate with other cells (see **Figure 4-1**). Neurons can form synapses with other nerve cells, with muscle cells, and with glands. Many disorders of the nervous system involve the synapses, including both physical and mental illnesses. In addition, many drugs that are prescribed to affect the nervous system affect the synapses, as do most drugs of addiction. Effective rehabilitation and therapy are designed to modify synapses in order to restore or improve function.

Synapse Structure

Two types of synapses are found in the nervous system: electrical synapses and chemical synapses. *Electrical synapses* are tiny channels called gap junctions that allow ions to flow from one neuron to the next. Electrical synapses produce very fast responses to stimuli and allow neurons to fire together in a coordinated way.

Most of the synapses found in the human nervous system are chemical synapses. At *chemical synapses,* one neuron communicates with another cell by releasing a chemical called a **neurotransmitter** that affects the function of the second cell.

At chemical synapses, there are always two cells: (1) a **presynaptic neuron** and (2) a postsynaptic cell (see **Figure 4-2**). The postsynaptic cell can be another neuron (a **postsynaptic neuron**), a muscle cell, or a gland cell. (If the postsynaptic cell is a muscle cell, the synapse is called a **neuromuscular junction.**) In between the presynaptic neuron and the postsynaptic neuron is a small space called the **synaptic cleft.** The cleft is about 30 nm wide and contains fluid.

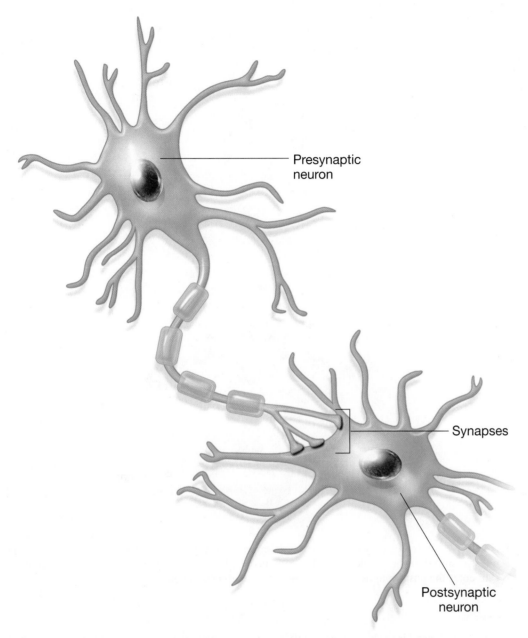

FIGURE 4-1   A presynaptic neuron synapsing with a postsynaptic neuron.

Inside each presynaptic axon terminal are several thousand small hollow spheres called **synaptic vesicles.** Each vesicle contains several thousand molecules of a chemical called a neurotransmitter. On the postsynaptic side of the synapse, each cell contains many small receptor proteins. These receptors are specific for the neurotransmitter found at that synapse. The neurotransmitter and its receptors must match in order for the synapse to function.

Synapse Function

Synapse function begins with an action potential in the presynaptic neuron. The action potential causes Ca^{+2} channels to open in the axon terminal, allowing Ca^{+2} ions to flow in. The Ca^{+2} influx allows synaptic vesicles to fuse with the presynaptic cell membrane. This results in **exocytosis** of the chemical neurotransmitter into the synaptic cleft (Rettig & Neher, 2002).

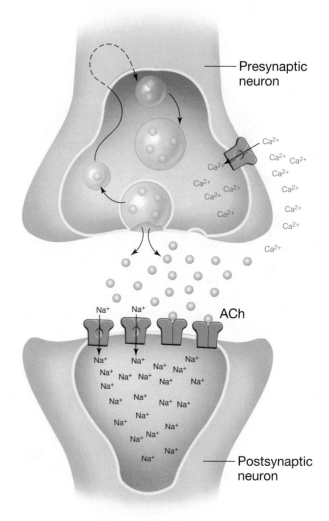

FIGURE 4-2   A chemical synapse. When Ca^{2+} enters the presynaptic neuron, acetylcholine (ACh) is released into the synaptic cleft. ACh binds to its receptors on the post-synaptic side. This allows Na^+ to enter the post-synaptic cell, triggering a new action potential.

Once released into the synaptic cleft, the neurotransmitter molecules diffuse across the cleft. The postsynaptic membrane contains neurotransmitter receptors. When a neurotransmitter molecule reaches the postsynaptic membrane, it binds to its receptor.

When a neurotransmitter binds to its receptor, ions flow either into, or out of, the postsynaptic cell (see below). Thus, neurotransmitter binding changes the postsynaptic cell's membrane potential (see **Figure 4-3**). This change is called the postsynaptic potential (PSP). The size of the PSP depends on how many neurotransmitter molecules bind to their **synaptic receptors;** more neurotransmitter means a stronger PSP.

At some synapses, neurotransmitter binding causes the interior of the postsynaptic neuron to become more positively charged; if this happens, the PSP will be an **excitatory postsynaptic potential (EPSP).** This type of synapse would be called a stimulatory synapse. If the post-synaptic cell becomes more negatively charged, the PSP will be an **inhibitory postsynaptic potential (IPSP).** A synapse with IPSPs is referred to as an inhibitory synapse. EPSPs are generated when neurotransmitter binding causes an inflow of positively charged ions (Na^+ or Ca^{+2}). IPSPs occur when binding of the neurotransmitter causes an outflow of positive ions (K^+), or an inflow of negatively charged ions (Cl^-).

Since each EPSP is about 0.2 to 0.4 mV, approximately 50 to 100 EPSPs are required to allow the postsynaptic cell to reach its threshold for depolarization. This means that either (1) one synapse must fire 50 to 100 times in order to stimulate an action potential in the postsynaptic neuron or (2) there must be firing of 50 to 100 separate synapses.

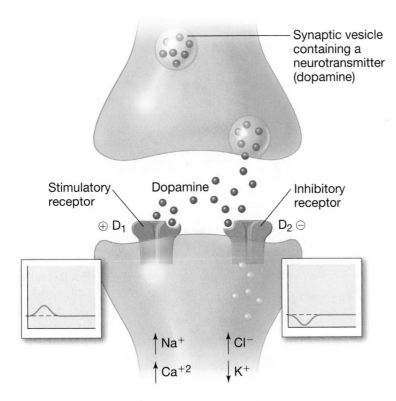

FIGURE 4-3 Postsynaptic potentials. When a neurotransmitter binds to a stimulatory receptor, the inside of the postsynaptic cell becomes more positively charged. This can occur if Na^+ or Ca^{+2} enter the cell. If the neurotransmitter binds to an inhibitory receptor, the inside of the postsynaptic cell becomes more negatively charged. This will occur if Cl^- ions enter the cell, or if K^+ ions leave the cell.

Every neuron in the human nervous system receives thousands of synapses. If the sum of all EPSPs and IPSPs reaches the depolarization threshold for that portion of the nerve cell, the cell will be stimulated; a new action potential will be generated. However, if the sum of EPSPs and IPSPs does not reach the threshold for the action potential, the postsynaptic neuron will be inhibited. Overall, the nervous system has about the same number of stimulatory (EPSPs) and inhibitory (IPSPs) synapses. Thus, whether a neuron depolarizes (generates an action potential) or not depends on the balance between excitatory/stimulatory synapses and inhibitory synapses at any particular moment.

The last step in synaptic function is inactivation. After a neurotransmitter has bound to its receptor, it detaches and returns to the synaptic cleft (see Figure 4-4). Once in the cleft, the neurotransmitter is available to bind to anther receptor. In order to inactivate the synapse, the neurotransmitter molecule must be removed from the cleft. This can occur in one of three ways: diffusion, degradation, or reuptake. All neurotransmitters are at least partially removed by diffusing out of the synaptic cleft. Degradation uses enzymes to break

Neuroscience Notes Box 4-1: Drugs and Synapses

Most drugs that people take for "recreational purposes" act at synapses. Some of these drugs stimulate synapses, whereas others inhibit them. For example, nicotine and cocaine are both stimulatory; heroin and alcohol are inhibitory. Overdose of a stimulatory drug can cause death because it will overactivate the nervous system: Cocaine can cause the heart rate to increase dramatically (tachycardia) and result in a heart attack. In contrast, overdose of an inhibitory drug may cause fatal respiratory arrest.

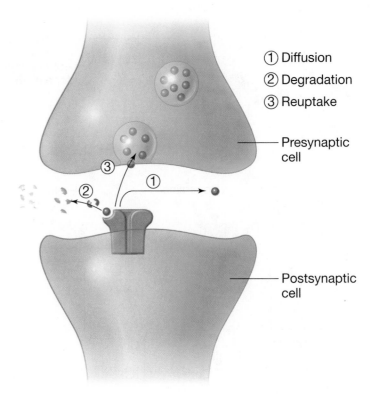

FIGURE 4-4 Neurotransmitter inactivation. Neurotransmitters are inactivated in one of three ways: they can diffuse out of the synapse (1), they can be broken down by enzymes (2), or they can be taken up by the presynaptic neuron (3).

down neurotransmitters into their component chemicals. In reuptake, transporter proteins pump the neurotransmitter molecules back into the presynaptic axon terminal. Once back inside the presynaptic terminal, the neurotransmitter can be destroyed by enzymes, or put into a new synaptic vesicle for reuse. Reuptake seems to be the most common mechanism for inactivating neurotransmitters.

Neurotransmitters and Receptors

A neurotransmitter is a chemical that acts at a synapse. Generally, neurotransmitters are organized into two categories: small-molecule neurotransmitters and large-molecule neurotransmitters (see **Tables 4.1** and **4.2**). Small-molecule neurotransmitters are either amines or amino acids. Amine neurotransmitters all have names that end in *-ine,* and

Review Concepts 4-1: Steps in Synapse Function

- Neurotransmitters are produced inside neurons and are released into the synaptic cleft after stimulation by an action potential.

- Neurotransmitters diffuse across the synaptic cleft and bind to their specific receptors.

- Receptor binding produces changes in the postsynaptic neuron, either stimulating or inhibiting it.

- Neurotransmitters detach from their receptors and are inactivated.

Table 4.1 Small Molecule Neurotransmitters

Name	Function	Associated Diseases	Drugs Affecting This Neurotransmitter or Its Receptors
Acetylcholine (Ach)	Skeletal muscle contraction; focus and attention	Myasthenia gravis, Alzheimer's disease	Botox, nicotine, curare
Dopamine (DA)	Movement initiation and inhibition; motivation and drive	Parkinson's disease, Tourette syndrome, schizophrenia, addiction, OCD	Nicotine, cocaine, alcohol, L-dopa, anti-psychotics
Norepinephrine (NE)	General arousal and alertness	Depression, mania, PTSD	Amphetamines
Glycine	Inhibition in spinal cord	Glycine encephalopathy	Strychnine
GABA (Gamma amino butyric acid)	Inhibition in brain	Huntington disease, spasticity, seizures	Valium, Baclofen, ethanol, Xanax, Phenobarbital, Neurontin, Topamax
Glutamate	Learning and memory	Seizures, ALS	
Serotonin	Mood, behavior, inhibits pain	Depression, anxiety	SSRIs (Prozac, Zoloft, Effexor)

include acetylcholine, dopamine, histamine, norepinephrine, and serotonin (5-hydroxytritamine). The amino acids include glycine, glutamate, and GABA (gamma-amino butyric acid). The large-molecule neurotransmitters are peptides (neuropeptides). Neuropeptides include substance P, endorphins, and enkephalins.

Each synaptic receptor is specific for a neurotransmitter. The neurotransmitter must have the correct chemical structure to fit into a binding site on its receptor. Every receptor has different subtypes, each of which can have a slightly different effect on the postsynaptic neuron. For example, the neurotransmitter dopamine can bind to a stimulatory (D1) receptor and to an inhibitory (D2) receptor. Thus, the same chemical neurotransmitter can have different effects on nervous system function based on the location and type of its receptors. It is the receptor that determines what effect the neurotransmitter will have on the postsynaptic cell (Klein et al., 2007).

A special type of synapse is located at the connection between a motor neuron and a skeletal muscle fiber. This is called a neuromuscular junction (see Figure 4-5). At neuromuscular junctions, the axon terminal always releases the neurotransmitter acetylcholine (Ach). Acetylcholine binds to its receptors on the muscle cell membrane and triggers

Table 4.2 Large Molecule Neurotransmitters

Name	Function	Associated Diseases	Drugs
Endogenous opioids (endorphins & enkephalins)	Decrease pain perception	Addiction	Morphine, heroin, Vicodin, Oxycontin
Substance P	Transmits pain	Pain and inflammation	

Neuromuscular Junction

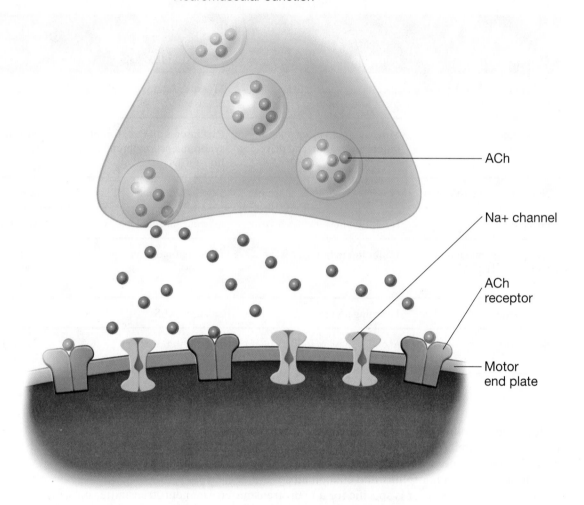

ACh

Na+ channel

ACh receptor

Motor end plate

FIGURE 4-5 The neuromuscular junction. When Ach (acetylcholine) is released from the axon terminal, it diffuses across the synaptic cleft and binds to its receptor on the motor end plate of the muscle cell. This causes a Na⁺ influx into the muscle cell. When the muscle cell is depolarized by the Na⁺ ions, the muscle will contract.

Clinical Box 4-1: Brain Disease and Neurotransmitters

Many diseases and conditions affecting the nervous system are associated with neurotransmitters and their receptors. For example, people with Parkinson's disease usually have a deficit of dopamine. Many mental illnesses (e.g., bipolar disorder, schizophrenia, and clinical depression) are actually biological conditions that affect the brain. These conditions are associated with changes in neurotransmitters, receptors, or both. For example, some cases of clinical depression are associated with abnormalities in the serotonin that is produced, or problems with dysfunctional receptors—that are unable to bind with the seratonin.

Challenge question: If you were designing a medication to treat the symptoms of Parkinson disease, what kind of receptors would you focus on?

Clinical Box 4-2: Denervation Hypersensitivity

Neurotransmitter receptors are found only at synapses. In a normal nervous system, receptors are never found on other parts of the cell membrane. It appears that the presynaptic axon terminal tells the postsynaptic neuron to put receptors into the cell membrane only at the synapses. When injury or disease damages a presynaptic neuron, the postsynaptic neuron loses some or all of its synapses, and is **denervated.** For unknown reasons, these neurons become hypersensitive and overreact to stimulation. This means that the denervated cell will respond too strongly to a "normal" amount of neurotransmitter. This phenomenon is referred to as denervation hypersensitivity.

Challenge question: If a patient has denervation hypersensitivity, what effect might this have on motor function? How might this affect sensory function?

contraction of the muscle cell. If Ach cannot be released from the motor neuron, or if the Ach receptors on the muscle cell membrane are damaged, the muscle cannot contract. There are several diseases, and a number of drugs, that can modify function of the neuromuscular junction. For example, curare (derived from South American frogs) blocks Ach receptors so that muscles are unable to contract. For this reason it is used as a poison. In myasthenia gravis, the immune system produces antibodies to Ach receptors, producing muscle weakness and fatigue.

Synaptic Plasticity

Neurons are connected by synapses into complex neural networks that perform many important functions in the nervous system. For example, these interconnected networks store memories, permit efficient movement, detect and respond to sensations, and allow thought, emotion, and communication. Synapse formation is believed to be the biological basis of long-term learning and memory. Throughout life, new synapses are created, and old ones are maintained or removed (pruned). Thus, the brain's network of connections is always changing. This is the basis of **neural plasticity,** which is the re-wiring of the brain's synaptic connections based on experience (Cohen-Cory, 2002; Sheng & Kim, 2002).

Synaptogenesis is the process of creating a new synapse. Synapses are formed throughout life, although they form more easily in younger people than in older ones. At birth,

Clinical Box 4-3: Botox

Botox (botulism toxin) prevents exocytosis of the neurotransmitter acetylcholine at the neuromuscular junction, preventing muscle contraction. It can be used clinically to decrease muscle contraction in patients with spastic muscles (for example, in people with torticollis or cerebral palsy). Injection of Botox results in temporary paralysis or paresis (weakening) of the muscles surrounding the injection site. Clinicians use this period of paresis to relax and elongate tight or spastic muscles in an effort to prevent or limit the progression of contractures and help restore normal posture. Some people have Botox injected into their facial muscles to paralyze them and temporarily minimize the appearance of wrinkles.

Botox wears off after a few months, so treatment must be repeated.

Challenge question: What could happen if a patient received a large overdose of Botox? (*Hint:* Suppose the phrenic nerve [supplying the diaphragm] were to receive a large quantity of this drug?)

Neuroscience Notes Box 4-2: Genes and Learning

In animals, including fruit flies and mice, scientists altered genes involved in synapse formation and have found that the animals' ability to learn and remember changed. For example, mice with more copies of a gene for a particular kind of glutamate receptor learned much faster than normal mice. In contrast, mice with fewer copies of this gene than normal were slow learners. In humans, several genetic conditions that produce cognitive disability are correlated with changes in this gene.

the human brain has a relatively small number of synapses already formed. After birth, stimulation promotes synaptogenesis. When synapses are activated sufficiently, synaptogenic genes in both presynaptic and postsynaptic neurons are expressed (turned on). Thus, sufficient sensory or motor stimulation can lead to the creation of new synapses in the CNS. In fact, appropriate stimulation is required for developing a normal pattern of synapses. An important function of therapy is to help patients acquire the synaptic connections most useful for regaining function.

Throughout life, some neurons will fail to form synapses. In addition, some synapses are seldom activated. These neurons are removed from the CNS via a process called **synaptic pruning.** Pruning of little-used neurons and synapses helps to explain why memories may fade with time; unless the synapses are fired regularly, they will be gradually pruned away and removed. Regular synaptic firing is required to activate genes coding for proteins that maintain the synapses.

In childhood, many synapses are established during certain developmental stages. These are referred to as *sensitive* or *critical periods*. During a critical period, many new synaptic connections are established among neurons in specific regions of the brain. These new synapses require appropriate stimulation in order to form. This has been demonstrated within the visual system of animals. For example, if a newborn animal's eyelids are sewn shut at birth (so that the visual system cannot receive any visual stimuli), the animal's visual cortex will not form normal synaptic patterns. Even when the animal's eyelids are opened, the visual system is unable to organize itself correctly and establish synapses, so visual function is impaired.

As described earlier, synapses are continually being created, maintained, and removed (pruned away) (see Figure 4-6). This is one proposed mechanism for the phenomenon of neuroplasticity. Neuroplasticity is reorganization of the nervous system based on experience, and is the basis for healing and recovery of function after injury or disease. It is also the basis for much physical, occupational, and speech therapy treatment. Therapy provides the appropriate motor and sensory experiences for patients in order to facilitate the desired pattern of synaptic connections in the CNS.

Review Concepts 4-2: Neuroplasticity

- Neuroplasticity is the reorganization of synaptic connections in the central nervous system.
- Synapses are created in patterns that reflect life experiences.
- Synapses that are used frequently are strengthened and persist within the CNS.
- Synapses that are rarely used are removed (pruned).

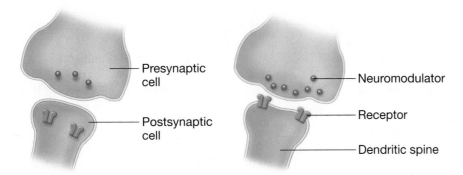

1) Synapse before activation

2) Synapse after activation:
beginning to grow dendritic spines

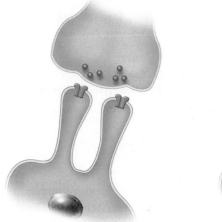 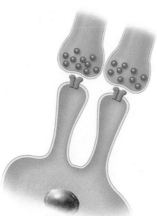

3) After continued activation,
new synapses begin organizing

4) Formation of new synapse
after repeated activation

FIGURE 4-6   Synaptic changes occur after a synapse is activated and include growth of new dendrites and axon terminals that can result in formation of new synaptic connections.

PATIENT SCENARIOS

Patient Case 2-1 (Andy)

Andy is 7 years old. He was born with cerebral palsy that affects both of his legs. Andy can walk with assistance but his gait is hampered by extreme spasticity and hypertonicity in his adductor compartment muscles. A physician recommends injection of Botulism toxin (Botox) to release the spasticity and permit Andy to walk more normally. Botox inhibits exocytosis of the neurotransmitter acetylcholine at the synapse between motor neurons and muscle cells (the neuromuscular junction).

Questions

a) How does inhibiting release of a neurotransmitter affect the function of a synapse?
b) How will the injection of Botox work to decrease contraction of Andy's adductor muscles?
c) What other methods can you think of to inhibit the function of a synapse?

Patient Case 4-2 (Johnnie)

Johnnie is a 33-year-old woman. She presents in your clinic with fatigue and muscle weakness on both sides of her body. This weakness affects all of her muscles, and is especially noticeable in the muscles that move her eyes (extraocular muscles) and face (muscles of facial expression). She also has trouble swallowing, and her eyelids droop. Her diagnosis is myasthenia gravis, an autoimmune disease. In myasthenia gravis, the immune system attacks and destroys receptors for acetylcholine at the synapse between motor neurons and muscle cells (the neuromuscular junction).

Questions

a) How does blocking acetylcholine receptors affect the function of a synapse (neuromuscular junction)?
b) What effect on muscle function will this disease have, since the nerve-muscle synapse is not functioning correctly?

Review Questions

1. Draw and label a synapse. Include the following in your diagram: axon terminal, synaptic vesicles, neurotransmitter molecules, synaptic cleft, and postsynaptic receptors.

2. Explain the process of synaptic transmission. What is the difference between excitatory (stimulatory) and inhibitory synapses?

3. Which neurotransmitter is found at the neuromuscular junction? Which one is deficient in people with Parkinson's disease? Which is associated with pain? With learning? With seizures? With addiction? With spasticity?

4. How are synapses affected when learning occurs? Why might a synapse be removed (pruned)?

References

1. Cohen-Cory, S. (2002). The developing synapse: Construction and modulation of synaptic structures and circuits. *Science, 298,* 770–776.

2. Rettig, J. & Neher, E. (2002). Emerging roles of presynaptic proteins in Ca^{+2} triggered exocytosis. *Science, 298,* 781–785.

3. Sheng, M., & Kim, M. J. (2002). Postsynaptic signaling and plasticity mechanisms. *Science, 298,* 776–780.

4. Klein, T. A., Neumann, J., Reuter, M., Hennig, J., von Cramon, D. Y., & Ullsperger, M. (2007). Genetically determined differences in learning from errors. *Science, 318,* 1642–1645.

Further Reading

1. Atwood, H. L. (2006). Gatekeeper at the synapse. *Science, 312,* 1008–1009.

2. Delkoe, D. L. (2002). Alzheimer's disease is a synaptic failure. *Science, 298,* 789–791.

3. Zoghbi, H. Y. (2003). Postnatal neurodevelopmental disorders: Meeting at the synapse? *Science, 302,* 826–830.

PEARSON
myhealthprofessionskit™

Use this address to access the Companion Website created for this textbook. Simply select "Physical Therapy" from the choice of disciplines. Find this book and log in using your username and password to access self-assessment questions, a glossary, and more.

Cerebral Cortex

CHAPTER OBJECTIVES

After completing this chapter, the reader will be able to:

1. Name the major types of neurons and axons (nerve fibers) found in the cerebral cortex.

2. Identify the major functional areas of each lobe of the cerebral cortex and state the role of each region.

3. Discuss the areas of the cerebral cortex responsible for movement, somatosensation, hearing, vision, smell and taste, and the reception and production of language.

4. Explain how the prefrontal cortex is involved in thinking, problem solving, and inhibition of impulsive behavior.

5. Describe the effect of injury or disease to each functional region of the cortex.

KEY TERMS

amnesia
amygdala
anosmia
aphasia
apraxia
auditory cortex
Broca's area
Brodmann's map
cerebral cortex
cerebral hemisphere
cerebrum
corpus callosum
frontal lobe
hemianopsia
hippocampus
internal capsule
limbic system
motor cortex
occipital lobe
olfactory cortex
parietal lobe
prefrontal cortex
prefrontal syndrome
somatosensory cortex
stereognosis
supplementary motor
    area (SMA)
temporal lobe
visual cortex
Wernicke's area

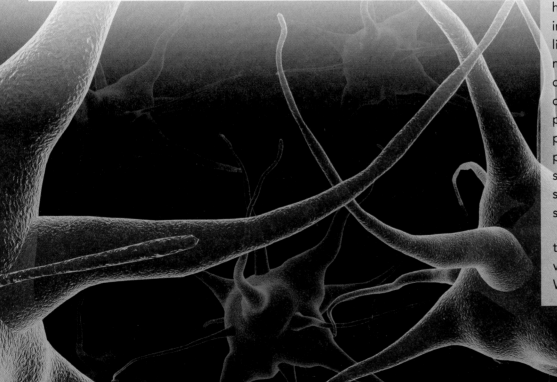

Essential Facts··

▶ The cerebral cortex is the outer part of the **cerebrum,** which makes up about 80% of the brain.

▶ The cerebral cortex is formed by right and left halves (hemispheres).

▶ Each cerebral hemisphere is divided into four lobes: frontal, parietal, occipital, and temporal

▶ The cortex has trillions of functional connections within each hemisphere, between

hemispheres, and to other areas of the nervous system.

▶ Memory, language, thought, emotion, problem solving, and sensation all take place in the cerebral cortex.

▶ Movement originates in the cortex, and also involves many other areas of the brain and spinal cord.

The cerebrum is the brain's largest subdivision; it makes up about 80% of the brain. It is divided into two halves called hemispheres (right and left). The outer shell of the cerebrum is called the **cerebral cortex,** and is subdivided into regions called lobes (see **Figure 5-1**). The cortex is the part of the brain where high-level processing occurs. Thought, emotion, language, memory, and sensory perception all occur in the cortex. Injuries to the cerebrum cause numerous functional difficulties, including paralysis and other movement disorders; loss of sensory perception, vision, and hearing; and problems with cognition, emotion, and language. Clinicians who treat patients with brain injury or disease will encounter disorders of the cerebrum.

Cellular Anatomy

The cerebral cortex is subdivided into two **cerebral hemispheres** (right and left). Together, they contain approximately 25 billion neurons that are interconnected by about 3×10^{14} synapses. This creates an amazing degree of complexity in the cortex. Cortical neurons are highly organized into distinct layers and columns; this organization is essential for normal cortical function.

Axons in the cerebral cortex are classified according to where they project (see **Figure 5-2**). Association fibers interconnect different parts of the same cerebral hemisphere. For example, some association fibers connect the right sensory cortex to the right motor cortex. Association fibers can be short (connecting nearby regions) or long (connecting distant regions). One group of long association fibers (the superior longitudinal fasciculus) connects all of the language areas within one hemisphere. Commissural fibers run between hemispheres (e.g., they connect the right motor cortex with the left motor cortex). The largest bundle of commissural fibers is called the **corpus callosum.** It interconnects the two hemispheres and contains about 300 million axons. Finally, projection fibers connect the cortex with other areas of the central nervous system (CNS). Many of these form a structure called the **internal capsule,** which contains axons that connect the cortex with the thalamus and with the spinal cord. The internal capsule is a small region that is tightly packed with axons. For this reason, a small lesion (stroke) in the internal capsule can have a serious negative effect on function.

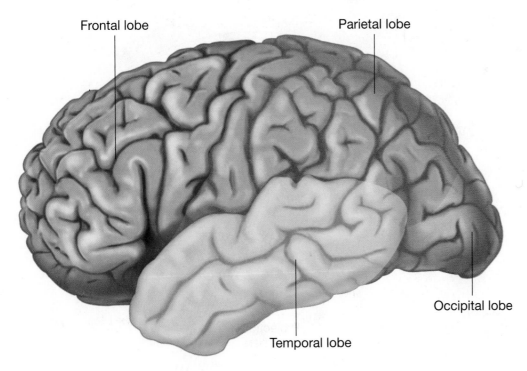

Frontal lobe

Parietal lobe

Occipital lobe

Temporal lobe

FIGURE 5-1 The cerebral cortex (lateral view) is divided into four lobes.

Regional Cortical Anatomy

Each cerebral hemisphere is divided into regions called lobes that are named for adjacent skull bones. In addition, a fifth "limbic lobe" is located on the internal surface of the brain. The cortex can be divided functionally into cortical regions according to **Brodmann's map.** Korbinian Brodmann was a German neurologist who identified and numbered 47 distinct regions. His map provides a handy way to identify specific functional areas (see Figure 5-3).

Frontal Lobe

The **frontal lobe** has two major functions: controlling voluntary movement and thinking/problem solving (see Figure 5-4). It is the largest cortical lobe and is located at the anterior aspect of the brain directly beneath the frontal bone.

The primary **motor cortex** (Brodmann area 4) is located on the precentral gyrus. Primary motor cortex contains the cell bodies of motor neurons that control voluntary movements of the opposite side (contralateral) head and body. They are often referred to as upper motor neurons, and have axons that form the corticospinal and corticobulbar tracts (see chapters 7 and 8 for more information on these tracts).

The neurons located on the primary motor cortex are precisely organized according to the region of the body that they control. For example, all neurons that move the thumb are clustered together in one place. If that specific part of the motor cortex were stimulated, the thumb would move. This arrangement creates a map of the body across the motor cortex that is called the motor homunculus (also known as "little man"; see Figure 5-5). Parts of the body that perform small, precise movements (e.g., lips, tongue, fingers) take up substantial space on the motor cortex, whereas body parts that are less precisely controlled (e.g., back, hips, knees) take up relatively little space. This is because more neurons are needed to control the small, exact movements of the mouth and fingers.

An injury to the primary motor cortex causes paralysis of the contralateral (opposite) side of the body, and of the muscles of facial expression on the bottom portion of the face. This is due to destruction of the neurons that control these muscles. This type of lesion can result from a stroke, an injury to the brain, or a disease that targets motor neurons such as ALS (Lou Gehrig's disease).

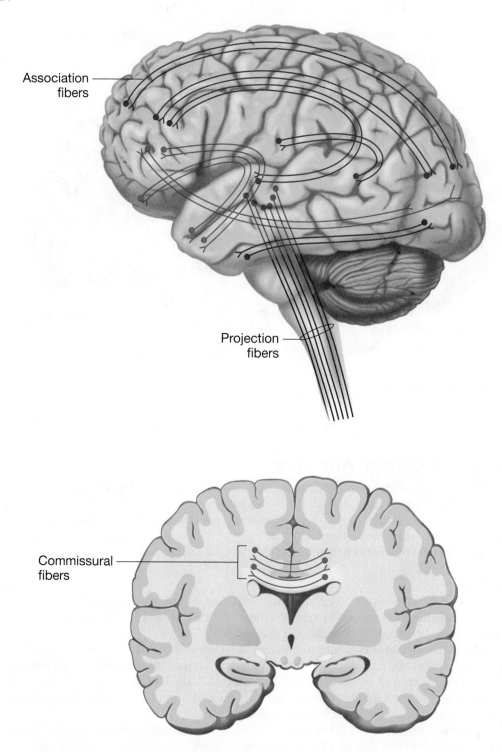

FIGURE 5-2 Axons (nerve fibers) in the cerebral cortex. Association fibers interconnect parts of the same hemisphere, commissural fibers interconnect the right and left hemispheres, and projection fibers connect the cortex to other brain regions. The top figure is a lateral view, and the bottom figure is a frontal section of the brain.

The premotor cortex (Brodmann area 6) is located just anterior to the primary motor cortex. Neurons in the premotor cortex connect to the spinal cord and brainstem, where they control the action of trunk and proximal limb muscles (via the reticulospinal and vestibulospinal tracts; see Chapter 8 for more on these pathways). The premotor cortex is also responsible for the experience of "body part ownership." Lesions to premotor cortex are part of a syndrome called unilateral neglect, in which people are unaware that their own body belongs to them.

Brodmann areas

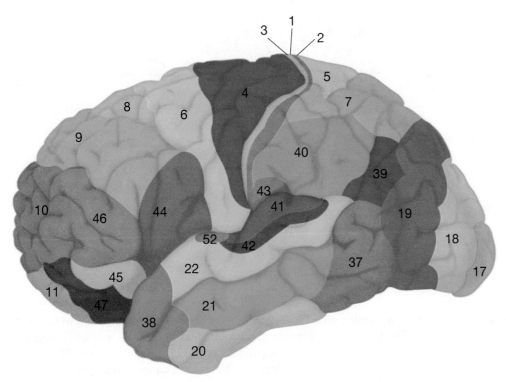

FIGURE 5-3   Brodmann's map of the cortex.

Motor areas (Frontal lobe map)

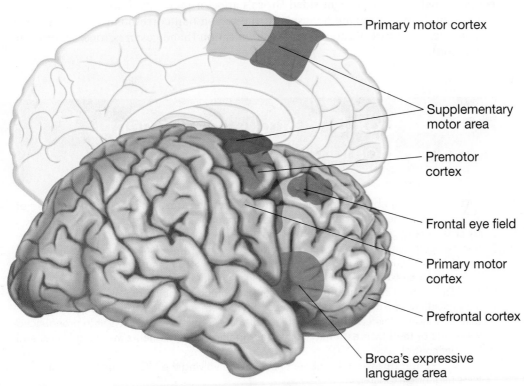

Primary motor cortex

Supplementary motor area

Premotor cortex

Frontal eye field

Primary motor cortex

Prefrontal cortex

Broca's expressive language area

FIGURE 5-4   Major functional regions of the frontal lobe.

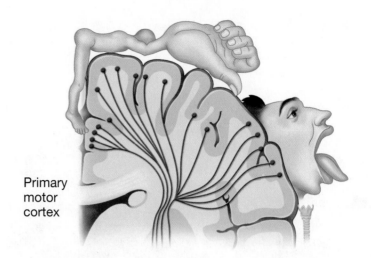

Primary
motor
cortex

FIGURE 5-5 Motor cortex: the motor homunculus represents cortical areas that control specific body regions. Body regions with large representation on the motor homunculus are under fine control and have muscles with small motor units.

The **supplementary motor area** (SMA; Brodmann area 8) is found medial to the premotor cortex. The SMA is a motor planning region. It stores motor memories (programs of movement) and directs the activity of the primary motor cortex. Lesions to SMA cause a motor planning deficit called **apraxia.** People with apraxia cannot "remember" how to perform normal motor tasks, but they are not paralyzed and have no sensory loss.

The fourth important motor area of the frontal lobe is the motor (expressive) speech area, also known as **Broca's area** (Brodmann area 44). This region contains the motor programs for speech and language. It has many connections to the portion of the primary motor cortex that controls muscles of the face, lips, tongue, and larynx used for speech. In most people (90%), Broca's area is located only in the left hemisphere. (For this reason the left side of the brain is often referred to as the "dominant" hemisphere.) Left-handed people sometimes have a right-sided Broca's area, or may have it located in both hemispheres. In the nondominant hemisphere, the region that corresponds to Broca's area is responsible for expressive nonverbal communication (hand gestures, tone of voice, facial expression).

Clinical Box 5-1: Stroke Impairments and the Homunculus

A stroke—or cerebral vascular accident (CVA)—results from a lack of blood flow to part of the brain. The motor deficits produced by damage to these regions can be predicted by cross-referencing the damaged region with the motor homunculus. For example, the middle cerebral artery (MCA) supplies blood to much of the lateral aspect of the frontal cortex. A stroke involving the MCA will therefore likely result in paralysis or paresis of the face and upper extremity—structures that map to the lateral aspect of the cortex (see Figure 5-5). The anterior cerebral artery (ACA), supplies blood to the medial aspect of the frontal lobe, including the motor neurons that control movement of the lower extremity and genitalia. Damage or disruption to blood flow of the ACA will therefore result in pronounced weakness of the lower extremity as well as significant impairments involving bowel and bladder control.

Challenge question: If a patient has a CVA involving the MCA, what functional problems might be expected?

Clinical Box 5-2: Unilateral Neglect

Unilateral neglect is a relatively common impairment following a CVA that affects premotor cortex. A patient suffering from unilateral neglect will commonly look only to one side, use only the unaffected arm, and bear weight only on the unaffected side. If this type of neglect and (lack of) muscular activation continues, significant changes in the individual's posture may occur. To help reduce the effects of neglect and stimulate the effects of neuroplasticity, clinicians will often incorporate the following types of activities into their treatment:

- Begin therapeutic interventions with proper postural alignment.
- Design weight-bearing activities through the affected upper extremity.
- Position the clinician toward the affected side of the patient to encourage scanning of the neglected visual field.
- Encourage activities that involve the use of the affected upper extremity (two-handed activities).
- Add visual cues to the affected upper extremity (such as a colorful bracelet).

Challenge question: Since the premotor cortex is located on the lateral aspect of the frontal lobe, which artery supplies blood to this region?

In addition to motor regions, the frontal lobe contains areas that are important for thinking, planning, and emotional responses (see **Figure 5-6**). Orbitofrontal cortex (Brodmann areas 11 and 47) is involved in impulse control, inhibition of inappropriate behavior, and carrying out plans. Damage to the orbitofrontal cortex causes patients to behave in an irresponsible, impulsive way. They cannot make realistic plans or carry out the plans

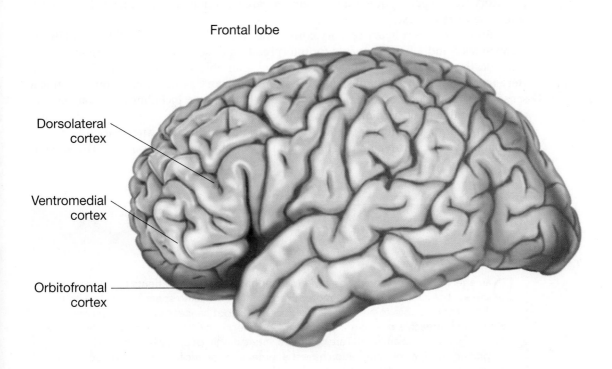

FIGURE 5-6 Frontal lobe regions involved in cognition and emotion include the dorsolateral prefrontal cortex (problem-solving), the ventromedial prefrontal cortex (emotion), and the orbitofrontal cortex (impulse control).

they make, and they tend to have trouble with focus, organization, and inhibition of their impulses. This condition is known as **prefrontal syndrome.**

The dorsolateral frontal cortex (Brodmann areas 45 and 46) is involved in analytical thinking, problem solving, and planning. It is also important for attention and focus (the ability to hold a thought in the "front" of the mind), and is correlated with general intelligence. Injury to this region results in disordered thinking and behavior; patients become disorganized and easily distracted.

The ventromedial frontal cortex (Brodmann areas 11, 12, and 25) is part of the limbic system. This region helps to connect emotions with thoughts, and attaches emotional meaning to life experiences. People with lesions to the ventromedial cortex are described as apathetic with a flat emotional affect. They have few preferences and display little or no interest in life. This region appears to be underactive in patients with depression, and overactive in people suffering from mania. In the past, this area was destroyed surgically in a procedure called a prefrontal lobotomy.

The anterior cingulate gyrus is visible on a mid-sagittal section of the brain (Brodmann areas 24 and 32). It is part of the limbic system and helps to integrate thought, motivation, attention, and behavior. It could be described as allowing a person to tune into his or her own thoughts. When it is overactive, people feel anxious; underactivity produces feelings of apathy.

Parietal Lobe

The **parietal lobe** is involved with perception and processing of sensation (see **Figure 5-7**). The primary **somatosensory (sensory) cortex** is located on the postcentral gyrus (Brodmann areas 3, 1, and 2). Sensations such as pain, temperature, pressure, touch, vibration, and proprioception (position sense) are perceived on the primary somatosensory cortex. Sensory nerves from each body region project to specific locations on the postcentral gyrus. This arrangement creates a sensory map of the body called the sensory homunculus (see **Figure 5-8**). Body parts that are very sensitive (e.g., lips, face, fingertips) have a large amount of space on primary sensory cortex, whereas less sensitive regions (e.g., back, arms, legs) take up less space. Taste sensations are perceived in a gustatory (taste) perception area (Brodmann area 43) that is located near the primary somatosensory cortex.

Posterior to the primary sensory cortex, the somatosensory association area (Brodmann areas 5 and 7) is responsible for interpretation of somatosensory information. For example, this region allows someone to recognize an object by touching it; this is called **stereognosis.** In the right hemisphere, the somatosensory association cortex contains a sensory representation of the body. Disorders of body image, including anorexia nervosa and unilateral neglect, are linked to dysfunction of this region.

The posterior and inferior portions of the parietal lobe are known as parietotemporal association cortex. This region overlaps both the parietal and temporal lobes (Brodmann

Clinical Box 5-3: Expressive Aphasia

Damage to Broca's area causes expressive **aphasia,** in which patients can understand speech but cannot access the motor program for producing speech. People with this condition may be able to articulate individual words, but cannot assemble complex sentences. Their speech is described as "hesitant and telegraphic." Sometimes, people can say only a single word (*no* and *damn* are common). Interestingly, people who use sign language as a primary form of communication have the same hemispheric localization as people who use spoken language (Hickok, Kirk, & Bellugi, 1998).

Challenge question: Identify the part of the primary motor cortex responsible for controlling muscles used for speech production.

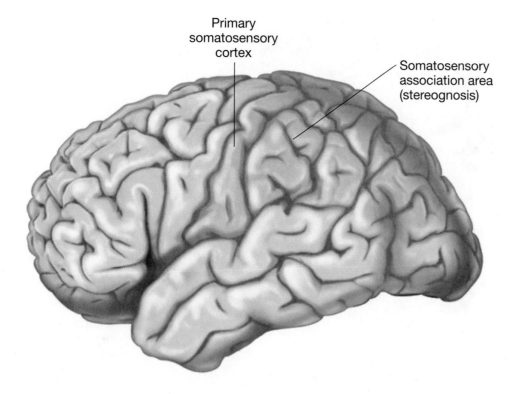

Primary somatosensory cortex

Somatosensory association area (stereognosis)

FIGURE 5-7 Major functional regions of the parietal lobe.

area 40). It is involved with abstract thought, reading and writing, mathematics, and spatial perception. The angular gyrus (area 39) is particularly important for understanding written language, and has numerous connections to other language centers. Interestingly, Albert Einstein had an unusually large parietotemporal association area.

Occipital Lobe

The **occipital lobe** is located at the back of the brain, beneath the occipital bone (see Figure 5-9). It contains two important regions: primary visual cortex and visual association cortex. The primary visual cortex (Brodmann area 17) is the site of visual perception. Neurons carrying visual information from the eyes project here. The primary visual cortex in each hemisphere receives visual input from the contralateral visual field. Injury to the

Neuroscience Notes Box 5-1:
Prefrontal Lobotomy

The prefrontal lobotomy originated with Portuguese neurologist Antonio Moniz, who drilled holes into patients' skulls and used a small wire loop to destroy tissue in the prefrontal cortex. Moniz won a Nobel Prize in 1949 for this technique. In the United States, neurologists Walter Freeman and James Watts modified the technique in order to make the surgery cheaper and easier to perform. Instead of drilling into the scalp, they lifted the upper eyelid and used a small hammer to drive an ice pick through the bone above the eye socket and into the frontal lobe. The ice pick was then moved laterally or rotated to cut axons. This surgery was performed on at least 20,000 people in the United States, and was developed as a means to make people with serious mental illness calmer and more "tractable." Since the development of medications that treat diseases such as schizophrenia and clinical depression, lobotomies are no longer being performed (Jones and Shanklin, 1950).

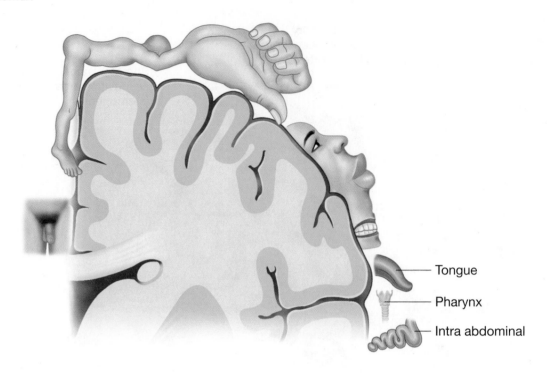

Tongue

Pharynx

Intra abdominal

FIGURE 5-8 Sensory cortex: the sensory homunculus represents a sensory map of the body. Regions with more sensory receptors occupy a larger amount of space on the sensory cortex compared to less sensitive regions.

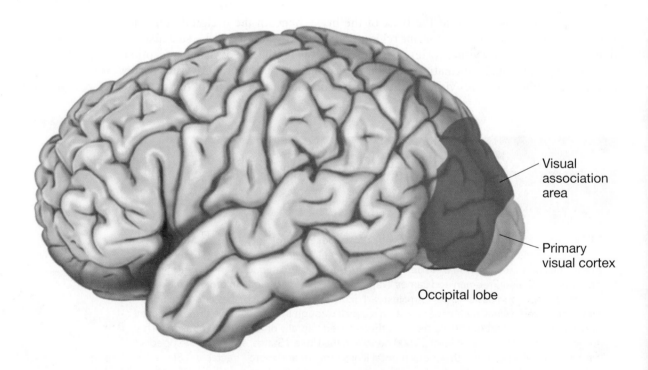

Visual association area

Primary visual cortex

Occipital lobe

FIGURE 5-9 Major functional regions of the occipital lobe include primary visual cortex (visual perception) and visual association cortex (interpretation of visual information).

visual cortex on one side causes loss of vision in the opposite visual field, a condition known as **hemianopsia.** Bilateral injury to the visual cortex causes cortical blindness. (See Chapter 12 for more information on visual field deficits.)

The visual association area is located anterior to the primary visual cortex (Brodmann areas 18 and 19). This region is responsible for interpreting visual stimuli. Damage to the visual association cortex causes visual agnosia, in which patients can see but are unable to recognize objects by sight. The visual association cortex has many connections to areas for spatial perception and recognition of faces.

Temporal Lobe

The **temporal lobes** are located on the lateral aspect of the brain, just above the ears (see **Figure 5-10**). They contain regions that are part of the **limbic system** (responsible for emotion and memory), the auditory system, the olfactory system, and a specific area for recognizing faces.

The primary **auditory cortex** (Brodmann area 41) is where sounds are perceived. It is organized by sound frequency. The auditory cortex on each side of the brain gets input from both ears. Part of the primary auditory cortex is devoted specifically to perception of music. This region is usually larger on the right side, and has many connections to emotional centers. The auditory association cortex is located posterior to the primary auditory cortex (Brodmann area 42) and is responsible for interpretation and understanding of sounds.

Wernicke's receptive speech/language area is also located in the temporal lobe. **Wernicke's area** (Brodmann area 22) is important for understanding language. This includes verbal/spoken language, sign language, and written language. In most people, Wernicke's area is located only in the left (dominant) hemisphere, but it is bilateral in 5 to 10% of people. The corresponding area in the nondominant hemisphere is responsible for interpretation of nonverbal communication, including hand gestures, facial expressions, body language, and tone of voice.

A large region on the lateral aspect of the temporal lobe is the inferotemporal cortex (Brodmann area 21). This area is responsible for recognition of faces, objects, and colors. Damage to this region can cause a condition called prosopagnosia, in which patients cannot recognize faces even of people they know well. Prosopagnosia can be an early sign of Alzheimer disease.

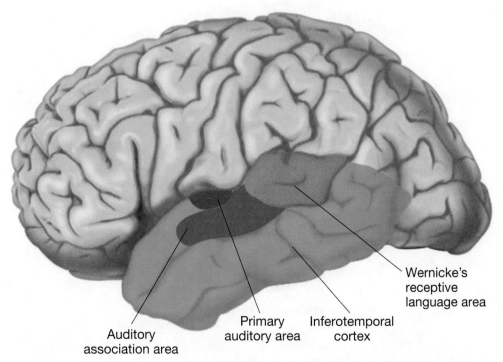

FIGURE 5-10   Major functional regions of the temporal lobe include primary auditory cortex (perception of sound), auditory association area (interpretation of sound), Wernicke's receptive language area, and the inferotemporal cortex (recognition of faces, objects, and colors).

Clinical Box 5-4: Receptive Aphasia

Lesions to Wernicke's area cause a condition called receptive **aphasia,** in which patients are unable to understand any form of language. People with this condition can speak in a flowing manner but what they say does not make sense because they cannot select the correct words to convey meaning, and also cannot understand what they themselves are saying. Wernicke's area has many connections to the other major language center (Broca's expressive language area in the frontal lobe). Some lesions damage both Broca's and Wernicke's language areas; this affects both expressive and receptive speech and is called global aphasia.

Challenge question: How might a clinician communicate with a patient who has receptive aphasia?

The medial part of the temporal lobe contains several areas that are part of the limbic system (see **Figure 5-11**). The primary **olfactory cortex** is responsible for perceiving odors. Destruction of this region bilaterally can cause **anosmia** (loss of the sense of smell). If seizures or tumors irritate the primary olfactory cortex, people smell things that are not actually there (olfactory hallucinations). Unfortunately, the odors they hallucinate are usually unpleasant (e.g., burning rubber).

The **amygdala** is a small, almond-shaped structure located on the medial side of the temporal lobe. It is part of the limbic system and is involved in strong negative emotions (fear and anger). It has connections to the hypothalamus, which causes physiological responses, including increased heart rate, breathing rate, and blood pressure.

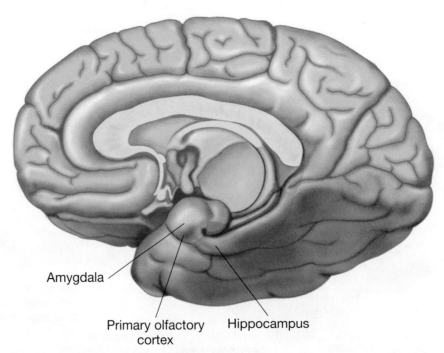

Amygdala

Primary olfactory cortex

Hippocampus

FIGURE 5-11 Temporal lobe: functional regions on the medial aspect of the brain include the primary olfactory cortex (perception of odors), the amygdala (emotions), and hippocampus (long-term memory).

Near the amygdala is another small structure called the **hippocampus** (Gardner and Hogan, 2005). The hippocampus is named for its shape (supposedly it resembles a sea horse). It is involved in creating new long-term memories. If both hippocampi are damaged, the patient will be unable to establish any new, long-term memories and will have anterograde **amnesia.** The hippocampus is one of only two regions in the adult human brain that can generate new neurons throughout life (Eriksson et al., 1998). These new neurons are correlated with learning and memory. When animals are exposed to extreme stress, the hippocampus shrinks and learning becomes more difficult. Animals that exercise and that are asked to perform challenging learning tasks have larger hippocampi. Some evidence suggests that the human hippocampus behaves in a similar manner.

PATIENT SCENARIOS

Patient Case 5-1 (Henry)

Henry is a 23-year old male who was involved in a serious car accident. He was in a coma for 4 weeks, and since regaining consciousness has been treated at a facility that specializes in traumatic brain injury. Henry suffered damage to his occipital lobes and the anterior part of his frontal lobes. He displays symptoms including verbal outbursts; socially inhibited behavior; a flat, blunted affect; and the inability to plan and to carry out his plans. In addition, he cannot see.

Questions

a) What is the term for the behavioral symptoms that Henry displays? Which part(s) of his brain have been injured to cause these symptoms?

b) Given the occipital lobe injury, what is the term for Henry's loss of vision?

Patient Case 5-2 (Georgia)

Georgia, age 78, suffered a cerebrovascular accident (CVA) 3 weeks ago. Now she is unable to speak more than one or two words at a time. She seems able to understand what is said to her, but she can talk only in short bursts. Most of the time, the only word she can get out is *no*,

even though it is clear that isn't really what she means. She has no trouble communicating with gestures, facial expressions, and body language.

Questions

a) What is the term for this condition? Which part of the cortex has been affected?

b) Which side of Georgia's brain was most likely affected by this CVA? (*Hint:* She is right-handed.)

Patient Case 5-3 (Mary Anne)

Mary Anne is a 56-year old woman who suffered a CVA. She now displays paralysis of the left side of her body and has sensory loss on the same side. In addition, she seems unaware of her left side. For example, she tends to look toward the right, eats food on the right side of her plate, and combs only the hair on the right side of her head. She seems not to know that she has a left side.

Questions

a) What is the term for this condition (lack of awareness of the left side of the body)? What region of the brain is damaged?

b) What region of the brain is damaged to cause the paralysis of her left side?

Review Questions

1. On a map of the cerebral cortex, label each lobe and identify all functional regions. For each region, be able to describe the primary function of that area and state the results of a lesion to that specific area.

2. Which functions are generally located in the right hemisphere? Which are usually found on the left side?

3. Name the cortical regions involved in each of the following functional activities:

- Speech/language
- Vision
- Thinking and problem solving
- Movement
- Sensory perception

4. Which areas of the body occupy the largest areas on the precentral gyrus? Which areas of the body take up the most space on the postcentral gyrus? Why?

References

1. Eriksson, P. S., Perfilieva, E., Bjork-Eriksson, T., Alborn, A. M., Nodborg, C., Peterson, D. A., & Gage, F. E. (1998). Neurogenesis in the adult human hippocampus. *Nature Medicine, 4*(11), 1313–1317.

2. Gardener, R., & Hogan, R. E. (2005). Three-dimensional deformation-based hippocampal surface anatomy, projected on MRI images. *Clinical Anatomy, 18,* 481–487.

3. Hickok, G., Kirk, K. & Bellugi, U. (1998). Hemispheric organization of local and global-level visuospatial processes in deaf signers and its relation to sign language aphasia. *Brain and Language, 65,* 276–286.

4. Jones, C. H., & Shanklin, J. G. (1950). Transorbital lobotomy in institutional practice. *American Journal of Psychiatry, 107*(2).

Further Reading

1. Cahill, L. (2005, May). His brain, her brain. *Scientific American,* 40–47.

2. Ramachandran, V. S., & Rogers-Ramachandran, D. (2007, December/2008, January). Touching illusions. *Scientific American Mind,* 14–16.

3. Rakic, P. (2006). No more cortical neurons for you. *Science, 313,* 928–929.

4. Schacter, D. L., & Wagner, A. D. (1999). Remembrance of things past. *Science, 285,* 1503–1504.

PEARSON

myhealthprofessionskit™

Use this address to access the Companion Website created for this textbook. Simply select "Physical Therapy" from the choice of disciplines. Find this book and log in using your username and password to access self-assessment questions, a glossary, and more.

Diencephalon

CHAPTER OBJECTIVES

After completing this chapter, the reader will be able to:

1. Describe the structure and function of each part of the thalamus and hypothalamus, and explain the effect of a lesion to each region.

2. Discuss connections between the hypothalamus and the endocrine system, as well as connections between the hypothalamus and the autonomic nervous system.

KEY TERMS

association nuclei
central autonomic
 fibers
diencephalon
epithalamus
hypothalamus
intralaminar nuclei
melatonin
oxytocin
pineal gland
pituitary gland
relay nuclei
reticular nucleus of the
 thalamus
subthalamic nucleus
thalamic syndrome
thalamus
vasopressin

Essential Facts···

▶ The thalamus and hypothalamus are part of the diencephalon, located in the center of the brain.

▶ The thalamus processes signals traveling to many parts of the cerebral cortex.

▶ Emotional centers in the thalamus are part of the limbic system.

▶ The hypothalamus controls the autonomic nervous system and regulates heart rate, respiration, appetite, thirst, sleep, and reproduction.

▶ The hypothalamus has connections to the pituitary gland and controls the body's hormones (endocrine system).

The thalamus and hypothalamus are part of the **diencephalon,** a subdivision of the forebrain. It is located just above the brainstem. The diencephalon has four parts: the thalamus, hypothalamus, epithalamus, and subthalamus (see **Figure 6-1**). The four parts function independently, and are grouped together based on their location in the brain. The thalamus is the largest portion, and the epithalamus and subthalamus are quite small. Disorders of the diencephalon are relatively uncommon, but have serious consequences for patients.

Thalamus

The **thalamus** is the largest part of the diencephalon. The right and left thalami are located on either side of the third ventricle, in the center of the brain. The overall function of the thalamus is to serve as a kind of "executive assistant" to the cerebral cortex. Almost all information that eventually reaches the cortex passes through the thalamus first. General sensory (i.e., pain, temperature, pressure, touch), auditory, visual, taste, and vestibular sensations all synapse in the thalamus before they reach the cortex. A general awareness of these sensations takes place in the thalamus, along with a determination about whether a sensation is pleasant or unpleasant. This contributes to the perception of general body well-being. In addition, the thalamus is involved in maintaining consciousness and alertness.

The thalamus can be subdivided into individual nuclei that are organized into three functional categories: relay nuclei, association nuclei, and intralaminar nuclei (also called nonspecific nuclei) (see **Figure 6-2**). A fourth region is called the reticular nucleus of the thalamus; this region controls the function of other thalamic nuclei. (In spite of its name, it is not related to the brainstem reticular formation.)

The six **relay nuclei** each receive input from a specific area of the nervous system and convey (relay) those signals to the cerebral cortex (see **Figure 6-3**). Two are general sensory, two are special sensory, and two are motor nuclei. The two general sensory nuclei receive input from the opposite (contralateral) side of the body and send it to the primary somatosensory cortex. The special sensory nuclei send visual and auditory information to the cortex. Finally, the two motor nuclei of the thalamus convey motor information to the motor areas of the cerebral cortex.

Association nuclei of the thalamus receive action potentials from all over the CNS. They send projections to limbic regions of the cortex, where they connect sensory input to emotional responses.

The **intralaminar nuclei** have many reciprocal connections with the basal ganglia and the limbic system. They project to widespread areas of the cortex and are highly

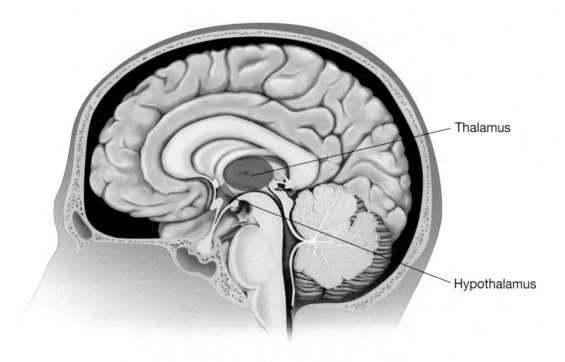

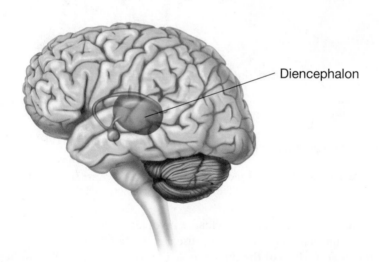

FIGURE 6-1 The diencephalon includes the thalamus and the hypothalamus. The top view is a mid-sagittal section, and the bottom view is a lateral view of the brain.

Neuroscience Notes Box 6-1: Coma

One of the first legal "right to die" cases in the United States involved a young woman named Karen Quinlan. She was in a coma for many years following an overdose of prescription drugs. Her parents won a court battle to remove her mechanical ventilator, after which she lived for another 10 years breathing on her own but unresponsive to stimuli (this is referred to as a "persistent vegetative state.") When Karen died, an autopsy of her brain showed that the injury causing her condition was located in the thalamus, specifically in the intralaminar nuclei.

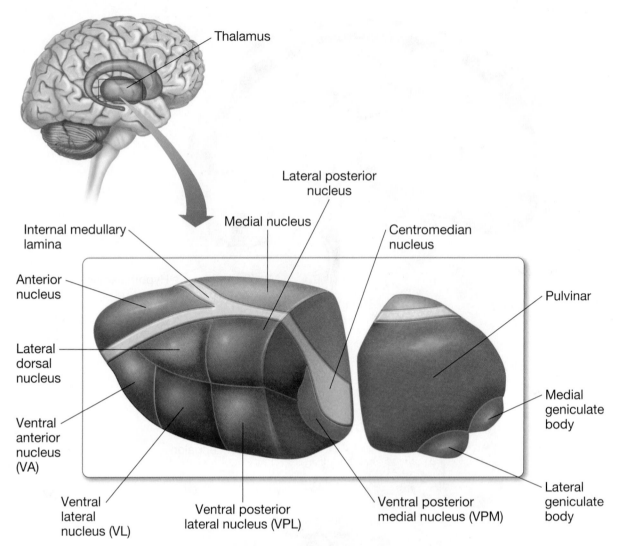

FIGURE 6-2 Anatomy of the thalamus. The medial and lateral geniculate bodies are special sensory relay nuclei, the VPM and VPL are general sensory relay nuclei, and the VA and VL are motor relay nuclei.

interconnected. The intralaminar nuclei are involved in maintaining conscious awareness. Lesions to the intralaminar nuclei can cause a coma (a prolonged loss of consciousness).

The **reticular nucleus of the thalamus** is a narrow band of cells that lies anterior and lateral to the thalamus. Its function is to determine which signals will be conveyed to the cerebral cortex. When we are awake and alert, relay nuclei neurons provide the cortex with

Review Concepts 6-1: Thalamic Nuclei

Relay nuclei

- Somatosensory nuclei convey somatosensation to somatosensory cortex.

- Special sensory nuclei convey visual or auditory signals to cortex.

- Motor nuclei convey motor signals to motor cortex.

- Association nuclei convey input to limbic (emotional) areas of cortex.

- Intralaminar nuclei maintain consciousness.

- Reticular nucleus controls relay nuclei.

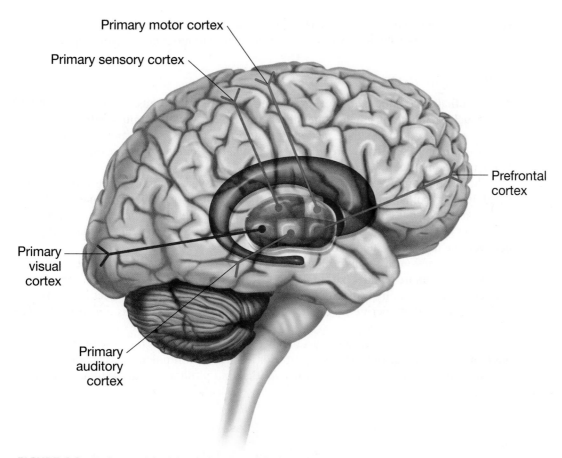

Primary motor cortex

Primary sensory cortex

Prefrontal cortex

Primary visual cortex

Primary auditory cortex

FIGURE 6-3 Relay nuclei of the thalamus and their projections.

detailed information about events going on around us. During sleep, the thalamus forwards very little information to the cortex. The reticular nucleus controls the activity of the relay nuclei. This likely helps improve the overall efficiency of the brain by limiting the flow of "unimportant" sensory information to the cortex. (For example, the cortex does not need to focus on the feel of your socks against your ankles, but may need to be made aware of a

Neuroscience Notes Box 6-2: Thalamic Syndrome

The thalamus receives most of its blood supply from branches of the posterior cerebral artery (reviewed in Schmahmann, 2003). CVAs and other lesions that damage the thalamus produce **thalamic syndrome.** The syndrome consists of three symptoms: hemianesthesia, sensory ataxia, and thalamic pain. Hemianesthesia is a profound, sometimes total, loss of somatosensation to one side of the body, contralateral to the lesion side. Pain, temperature, and crude touch usually return after a period of time. A patient with sensory ataxia displays motor incoordination due to loss of proprioceptive information from muscles, joints, and tendons. Without information about muscle length, joint position and velocity of limb movement, the motor structures cannot successfully plan, coordinate, and execute movement. **Thalamic pain** is intense and very unpleasant. Often, it does not diminish when treated with pain medications, and it can be triggered by stimuli that do not usually cause pain (e.g., touching the skin). Thalamic pain is probably caused by abnormal pain modulation in the damaged thalamus. Thalamic pain is known as *intractable* or *central pain* because it is resistant to treatment with therapy and medication. This pain cannot be localized to any specific part of the thalamus. It usually does not get better with time.

spider crawling up your leg.) There is evidence that dysfunction of the reticular nucleus is linked to disorders such as autism that limit the ability to modulate sensory input.

Hypothalamus

The **hypothalamus** is located inferior and anterior to the thalamus, and its right and left sides touch each other just below the third ventricle. The hypothalamus controls the autonomic nervous system, regulates activity of endocrine glands, and connects physiological responses to emotions. It also regulates water balance, hunger, thirst, sexual drive, body temperature, and sleep/wake cycles.

The hypothalamus receives information from all over the brain and the spinal cord. In addition, hypothalamic neurons respond to blood glucose levels, hormones, and blood temperature. Changes in the chemical composition of the cerebrospinal fluid are also conveyed to the hypothalamus. This makes the hypothalamus an important connection point between the nervous system and the blood system.

A vital function of the hypothalamus is control of the hypophysis **(pituitary gland).** Because the pituitary gland is part of the endocrine system and directs function of the other endocrine glands, the hypothalamic-pituitary connection provides a direct link between brain activity and endocrine function; this is sometimes referred to as a *neuroendocrine connection* (see **Figure 6-4**).

The pituitary gland is located just below the hypothalamus at the base of the brain. It has two parts: an anterior lobe and a posterior lobe. The hypothalamus is connected to the anterior lobe by a set of veins called the hypothalamo-pituitary portal system. Neurons in

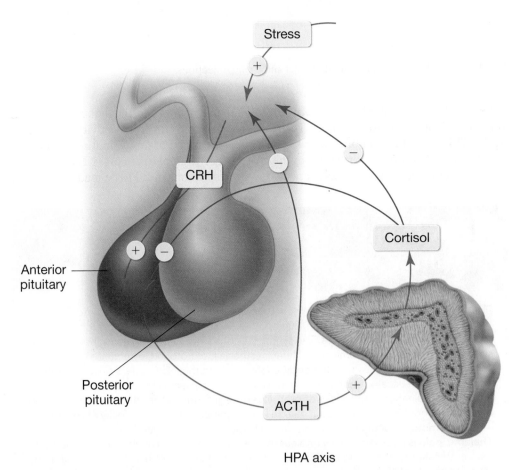

FIGURE 6-4   Hypothalamus, pituitary gland, and the endocrine system. In this example, the hypothalamus releases corticotrophin releasing hormone (CRH) to stimulate secretion of adrenocorticotropic hormone (ACTH, corticotropin). ACTH acts on the adrenal gland and causes release of cortisol. Cortisol then has a negative feedback effect on both the hypothalamus and on the anterior pituitary.

the hypothalamus release hormones that flow through these portal veins to the anterior lobe of the pituitary, where they affect the release of pituitary hormones into the bloodstream. In this way, the brain can regulate the secretion of many hormones.

Part of the hypothalamus contains specialized neurons that release two hormones from their axon terminals: **vasopressin** (also called antidiuretic hormone or ADH) and **oxytocin.** Both hormones are released in the posterior lobe of the pituitary gland, and then diffuse into the blood. Vasopressin controls water balance in the body by increasing reabsorption of water in the kidney, decreasing urine production. It also causes constriction of blood vessels, raising the systemic blood pressure. Oxytocin causes contraction of smooth muscle in the uterus and mammary glands. It is released after orgasm and produces a feeling of relaxation; for this reason, it is sometimes called the "cuddle hormone."

Some neurons from the hypothalamus descend directly to the brainstem and spinal cord in the reticulospinal tracts, forming the **central autonomic fibers** (see Figure 6-5).

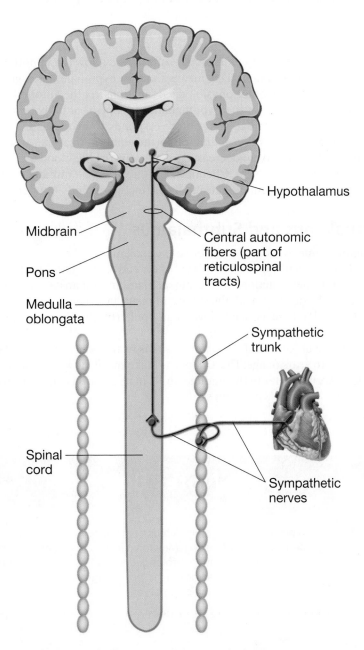

FIGURE 6-5 Central autonomic fibers control the autonomic nervous system and travel in the spinal cord reticulospinal tracts. Central autonomic fibers synapse onto sympathetic and parasympathetic neurons and control the function of visceral organs.

Neuroscience Notes Box 6-3: Diabetes Insipidus

Diabetes insipidus (DI) results from decreased production of vasopressin (antidiuretic hormone; ADH) by the hypothalamus and posterior pituitary gland. ADH acts on the kidney to increase water reabsorption and decrease urine volume. Without ADH, the kidney cannot reabsorb water, and the urine becomes very watery (dilute and copious). This causes excessive urine production and urination (polyuria) that, in turn, leads to excessive thirst and drinking (polydipsia). Diabetes insipidus different from diabetes mellitus, which is a disorder involving blood sugar regulation. However, both conditions can cause polyuria.

These fibers synapse onto autonomic neurons and allow the hypothalamus to control the autonomic nervous system. This means that the hypothalamus regulates blood pressure, blood flow, and many other physiological functions via the autonomic nerves.

A critical function of the hypothalamus is control of body temperature. In the anterior hypothalamus, a "heat-loss center" responds to increases in blood temperature by stimulating sweating and vasodilation in the skin. A "heat-gain center" in the posterior hypothalamus responds to decreased temperature of the blood by initiating shivering and vasoconstriction in the skin. Chemicals produced by the immune system can affect these temperature control centers, causing fever (increased body temperature) during illness.

Epithalamus and Subthalamus

The **epithalamus** is located just above the thalamus, and consists of the **pineal gland** and several other small nuclei. The pineal is an endocrine gland that secretes the hormone **melatonin.** Other functions of the pineal gland in humans are not well defined. Tumors involving cells of the pineal gland tend to result in delayed puberty, whereas lesions that destroy the gland are associated with early puberty. Thus, the pineal gland probably plays some role in sexual development.

An unusual feature of the pineal gland is its tendency to accumulate calcium deposits after about 16 years of age. These deposits make the gland visible in brain imaging. Because the gland normally lies in the midline, shifts in its position can be useful in the diagnosis of tumors and bleeding within the skull.

Neuroscience Notes Box 6-4: Melatonin

Melatonin is produced in the epithalamus from the neurotransmitter serotonin, and helps to regulate sleeping and waking. Melatonin levels are sometimes decreased in people with chronic depression. In addition, prolonged stress has been shown to lower melatonin levels. Melatonin supplements can be purchased in drugstores as a supposed cure for insomnia, although this has not been clinically proven to work.

The subthalamus is a small subdivision of the diencephalon located between the thalamus and the midbrain. Its most important part is the **subthalamic nucleus,** part of the basal ganglia circuitry. The function of the subthalamic nucleus is discussed in chapter 13.

PATIENT SCENARIO

Patient Case 6-1 (Ted)

Ted is a 24-year old man who was injured in an auto accident. He suffered a traumatic brain injury that affected his thalamus and caused him to experience thalamic syndrome. Whenever his nurses or therapists try to touch or position him, he cries out and appears to be in extreme pain. Ted also shows ataxia (lack of motor coordination) and hemianesthesia (sensory loss) on the right side of his body.

Question

a) What challenges would there be for a clinician treating a patient suffering from thalamic syndrome, given that many kinds of touch and movement can trigger intense pain?

Review Questions

1. Name the function of each thalamic nucleus.

2. Describe the functions of the hypothalamus, and how the hypothalamus and hypophysis (pituitary) work together to regulate secretion of hormones, the autonomic nervous system, and water balance in the body.

3. Explain the symptoms and signs of thalamic syndrome.

Reference

1. Schmahmann, J. D. (2003). Vascular syndromes of the thalamus. *Stroke, 34,* 2264–2278.

Further Reading

1. Broggi, G. (2008). Pain and psycho-affective disorders. *Neurosurgery, 62*(6), 901–919.

2. Brooks, D., & Halliday, G. M. (2008). Intralaminar nuclei of the thalamus in Lewy body disease. *Brain Res. Bull.* (e-publication).

3. Chen, F. Y., Tao, W., & Li, Yong-Jie. (2008). Advances in brain imaging of neuropathic pain. *Chinese Medical Journal, 121*(7), 653–657.

4. Henderson, J. M., Carpenter, K., Cartwright, H., & Halliday, G. M. (2000). Loss of thalamic intralaminar nuclei in progressive supranuclear palsy and Parkinson's disease: clinical and therapeutic implications. *Brain, 123*(7), 1410–1421.

5. Houtchens, M. K., Benedict, R. H. B., Killiany, R., Sharma, J., Jaisani, Z., Singh, B., Weinstock-Guttman, B., Guttman, R. G., & Bakshi, R. (2007). Thalamic atrophy and cognition in multiple sclerosis. *Neurology, 69,* 1213–1223.

6. Mesaros, S., Rocca, M. A., Absinta, M., Ghezzi, A., Milani, N., Moiola, L., Veggiotti, P., Comi, G., & Filippi, M. (2008). Evidence of thalamic gray matter loss in pediatric multiple sclerosis. *Neurology, 70,* 1065–1066.

7. Schiff, N. D. (2008). Central thalamic contributions to arousal regulation and neurological disorders of consciousness. *Ann. N.Y. Acad. Sci., 1129,* 105–118.

PEARSON
myhealthprofessionskit™

Use this address to access the Companion Website created for this textbook. Simply select "Physical Therapy" from the choice of disciplines. Find this book and log in using your username and password to access self-assessment questions, a glossary, and more.

Brainstem and Cranial Nerves

CHAPTER OBJECTIVES

After completing this chapter, the reader will be able to:

1 Describe the structure and function of each portion of the brainstem, including major tracts, nuclei, and relevant cranial nerves.

2 Discuss the organization and functions of the reticular formation.

3 List the function of each cranial nerve, and state the consequences of injury to each nerve.

4 Explain the neuroanatomy of major brainstem pathologies.

KEY TERMS

abducens nerve
amygdala
ascending reticular activating system (ARAS)
colliculi
coma
diplopia
dorsal respiratory nucleus
dysarthria
dysphagia
facial nerve
glossopharyngeal nerve
hypoglossal nerve
locked-in syndrome
medulla oblongata
oculomotor nerve
olfactory nerve
optic nerve
pons
reticular formation (RF)
spinal accessory nerve
substantia nigra
trigeminal nerve
trochlear nerve
vagus nerve
vestibular apparatus
vestibular nuclei
vestibulocochlear nerve

Essential Facts··

▶ The brainstem consists of three regions: midbrain, pons, and medulla oblongata.

▶ Many essential life functions are controlled by the brainstem, including heart rate, breathing, and sleeping and waking.

▶ Most of the cranial nerves originate in the brainstem; they mainly control functioning of structures in the head and neck.

The brainstem connects the spinal cord with the rest of the central nervous system, and is the connection point for nerve fibers running to and from the cerebellum. The brainstem controls basic life functions (sometimes called "vegetative" functions), and contains 10 of the 12 pairs of cranial nerves. It also has a complex network of neurons known as the reticular formation. Because so many vital structures are located in the brainstem, damage to this region is often fatal. However, clinicians will likely treat patients who have pathologies involving the cranial nerves, most of which arise from the brainstem.

Brainstem Regions

The brainstem has three parts: midbrain, pons, and medulla oblongata (see Figure 7-1). The midbrain is very small and is located between the diencephalon and the pons. It is easiest to view the midbrain in a mid-sagittal section. The pons and medulla oblongata are both subdivisions of the embryonic hindbrain. They can be seen in a ventral view of the brain.

Midbrain

The midbrain is the smallest subdivision of the brainstem and contains four important paired structures: the red nucleus, the substantia nigra, the superior colliculus, and the inferior colliculus (see Figure 7-2). The red nucleus is involved in motor coordination, primarily of the upper extremity. It is named for its color; it appears red in a fresh brain.

The **substantia nigra** ("black substance") is also named for its color. This nucleus contains neurons that make the neurotransmitter dopamine. A black pigment, melanin, is a

Clinical Box 7-1: Parkinson Disease

Parkinson disease results from death of dopamine-producing neurons in the substantia nigra. The signs and symptoms of Parkinson's begin to appear when about 80% of the substantia nigra neurons have been lost. These include a tremor evident at rest (resting tremor), bradykinesia (slowness of movement), and postural instability. People with Parkinson's also display a flexed, stooped posture. As more and more substantia nigra cells die, the disease gets progressively worse. It can be treated with medications that replace or augment the effects of the missing dopamine.

Challenge question: Would the substantia nigra in the midbrain appear black in a patient with advanced Parkinson disease?

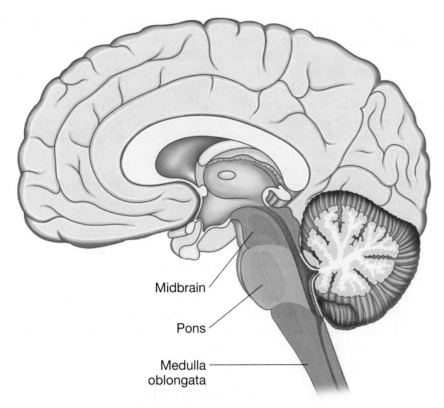

FIGURE 7-1 Brainstem (lateral view) shown in a mid-sagittal section. The brainstem consists of the midbrain, the pons, and the medulla oblongata.

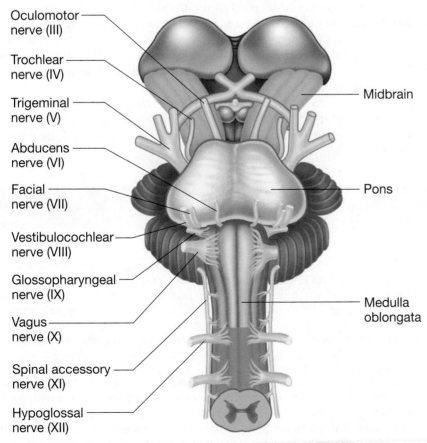

FIGURE 7-2 Brainstem (ventral view) with cranial nerves III–XII.

by-product of dopamine synthesis so the substantia nigra appears black. Neurons in the substantia nigra project to a part of the forebrain called the basal ganglia. The basal ganglia regulate movement initiation and inhibition, as well as thought, emotion, and cognition.

The superior and inferior **colliculi** are visible on the dorsal/posterior surface of the midbrain as four small bumps. The superior colliculi are visual relay nuclei. They connect the eyes to the cranial nerves that control eye movements. This allows the eyes to track a moving object, and to scan across a surface such as when reading. The inferior colliculi are auditory relay nuclei. They receive input from the cochlear (hearing) portion of the inner ear and project to other structures in the auditory system of the brain. Each inferior colliculus receives auditory signals from both ears.

Two cranial nerves are found in the midbrain: the oculomotor nerve (CN III) and the trochlear nerve (CN IV). These nerves control muscles that move the eyes.

Pons

The **pons** is the largest subdivision of the brainstem. It is visible as a large bulge on the brain's ventral surface and contains important cranial nerves (V–VII) described later in this chapter.

The pons contains many connections to and from the cerebellum. Axons traveling in and out of the cerebellum pass through one of three large fiber bundles called the cerebellar peduncles. Because of these connections, injury to the pons can mimic cerebellar lesions and result in coordination and balance deficits.

Motor nerve fibers are also found in the pons. They are located in the ventral/anterior region that receives its blood supply from the basilar artery and its small pontine branches. These axons connect motor areas of the cerebral cortex to the spinal cord, and allow voluntary control of movement. Injury to these nerves can result in a condition called *locked-in syndrome.*

Medulla Oblongata

The **medulla oblongata** connects the spinal cord with the rest of the CNS. The medulla contains the **dorsal respiratory nucleus** that controls breathing. The dorsal respiratory nucleus receives projections from the motor cortex, and sends axons to spinal cord segments C3 to C5 that form the phrenic nerves. Thus, the dorsal respiratory nucleus stimulates contraction of the diaphragm so that we can breathe without conscious effort and while sleeping. Injury to the respiratory nucleus usually results in death.

The medulla oblongata also contains the inferior olivary nucleus (olive), part of the brain's motor system that is involved in detecting movement errors and may also play a role in motor learning. It is named for its appearance, which supposedly resembles a wrinkled olive.

Clinical Box 7-2: Locked-In Syndrome

A basilar artery infarct can result from compression of the artery after a motor vehicle accident, from a stroke (CVA), or from certain types of spinal manipulations. The injury can selectively damage all motor neurons in the pons, which creates a condition known as **locked-in syndrome.** This extremely debilitating condition typically results in complete paralysis of all four extremities, the diaphragm, and the face. Because of the extreme paralysis of locked-in syndrome, patients may initially appear to be in a vegetative (unresponsive) state. However, people with this condition are fully alert and oriented, have full sensation, and maintain control of eye movement. Innovative therapists have capitalized on eye control, and have developed ways for the patient to communicate using an "alphabet board" combined with blinking to spell out words, and express various wants and needs.

Challenge question: Why would eye movement usually be spared in patients with locked-in syndrome? (*Hint:* Which part of the brainstem contains the cranial nerves that control most eye movements?)

Brainstem Tracts

There are four major ascending (sensory) tracts found in the brainstem (see Figure 7-3):

1. The anterior spinothalamic tract (light touch and pressure)
2. The lateral spinothalamic tract (pain and temperature)

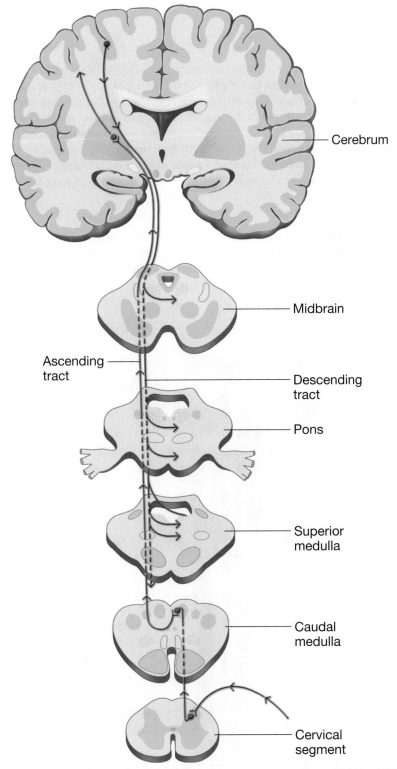

FIGURE 7-3 Ascending brainstem tracts (red) and descending brainstem tracts (blue).

3. The dorsal column tracts (two-point discrimination—vibration and conscious proprioception)
4. The spinocerebellar tracts (unconscious proprioception)

All of these tracts contain neurons that convey somatosensory action potentials to the brain. They are described in detail in chapter 8 of this textbook. Brainstem injuries can damage these tracts and result in sensory loss.

Three major descending (motor) tracts run through the brainstem to the spinal cord:

1. The lateral corticospinal tract
2. The reticulospinal tracts
3. The vestibulospinal tracts

These tracts all contain neurons that connect motor areas of the brain with lower motor neurons in the spinal cord. This means that the tracts contain upper motor neurons. The *lateral corticospinal tract* is the major tract controlling muscles of the entire body. Axons in this tract cross over to the other side of the brain in the medulla oblongata. If they are injured, patients will experience spastic paralysis. The *reticulospinal tracts* have a strong inhibitory effect on muscle tone. Injury to the reticulospinal tracts can cause hypertonicity and spasticity. The *vestibulospinal tracts* receive input from the **vestibular apparatus** in the inner ear, and help to maintain balance and posture. More detail concerning these tracts is found in chapter 8 of this textbook.

Reticular Formation

The **reticular formation (RF)** forms the core of the brain stem (see **Figure 7-4**). It is a complicated network of neurons and nerve fibers traveling in all directions (each RF neuron may synapse onto 25,000 other neurons). The RF is involved in motivation, decision making, mood, sleeping and waking, and pain modification.

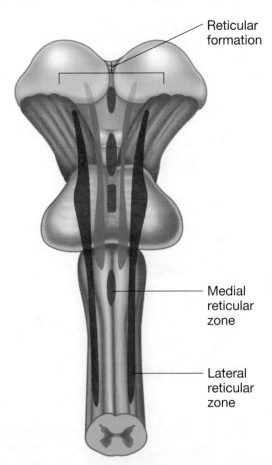

FIGURE 7-4 The reticular formation is a complex network of neurons in the brainstem.

Neuroscience Notes Box 7-1: Coma versus Vegetative State

The term *coma* describes a state of unconsciousness in which the eyes remain closed, and the patient is unable to be aroused by either internal or external stimuli. When a person is in a coma, brainstem reflexes are absent, and sleep/wake cycles cannot be distinguished on an electroencephalogram (EEG). A vegetative state is similar to a coma but is characterized by spontaneous eye opening and the return of brainstem reflexes and sleep/wake cycles. Patients in a vegetative state may display physiological responses to pain stimuli, such as increased blood pressure and heart rate, but they remain unconscious. Comas are often caused by traumatic brain injuries.

The Glasgow Coma Scale is used to assess the initial state of the patient and track the level of impairment. Patients receive scores in three significant areas related to consciousness: eye opening (1–4 points), motor responses (1–6 points), and verbal responses (1–5 points). Low scores indicate more serious brain damage and decreased consciousness, whereas higher scores mean less neural damage.

The reticular formation contains the **ascending reticular activating system (ARAS)** that sends input to the thalamus from all parts of the sensory system. A constant upward flow of input from sensory systems through the ARAS to the thalamus and cortex is necessary in order to maintain conscious awareness; damage to this system can result in a **coma**.

Cranial Nerves

The cranial nerves provide all sensory and motor innervation for structures of the head and neck. There are 12 pairs of cranial nerves in the human nervous system (see **Figure 7-5** and **Table 7.1**). Ten of them (III through XII) emerge from the brainstem and are considered part of the peripheral nervous system; the other two (I and II) are actually tracts of the central nervous system although they are still described as cranial nerves. (The term *cranial* refers to the fact that the nerves exit the skull, or cranium.)

Cranial Nerve I: Olfactory Nerve

The **olfactory nerve** is a special sensory nerve whose function is detection and transmission of odors. Although it is described as a cranial nerve, it is actually a tract of the brain and part of the CNS. It is not associated with the brainstem.

When a molecule to be smelled (an odorant) enters the nose, it dissolves in the nasal mucus and then binds to an olfactory receptor cell located in the top of the nasal cavity. The olfactory cells convert the chemical signal (molecule of odorant) into an electrical one (action potential). In order to create an action potential, the molecule of odorant usually must bind to the olfactory neuron receptor many times, since each binding is extremely brief (Bhandawat, Reisert, & Yau, 2005).

Olfactory receptors form synapses with the olfactory nerves. Each olfactory nerve has three major connections in the cerebral cortex. One connection is to the primary olfactory cortex

Neuroscience Notes Box 7-2: Central and Peripheral Cranial Nerves

Cranial nerve I (the olfactory nerve) and cranial nerve II (the optic nerve) are considered part of the central nervous system based on their anatomy. If either of these nerves is injured, it will not regenerate (grow back). The remaining cranial nerves (III through XII) all emerge from the brainstem and are anatomically part of the peripheral nervous system. Like other peripheral nerves, they can regenerate if damaged.

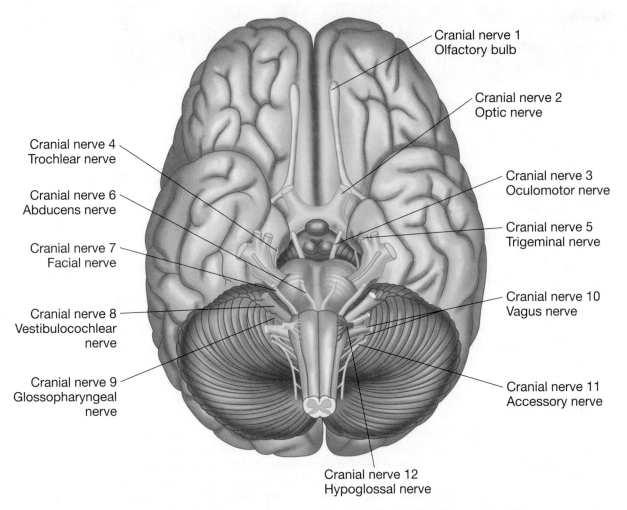

FIGURE 7-5 Cranial nerves are shown in an inferior view of the whole brain. Cranial nerves I and II are not associated with the brainstem, whereas cranial nerves III–XII are derived from the brainstem.

in the temporal lobe, for awareness and recognition of the smell. Another connection is to the **amygdala,** also located in the temporal lobe. The amygdala is part of the limbic system, and is responsible for emotional and visceral responses to odors (i.e., pleasure or disgust). Finally, the olfactory nerve connects to the hypothalamus, which can produce salivation (drooling) in response to pleasant food odors, and is responsible for nausea in response to unpleasant odors.

Cranial Nerve II: Optic Nerve

The **optic nerve** is a special sensory nerve that functions to detect and transmit visual information to the brain. Like the olfactory nerve, it is actually a tract of the brain and part of the CNS. The optic nerve does not regenerate if it is injured.

Neuroscience Notes Box 7-3: Anosmia

A lost sense of smell is called anosmia, and can result from compression of the olfactory nerve due to tumors or infections, or from tearing of olfactory nerve fibers. Temporary anosmia can occur when olfactory receptors are blocked with mucus (e.g., when suffering from a bad head cold). Also, food will lose much of its flavor without the olfactory component. With increased age, cells in olfactory epithelium are progressively lost; the sense of smell and therefore taste decline as one gets older. However, olfactory epithelial cells can regenerate throughout life, unlike almost all other nerve cells in the body (Gage, 2000). Anosmia can also be an early sign of degenerative brain disease—for example, it is often found in people with Parkinson disease.

Table 7.1 Cranial Nerves

Number	Name	Components	Structures innervated	Function
1	Olfactory	Special sensory (smell)	Olfactory epithelium (nasal cavity)	Olfactory perception
2	Optic	Special sensory (vision)	Retina (eye)	Visual perception
3	Oculomotor	Voluntary motor	4 extraocular muscles, levator palpebrae muscle	Move eyeball; open eyelid
		Parasympathetic	Pupillary constrictor muscle and ciliary muscle of lens	Constrict pupil; accommodate lens (close vision)
4	Trochlear	Voluntary motor	Extraocular muscle (superior oblique)	Move eyeball
5	Trigeminal	Somatosensory	Face, scalp, teeth, lips, anterior 2/3 tongue	Somatosensation from face & head
		Voluntary motor	Muscles of mastication & muscles of palate	Move jaw and palate
6	Abducens	Voluntary motor	Extraocular muscle (lateral rectus)	Move eyeball
7	Facial	Voluntary motor	Muscles of facial expression; stylohyoid and posterior belly of digastric; stapedius muscle (inner ear)	Move facial muscles (facial expression); move hyoid bone (swallowing); dampen loud noise
		Special sensory (taste)	Anterior 2/3 tongue & palate	Taste
		Parasympathetic	Salivary glands (sublingual & submandibular); lacrimal (tear) gland of eye; glands of nose and palate	Salivation; tears
		Somatosensory	Skin of external acoustic meatus	Somatosensation to external acoustic meatus
8	Vestibulo-cochlear (acoustic)	Special sensory (balance & hearing)	Semicircular canals, utricle and saccule of inner ear (vestibular apparatus) Cochlea of inner ear (hearing)	Vestibular sensation Hearing

(continued)

Table 7.1 *Continued*

Number	Name	Components	Structures innervated	Function
9	Glosso-pharyngeal	Somatosensory	Pharynx, palate, posterior 1/3 tongue, carotid sinus & carotid body, middle ear & external ear	Somatosensation; detection of blood pressure and blood O_2
		Special sensory (taste)	Posterior 1/3 tongue	Taste
		Voluntary motor	Stylopharyngeus muscle (swallowing)	Swallowing (assists)
		Parasympathetic	Parotid gland (salivary gland)	Salivation
10	Vagus	Somatosensory	Larynx, dura mater, ear, thoracic & abdominal viscera	Somatosensation
		Voluntary motor	Muscles of pharynx & larynx	Swallowing; vocalizing
		Parasympathetic	Viscera of thorax & abdomen	Slows heart; decreases bronchial diameter, stimulates digestion
		Special sensory (taste)	Back of throat	Taste
11	Spinal accessory	Voluntary motor	Sternocleidomastoid & trapezius muscles	Movement of head, neck, shoulder
12	Hypoglossal	Voluntary motor	Muscles of tongue (intrinsic & extrinsic)	Movement of tongue

Sources:
1. Marieb, E. N. and Mallatt, J. (2001). *Human Anatomy*, 3rd ed. San Francisco: Benjamin Cummings.
2. Moore, K. L and Dalley, A. F. (1999). *Clinically Oriented Anatomy*, 4th ed. Philadelphia: Lippincott Williams and Wilkins.
3. Snell, R. S. (2006). *Clinical Neuroanatomy*, 6th ed. Philadelphia: Lippincott Williams and Wilkins.

Neuroscience Notes Box 7-4: Blindness (Retinopathy of Prematurity)

When babies are born prematurely, they may need to be given supplemental oxygen because their lungs are not always fully developed. If too much oxygen is given to the child, the small blood vessels in the retinas can rupture, resulting in blindness of one or both eyes. This is called retinopathy of prematurity.

Visual perception begins with photoreceptor cells located in the retina at the back of each eye. There are two types of photoreceptors: rods for detecting black and white, and cones for detecting color. When light strikes the rods and cones, they convert the light waves into action potentials via a complex series of chemical reactions. The action potentials then travel through the optic nerves to the brain.

Cranial Nerve III: Oculomotor Nerve

The **oculomotor nerve** is located in the midbrain. The nerve contains motor neurons that innervate most of the muscles that move the eyeball (extraocular muscles). In addition, each oculomotor nerve supplies the levator palpebrae superioris muscle in both eyes. This muscle is responsible for voluntarily opening the eye.

The oculomotor nerve also contains parasympathetic neurons that control smooth muscle within the eye: the pupillary sphincter muscle and the ciliary muscle (ciliary body). The pupillary sphincter constricts the pupil in response to light. The ciliary muscle changes the shape of the lens to allow the eye to focus on nearby objects.

Cranial Nerve IV: Trochlear Nerve

The **trochlear nerve** is also located in the midbrain and innervates one extraocular muscle (the superior oblique) that moves each eye medially and downward. It is the only cranial nerve to exit the brainstem on its dorsal side. Before leaving the midbrain, its axons cross to the opposite side, so that the left trochlear nerve innervates the superior oblique muscle in the right eye, and vice versa. Trochlear nerve injury causes **diplopia** (double vision) and trouble looking down and inward.

Cranial Nerve V: Trigeminal Nerve

The **trigeminal nerve** is the largest cranial nerve and emerges from the pons. It has three subdivisions: the ophthalmic division (V_1), the maxillary division (V_2), and the mandibular division (V_3). The *ophthalmic division* (V_1) supplies sensation to the eyes (including the corneas) and eyelids, forehead, nose, and the top of the head/scalp. The *maxillary division* (V_2) supplies the lower eyelid, cheeks, upper lip, upper jaw, gums, teeth, and the palate, as

Neuroscience Notes Box 7-5: Oculomotor Nerve Palsy

The oculomotor nerve is especially vulnerable to compression against the temporal bone whenever there is swelling or bleeding within the skull. Therefore, oculomotor nerve signs and symptoms are an early indicator of serious injury to the skull or the brain after traumatic injury. In particular, oculomotor nerve injury can paralyze the pupillary sphincter muscle so that the pupil no longer constricts in response to light. This is known as a *fixed, dilated, nonreactive pupil,* and it can be the first indicator of a potentially serious head injury. This is one reason that a doctor may shine a light into the eyes when checking for head trauma.

Clinical Box 7-3: Lid Drop (ptosis)

Damage to CN III will produce a condition known as *ptosis* or *lid drop,* in which the upper eyelid droops. In addition, loss of extraocular muscles will result in diplopia (double vision), since movement of the two eyeballs will no longer be precisely coordinated.

Challenge question: What would be a good clinical test for oculomotor nerve function?

well as part of the external ear. Finally, the *mandibular division* (V_3) supplies sensation to the lower jaw, floor of the mouth, lower lip, gums and teeth, as well as to the chin, side of the head and part of the external ear, and the anterior two-thirds of the tongue. All three divisions innervate the dura mater, which is richly supplied with pain receptors.

The mandibular division of the trigeminal nerve also innervates eight skeletal muscles. These include the four muscles of mastication that move the jaw and allow chewing. The other four muscles are small and are involved in movement of the palate, and one of them (tensor tympani) is found in the middle ear and contracts to prevent damage to the eardrum.

Cranial Nerve VI: Abducens Nerve

The **abducens nerve** emerges from the pons and supplies one extraocular muscle: the lateral rectus. The lateral rectus muscle abducts the eyeball, so damage to the abducens nerve can cause diplopia and inability to move the eye laterally. The nerve is vulnerable to injury because it becomes stretched over a ridge on the temporal bone whenever there is a rise in intracranial pressure.

Cranial Nerve VII: Facial Nerve

The **facial nerve** contains four different kinds of neurons, making it a complex, mixed nerve. It emerges from the pons. The facial nerve innervates the muscles of facial expression, a group of delicate skeletal muscles that move the facial skin to convey emotion. It also innervates a small muscle in the middle ear (stapedius muscle). Contraction of this muscle reduces the effect of loud noises by contracting when loud sounds enter one ear.

The facial nerve sends parasympathetic axons to the lacrimal gland of the eye that stimulate production of tears, and to the salivary glands to produce saliva. It transmits taste sensation from the tongue, and contains sensory nerve fibers that innervate the soft palate and part of the pharynx.

Cranial Nerve VIII: Vestibulocochlear Nerve

The **vestibulocochlear nerve** conveys vestibular (balance) and auditory (hearing) information from specialized receptors called hair cells in the inner ear. Because injury or illness affecting one part of the nerve can also affect the other portion, balance disorders and hearing impairments frequently occur together. Damage to the vestibular part of the nerve has an impact on balance and can cause vertigo (disequilibrium or a sense of spinning), whereas lesions to the cochlear portion can cause unilateral hearing loss. This nerve emerges from the medulla oblongata. (See chapter 12 for more information about the role of the vestibulocochlear nerve in balance and hearing.)

Neuroscience Notes Box 7-6: Corneal Reflex

V_1 is important for vision because it forms the sensory limb of the corneal reflex. The cornea of the eye is extremely sensitive; any foreign object touching the cornea produces an automatic blinking and watering of the eye to flush it out. If the corneal reflex is absent, damage to the cornea is likely; in extreme cases this can result in loss of vision due to scarring.

Neuroscience Notes Box 7-7: Trigeminal Neuralgia

Trigeminal neuralgia (tic douloureux) is a potentially disabling condition involving the **trigeminal nerve.** This disorder is characterized by brief episodes of excruciating pain that travel along one or more branches of the nerve (usually either the maxillary or mandibular divisions). The pain is described as extremely intense, "white-hot," and stabbing; it may be triggered by touching the face, chewing, yawning, brushing the teeth, or other normally painless stimuli. The most common cause of trigeminal neuralgia appears to be pressure on the nerve from a blood vessel; it is also seen in people with multiple sclerosis. In some cases, the pain can be relieved by surgery to separate and cushion the nerve from the artery (Kabatas, Karasu, Civeiek, Sabanci, Hepgul, & Teng, 2008), or by the use of Botox (Zuniga, Diaz, Piedimonte, & Micheli, 2008).

Cranial Nerve IX: Glossopharyngeal Nerve

The **glossopharyngeal nerve** emerges from the medulla oblongata and innervates structures in and around the pharynx. The nerve provides sensation to the palate, the pharynx, part of the external ear, and the posterior third of the tongue. In addition, the glossopharyngeal nerve innervates structures that are important for controlling heart rate and blood pressure (carotid sinus and carotid body). The nerve also contains special sensory fibers for taste from the posterior part of the tongue, and parasympathetic neurons that supply the parotid salivary gland. Finally, it contains motor neurons to one small pharyngeal muscle—the stylopharyngeus.

Lesions to the glossopharyngeal nerve can affect regulation of blood pressure and blood oxygen levels. In addition, since the nerve provides part of the afferent (sensory) limb of the gag reflex, nerve damage creates a risk of choking. However, isolated lesions of the glossopharyngeal nerve are rare.

Cranial Nerve X: Vagus Nerve

The **vagus nerve** is one of two cranial nerves that leaves the head; its axons supply structures in the neck, thorax, and abdomen. It emerges from the medulla oblongata. The largest part of the vagus nerve consists of parasympathetic neurons that innervate smooth and

Clinical Box 7-4: Bell's Palsy

The most clinically obvious symptom of facial nerve damage is facial paralysis (also called Bell's palsy), in which muscles of facial expression on one side of the face, ipsilateral to the damaged nerve, are paralyzed. In addition, sounds may be perceived as too loud due to paralysis of the stapedius muscle. Bell's palsy is often caused by an infection (frequently the herpes simplex virus) that produces swelling and compresses the nerve. About 80% of the time, the nerve heals and begins to function again once the swelling reduces, usually within 8 weeks. In most cases, no treatment is necessary and recovery is complete. However, some physicians will treat Bell's palsy with a combination of corticosteroids and antiviral medications (Hato et al., 2007).

Facial paralysis that does not heal can be debilitating. In addition to the severe changes in appearance, the facial muscles are critical for normal function of the eyes and mouth. Because facial paralysis makes it impossible to close the eyes, and because the lacrimal glands cannot produce tears, the eyes can become dry and irritated. Changes in the ability to taste, as well as dry mouth due to the loss of some salivary glands and paralysis of muscles around the mouth, mean that eating can become challenging, with food getting caught inside the cheeks or dribbling down from the mouth. Facial rehabilitation therapy can be helpful in restoring normal nerve function.

Challenge question: Would general sensation to the face be affected by Bell's palsy?

cardiac muscle found in the thorax and abdomen. This includes the heart, where the vagus acts to slow the heart rate and decrease the force of heart contractions. It also innervates smooth muscle in the trachea and bronchial tree, the digestive tract from the inferior esophagus through the transverse colon as well as the pancreas, liver, and gall bladder.

The vagus nerve contains voluntary motor neurons that innervate most of the pharyngeal muscles and all muscles of the larynx. Thus, it is important for both swallowing and speech production. The vagus forms the motor arm of the gag reflex. This nerve also contains general sensory neurons that supply sensation to the larynx, trachea, esophagus, parts of the external and internal ear, part of the dura mater, some of the pharynx, and the thoracic and abdominal organs. In addition, the nerve contains a few special sensory nerve cells that are responsible for taste in the back of the throat.

Injury to the vagus nerve produces a range of symptoms. Its voluntary motor fibers are responsible for voluntary swallowing and for speech production; thus, nerve damage can result in **dysphagia** (difficulty swallowing) and **dysarthria** (difficulty speaking or a hoarse voice). Because the nerve forms the motor limb of the gag reflex, injury can result in increased chances of choking. If both vagus nerves are injured, the laryngeal muscles will be paralyzed and this will obstruct the airway, leading to asphyxia. Finally, vagal innervation of the digestive organs is necessary for normal functioning, especially for peristaltic contraction and for release of digestive juices and hormones from the liver and pancreas.

Cranial Nerve XI: Spinal Accessory Nerve

The **spinal accessory nerve** contains voluntary motor fibers that innervate two skeletal muscles: the sternocleidomastoid and the trapezius. The nerve is formed from two parts: one arises from the medulla oblongata (the cranial portion of the nerve), and the other arises from the upper cervical spinal cord (the spinal portion of the nerve). Injury to the spinal accessory nerve would produce flaccid paralysis of sternocleidomastoid and trapezius muscles, impairing neck and shoulder motion.

Cranial Nerve XII: Hypoglossal Nerve

The **hypoglossal nerve** comes from the medulla oblongata and contains voluntary motor neurons that supply all extrinsic and intrinsic muscles of the tongue. Injury to the hypoglossal nerve will cause an ipsilateral paralysis of the tongue; the tongue will atrophy (shrink) on the side of the lesion and if protruded it will deviate toward the paralyzed side.

Brainstem Reflexes

Brainstem reflexes include the blink reflex, jaw jerk reflex, and the swallowing reflex. Similar to those found in the spinal cord, each reflex consists of a sensory neuron and a motor neuron, with at least one connecting synapse. Brainstem reflexes allow rapid responses to sensory stimulation, and are clinically useful for assessing cranial nerve function (see **Figure 7-6**).

The blink reflex causes a bilateral reflex contraction of the orbicularis oculi muscles to close the eyes whenever something touches the cornea. The sensory part of the reflex is formed by the ophthalmic division of the trigeminal nerve (V_1). This nerve synapses in the pons onto several interneurons that in turn synapse onto the facial nerve, which forms the motor part of the reflex.

A delayed, abnormal, or absent blink reflex provides evidence of a problem with the trigeminal nerve, the facial nerve, or with the pons itself. Patients with Bell's palsy, tumors in the pons, and multiple sclerosis will often have an impaired blink reflex.

The jaw jerk is the simplest brainstem reflex and is the one most widely used in clinical neurology. The reflex tests the integrity of the mandibular division of the trigeminal nerve (V_3). The reflex is tested by placing a finger over the middle of the subject's chin when the jaw is relaxed, and gently tapping the finger with a reflex hammer to stretch the muscle spindles. This will produce bilateral contraction of the masseter muscles and closing of the jaw. Normally the jaw jerk is difficult to elicit, so when it is easily observed it is usually a sign of hyperreflexia.

The swallowing reflex is both complex and important. The first phase of swallowing is voluntary and uses muscles of the palate and the pharynx that are innervated by the

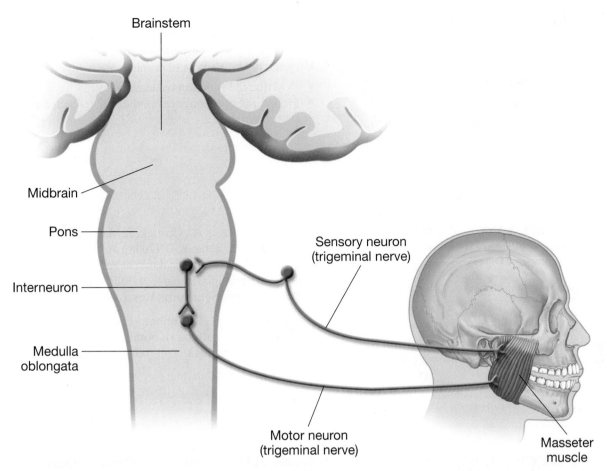

FIGURE 7-6 Brainstem reflexes: the jaw jerk reflex. Rapid stretching of the masseter muscle sends an action potential to the brainstem, where an interneuron connects to a motor neuron that causes contraction of the muscle.

glossopharyngeal (IX) and vagus (X) nerves. This is followed by an involuntary phase that is controlled by the vagus nerves, which pushes food down into the stomach. Damage to the cranial nerves can impair the swallowing reflex and cause patients to gag or choke; there is a risk of getting food or liquid into the lungs and causing pneumonia.

PATIENT SCENARIOS

Patient Case 7-1 (William)

William is a 96-year old man who had a CVA affecting the left side of the brainstem. It created an infarct (an area of dead neurons) in the ventral medulla oblongata. William displays paralysis of the right side of his body. After 4 weeks of physical therapy, he regains the ability to walk with assistance.

Questions

a) Which cranial nerves arise from the medulla oblongata? What symptoms might injury to these nerves cause?
b) Why will a left brainstem injury cause paralysis of arm and leg muscles on the patient's right side?

Patient Case 7-2 (Ann)

Ann, age 44, woke up one morning and was unable to move the left side of her face. Her diagnosis was Bell's palsy.

Questions

a) Which cranial nerve is affected in Bell's palsy?
b) What signs and symptoms could Ann expect in addition to the facial paralysis?

Patient Case 7-3 (David)

David has suffered a cranial nerve injury. His signs and symptoms include loss of sensation on the right side of his face and paralysis of his jaw muscles on the right.

Questions

a) Which cranial nerve is affected? On which side?
b) Will David still be able to move his facial muscles in order to smile, close his eyes, and raise his eyebrows?

Review Questions

1. List the major structures found in the midbrain, pons, and medulla oblongata, and state the function of each.

2. Describe the function of the reticular formation and of the ascending reticular activating system (ARAS). What effect will a severe lesion of the ARAS have?

3. For each of the 12 pairs of cranial nerves, be able to:
   - Describe the functions of each nerve.
   - Predict the consequences of damage to each nerve.

References

1. Bhandawat, V., Reisert, J., & Yau, K.-W. (2005). Elementary response of olfactory receptor neurons to odorants. *Science, 308,* 1931–1934.

2. Gage, F. H. (2000). Mammalian neural stem cells. *Science, 287,* 1433–1438.

3. Hato, N., et al (2007). Valacyclovir and prednisolone treatment for Bell's palsy: A multicenter, randomized, placebo-controlled study. *Otol. Neurotol., 28*(3), 408–413.

4. Kabatas, S., Karasu, A., Civeiek, E., Sabanci, A. P., Hepgul, K. T., & Teng, Y. D. (2008). Microvascular decompression as a surgical management for trigeminal neuralgia: Long-term follow-up and review of the literature. **Neurosurg. Rev**. (e-publication).

5. Zuniga, C., Diaz, S., Piedimonte, F., & Micheli, F. (2008). Beneficial effects of botulinum toxin type A in trigeminal neuralgia. *Arq. Neuropsiquiatr, 66*(3-A), 500–503.

Further Reading

1. Sugita, M., & Shiba, Y. (2005). Genetic tracing shows segregation of taste neuronal circuitries for bitter and sweet. *Science, 309,* 781–785.

2. Teixeira, L. J., Soares, B. G. O., Vieira, V. P., & Prado, G. F. (2008). Physical therapy for Bell's palsy (idiopathic facial paralysis). *Cochrane Database of Systematic Reviews, 3.*

3. Tiemstra, J. D., & Khatkhate, N. (2007). Bell's palsy: Diagnosis and management. *Am. Fam. Physician, 78*(3), 997–1002.

PEARSON
myhealthprofessionskit™

Use this address to access the Companion Website created for this textbook. Simply select "Physical Therapy" from the choice of disciplines. Find this book and log in using your username and password to access self-assessment questions, a glossary, and more.

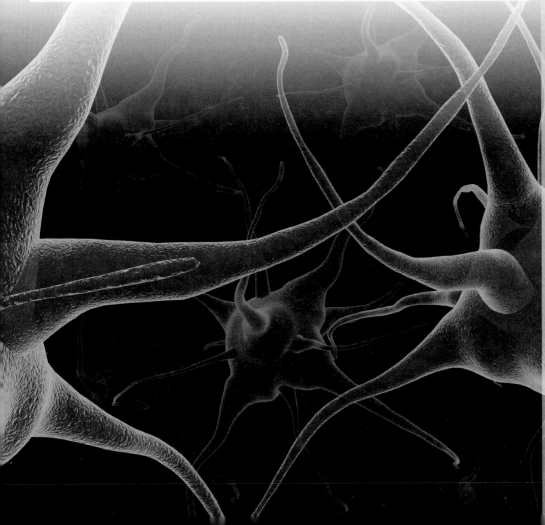

8

The Spinal Cord

CHAPTER OBJECTIVES

After completing this chapter, the reader will be able to:

1. Desribe the anatomy of the spinal cord and its meningeal coverings.

2. Discuss the role of the ascending/sensory tracts, and the functional implications of injury to each tract.

3. Explain the role of the descending/motor tracts in producing movement, and the functional effect of injury to each tract.

4. Describe the blood supply to the spinal cord and predict the functional consequences of damage to spinal cord arteries.

5. Classify spinal cord injuries according to their locations and functional effects

6. List common complications of spinal cord injury.

KEY TERMS

anterior cord syndrome
anterior corticospinal tract
anterior spinothalamic tract
ascending tracts
Babinski sign
Brown-Sequard syndrome
cauda equina
central cord syndrome
clonus
complete spinal cord injury
descending tracts
dorsal columns
dorsal (posterior) horn
grey matter
hemiplegia
incomplete spinal cord injury
hypertonicity
lateral corticospinal tract
lateral horn
lateral spinothalamic tract
lower motor neurons
monoplegia
paralysis
paraplegia
paresis
quadriplegia
reticulospinal tract
sacral sparing
spasticity
spinal cord segments
spinal meninges
spinal nerves
spinal shock
spinocerebellar tracts
spondylosis
tetraplegia
ventral (anterior) horn
vertebral column
vestibulospinal tracts
white matter

Essential Facts··

▸ The spinal cord connects the brain with the spinal nerves.

▸ The spinal cord conveys sensation from the body to the brain, and motor signals from the brain to the body.

▸ The spinal cord is subdivided into four anatomical regions (cervical, thoracic, lumbar, and sacral) and 30 individual segments.

▸ Each spinal cord segment gives rise to a pair of spinal nerves: one to the right side of the body, and one to the left side.

The spinal cord is the connection between the brain and the body. It transmits sensory information from the body to the brain, and carries motor signals from the brain to control muscle contraction and motor function. Damage to the spinal cord can have serious consequences, because normal movement and sensation depend on the flow of nerve signals (action potentials) to and from the brain. Spinal cord injury can occur due to pathologies such as tumors, arthritis of the spine, and bleeding into the cord. However, most spinal cord injuries result from trauma (for example, car accidents, falls, and sports injuries). This chapter addresses spinal cord anatomy and function as well as spinal cord injury.

Spinal Cord Anatomy

Spinal cord anatomy, including the structures that surround and protect the cord, is discussed in this section.

Bones and Meninges

The spinal cord is surrounded by the **vertebral column (spine),** formed by 33 bones called vertebrae (see **Figure 8-1**). The spine is composed of 7 cervical, 12 thoracic, 5 lumbar, and 5 sacral vertebrae. In addition, 3 to 5 small coccygeal vertebrae are found below the sacrum, forming the "tailbone." (See chapter 2 for more detail concerning the anatomy of the vertebrae and spinal column.)

Inside the vertebral column, the spinal cord is covered by three layers of connective tissue called **spinal meninges** (see **Figure 8-2**). The *pia mater* is the innermost layer. It is attached to the outside of the spinal cord. The *arachnoid* is outside of the pia mater and is formed by delicate connective tissue that is connected to the pia by tiny filaments. The *subarachnoid* space is found between the arachnoid and the pia mater and contains cerebrospinal fluid (CSF). Cerebrospinal fluid provides a watery protective cushion around the spinal cord. The outermost layer of meninges is the *dura mater*. The dura mater is a sturdy layer of connective tissue that is richly supplied with sensory nerve endings. Anything that presses against or stretches the dura (such as a bulging intervertebral disc or a tumor) can cause pain.

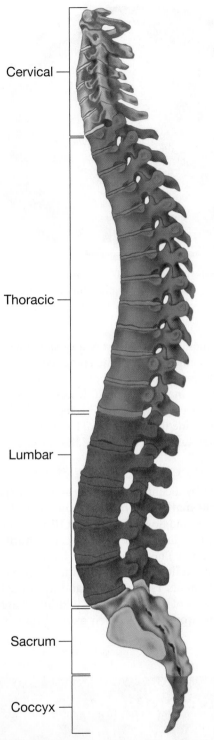

Cervical

Thoracic

Lumbar

Sacrum

Coccyx

FIGURE 8-1 The vertebral column (spine) consists of
31 individual vertebrae organized into 5 regions.

Segmental Organization

The spinal cord extends from the base of the skull to vertebral level L1. It is about 45 cm
long, and about 1 cm wide. The cord is organized segmentally, with 30 **spinal cord segments**
and 30 pairs of spinal nerves that can be grouped into four regions (see Figure 8-3). The
cervical region has 8 spinal cord segments, the thoracic region has 12 segments, the lumbar
region has 5 segments, and the sacral region has 5 segments. (Normally the coccygeal region
is considered to have 1 segment, although it has no functional significance.)

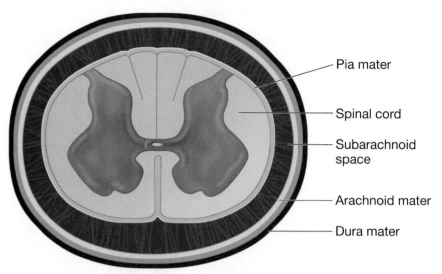

FIGURE 8-2 The spinal cord is surrounded and protected by the spinal meninges: dura mater, arachnoid, and pia mater. Cerebrospinal fluid circulates in the subarachnoid space.

Each spinal cord segment gives rise to a pair of **spinal nerves** (one right and one left). Each pair of spinal nerves emerges from the spinal cord and passes laterally through an intervertebral foramen. Because the spinal cord ends at vertebral level L1, and is shorter than the vertebral column, spinal nerves must descend within the vertebral canal in order to reach the correct intervertebral foramen. This means that the lumbar and sacral spinal nerve roots run inferiorly inside the spinal canal for up to 6 inches. These nerve roots form the **cauda equina** inside the lumbosacral part of the spine.

Internal Organization

The spinal cord is formed by a central core of **grey matter** (neuron cell bodies and dendrites) surrounded by **white matter** (axons) (see **Figure 8-4**). The white matter is formed by bundles of axons that run up and down the spinal cord, connecting the body with the brain.

Grey matter is organized into three regions called horns. The **dorsal (or posterior) horn** contains sensory (afferent) nerve fibers. The **lateral horn** contains the cell bodies of autonomic neurons (sympathetics and parasympathetics; see chapter 10). The lateral horn is found only in spinal segments T_1 through L_2 and S_2 through S_4. The **ventral (anterior) horn** contains the cell bodies of motor neurons that innervate skeletal muscle. These are considered **lower motor neurons** because their axon terminals synapse onto muscle cells.

Neuroscience Notes Box 8-1:
The Cauda Equina

The cauda equina is composed of spinal nerves that descend as a group from the level of the first lumbar vertebrae (L1) toward each nerve's respective intervertebral foramen. As a group, these nerves resemble a "horse's tail," the Latin translation of *cauda equina*. Interestingly, although these nerves travel within the spinal canal for some distance, they are actually peripheral nerves. Therefore, injuries to the spine at the L1 or L2 level and below result in injuries that are consistent with lower motor neuron injuries, displaying impairments such as flaccid paralysis, atrophy, and hyporeflexia. Injuries to the spine above the L1 level typically result in damage to the actual spinal cord, and therefore exhibit the signs and symptoms of upper motor neuron injuries: **spasticity** and hyperreflexia.

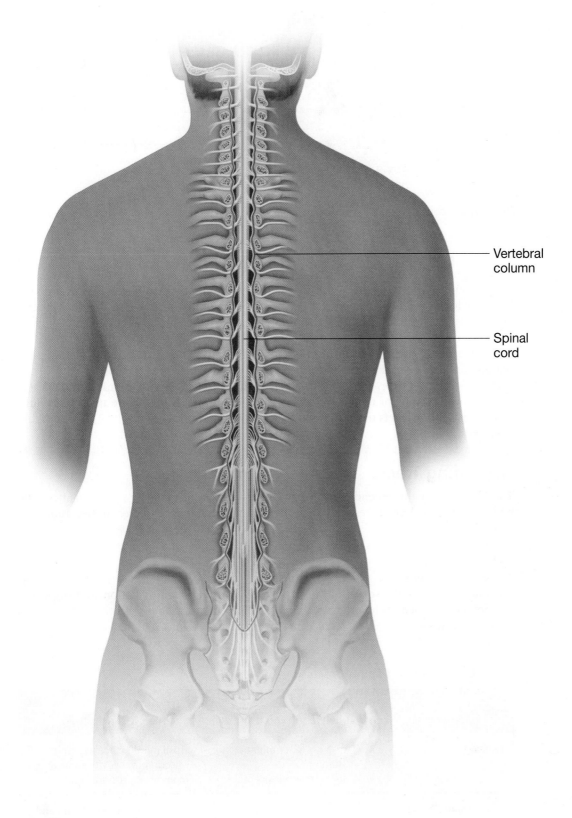

Vertebral column

Spinal cord

FIGURE 8-3 The spinal cord and spinal nerves within the vertebral column.

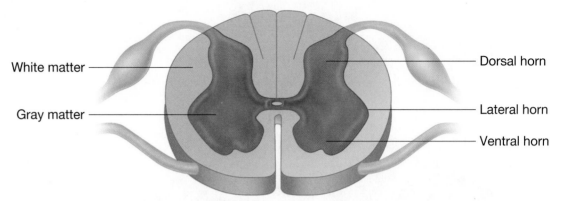

White matter

Gray matter

Dorsal horn

Lateral horn

Ventral horn

FIGURE 8-4 Spinal cord section: grey matter (neuron cell bodies) and white matter (axon bundles).

Each individual muscle is innervated by a group of lower motor neurons distributed over several segments of the spinal cord. The total number of motor neurons is correlated with the muscle's specific function. Muscles that perform precise movements are supplied by many lower motor neurons, whereas muscles that perform powerful but less precise movements are innervated by fewer motor neurons. Thus, the more precise the movements, the more motor neurons a muscle will have.

White matter is divided into three regions: anterior, lateral, and dorsal. Within each region there are several white matter columns, each of which is composed of many axons packed tightly together. These axons reciprocally connect the brain and body, and also interconnect regions of the spinal cord with one another. Some white matter columns contain **ascending tracts** that carry action potentials up to the brain, while others contain **descending tracts** that convey signals down from the brain to the body.

Ascending Tracts

There are four major ascending (sensory) tracts, all of which convey sensations from the body to the brain. Each ascending tract carries a different type (or types) of sensation (see **Table 8.1**).

Dorsal Columns

The **dorsal columns** are located in the posterior (dorsal) white matter. Axons in the dorsal columns convey the sensations of conscious proprioception, vibration, and two-point discriminative touch to the brain (see **Figure 8-5**). The information carried by these tracts comes from sensory receptors located in skin, muscles, tendons, and joints.

Table 8.1 Ascending Spinal Tracts

Tract	Functions	Effect of Unilateral Lesion in Spinal Cord
Dorsal columns	Two-point discrimination Vibration Conscious proprioception	Ipsilateral loss of two-point discrimination, vibration, and conscious proprioception
Lateral spinothalamic	Pain Temperature	Contralateral loss of pain and temperature
Anterior spinothalamic	Pressure Touch	Contralateral loss of pressure and touch
Spinocerebellar	Unconscious proprioception	Partial loss of unconscious proprioception

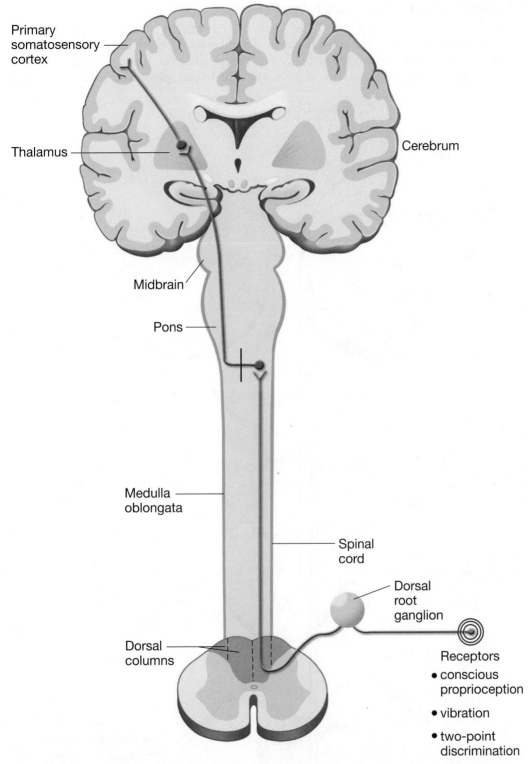

FIGURE 8-5 The dorsal columns convey vibration, two-point discriminative touch, and conscious proprioception to the brain. The dorsal columns cross in the brainstem and project to the contralateral primary somatosensory cortex.

Sensations carried in the dorsal columns are conveyed to the primary sensory cortex in the brain. This is where awareness of the sensation takes place, including knowledge of its specific location on the body, its duration, and its intensity. Damage to the dorsal column tracts results in loss of the ability to feel vibration, two-point discriminative touch, and conscious proprioception.

Spinothalamic Tracts (Antero-Lateral System)

The second and third major ascending tracts are the anterior and lateral spinothalamic tracts, which are sometimes called the anterolateral system (see Figure 8-6). The **anterior spinothalamic tract** contains axons that convey the sensations of pressure, texture, and light touch. It is located in the anterior white matter. The **lateral spinothalamic tract** is located

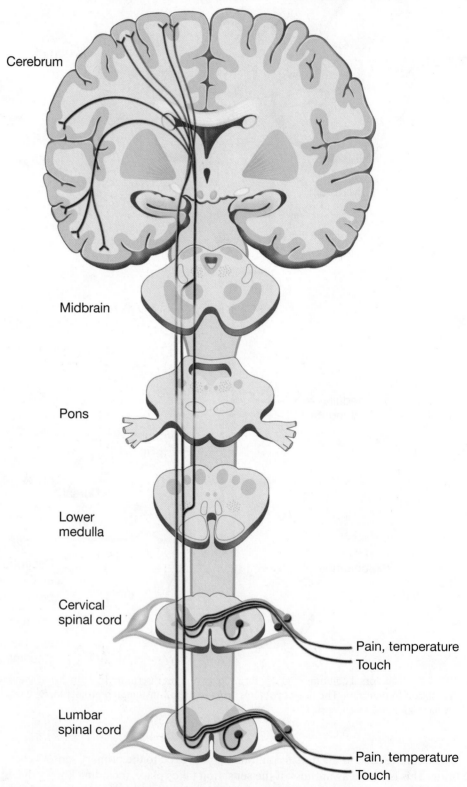

FIGURE 8-6 The anterior and lateral spinothalamic tracts convey touch, pressure, pain, and temperature sensations to the brain. The spinothalamic tracts cross in the spinal cord and project to the contralateral somatosensory cortex.

in the lateral white matter, and carries nerve fibers that convey pain and temperature. Sensation in both of these tracts comes from receptors located in the skin and subcutaneous tissue. These sensations are perceived in the primary sensory cortex, where perception and localization of the stimulus occur.

Damage to the anterolateral system in the spinal cord produces sensory changes on the side of the body contralateral (opposite) to the lesion. For example, injury to the right lateral spinothalamic tract will result in the inability to feel pain or temperature on the left side of the body (and vice versa). This occurs because the anterolateral tract axons cross to the opposite side of the spinal cord on their way to the brain.

Spinocerebellar Tracts

Spinocerebellar tracts convey unconscious proprioceptive information to the cerebellum from muscles and tendons, and monitor the activity of motor neurons (see Figure 8-7).

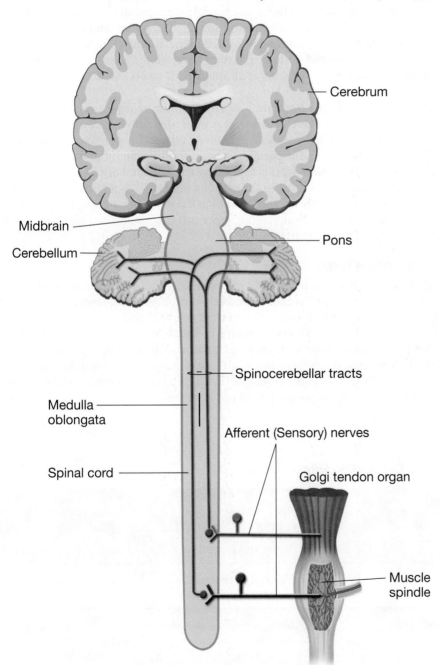

FIGURE 8-7 The spinocerebellar tracts convey unconscious proprioception to the brain (cerebellum). These tracts send axons to both sides of the cerebellum, and are described as partially crossed.

The cerebellum uses this input to coordinate movement. The spinocerebellar tracts can be damaged by demyelinating diseases such as multiple sclerosis, and are affected in people with Friedreich's ataxia, resulting in decreased muscle coordination (ataxia).

Descending Tracts

Descending (motor) tracts in the spinal cord connect the brain to lower motor neurons, and are responsible for controlling voluntary muscle contraction and movement. Neurons in these tracts are referred to as upper motor neurons (see **Table 8.2**).

Corticospinal (Pyramidal) Tracts

The corticospinal tracts are the largest tracts in the human nervous system; they contain more than 1,000,000 axons. Corticospinal tract fibers originate in the cerebral cortex and travel through the brainstem to the spinal cord. In the medulla oblongata, about 90% of the corticospinal fibers cross and enter the spinal cord as the **lateral corticospinal tract** (see **Figure 8-8**). In the cord, this tract is located in the lateral white matter. At each spinal cord level, axons exit the tract and synapse onto lower motor neurons that produce muscle contraction. This tract gives off fibers at all spinal cord levels and thus decreases in size as it descends.

The lateral corticospinal tract contains upper motor neurons that are responsible for control of voluntary movement. If this tract is injured, **paralysis** (loss of voluntary movement) or **paresis** (incomplete paralysis) will likely occur. If damage affects only the right or left half of the spinal cord, the paralysis or paresis is ipsilateral to the lesion.

The **anterior corticospinal tract** is formed by a small number (about 10%) of corticospinal tract fibers that do not cross in the medulla oblongata, but remain on the ipsilateral side of the brainstem and spinal cord. Neurons in the anterior corticospinal tract primarily innervate lower motor neurons supplying upper extremity muscles. This tract is located in the anterior (ventral) white matter.

Other Descending Tracts

Some upper motor neurons originate in the brainstem, rather than in the cerebral cortex. Together, these brainstem tracts control muscle tone, posture, balance, and gait. They are sometimes collectively referred to as the "extrapyramidal tracts."

The two **reticulospinal tracts** originate in the brainstem reticular formation (see **Figure 8-9**). Both tracts control rhythmic gait patterns. Reticulospinal tracts also contain the central autonomic fibers that control the autonomic nervous system. Damage to the reticulospinal tracts can impair autonomic function as well as posture and walking. Most neurons within these tracts are ipsilateral (do not cross).

Table 8-2 Descending Spinal Cord Tracts

Tract	Functions	Effect of unilateral lesion in spinal cord
Lateral corticospinal	Voluntary movement	Ipsilateral spastic paralysis
Anterior corticospinal	Voluntary movement, neck and shoulder muscles	Ipsilateral spastic paresis
Reticulospinal	Muscles used for gait (flexors); muscle tone	Loss of control, limb flexors; hypertonicity and muscle spasms
Vestibulospinal	Muscles used for balance and posture (extensors)	Loss of control, postural muscles

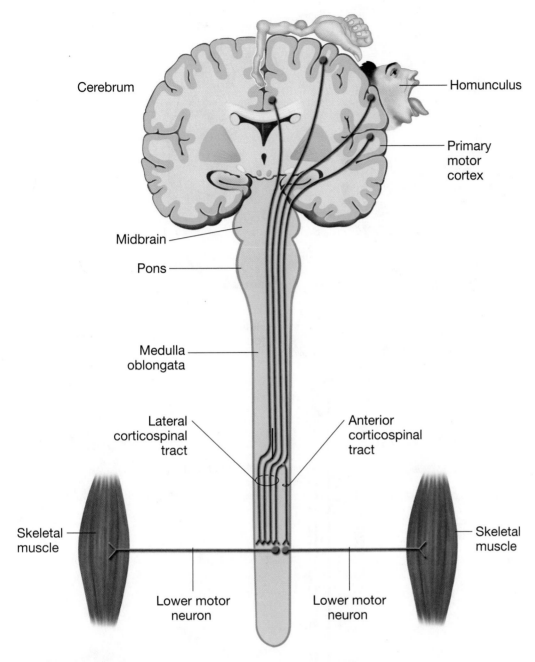

FIGURE 8-8   The lateral corticospinal tract is the primary tract controlling voluntary movement; the anterior spinothalamic tract is involved in control of the upper limbs.

Because the reticulospinal tracts tend to inhibit muscle tone, increased tone **(hypertonicity)** and spasticity are signs of damage to upper motor neurons in the descending tracts. Such damage results in hyperactive tendon (stretch) reflexes and a positive **Babinski sign.**

The **vestibulospinal tracts** begin in the brainstem vestibular nuclei, and descend through the brainstem and spinal cord. They connect to interneurons and lower motor neurons controlling proximal limb muscles responsible for maintaining balance. Vestibular nuclei receive inputs from the inner ear (vestibular apparatus), cerebellum, and other motor areas of the brain. They are bilateral tracts; some axons cross in the brainstem while others stay ipsilateral. Injury to the vestibulospinal tracts causes problems with balance (ataxia).

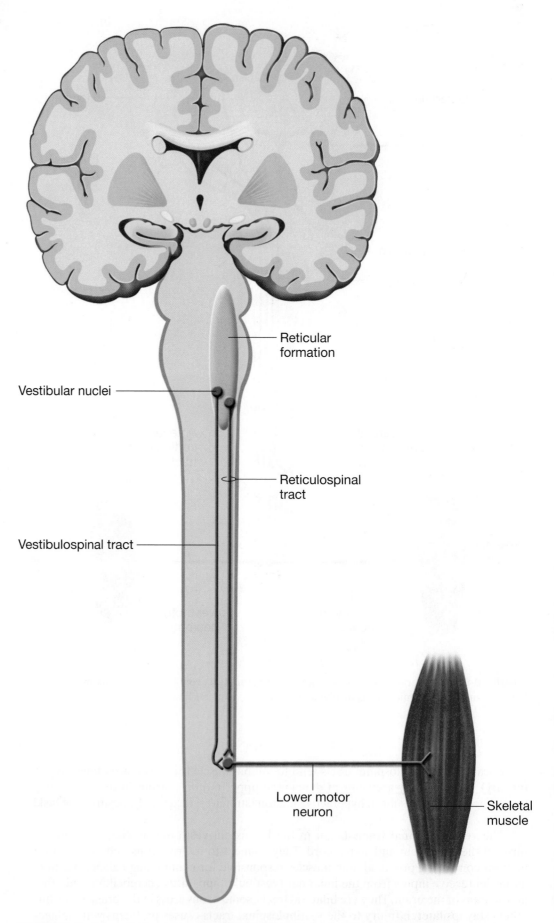

FIGURE 8-9 The reticulospinal tracts and vestibulospinal tracts control muscles involved in gait, posture, and muscle tone.

Clinical Box 8-1: Babinski Sign

A well-known sign of upper motor neuron injury is a positive Babinski sign. A Babinski sign is elicited by stroking the sole of the foot with a firm object such as the thumb or the back of a reflex hammer. The examiner begins at the heel and progresses up the outside of the foot and then crosses toward the base of the great (big) toe. A normal response to this stimulus is flexion of all five toes; however, individuals suffering from CNS damage will display extension of the great toe (instead of flexion; see **Figure 8-10**). Extension of the great toe resulting from this type of stimulation is considered a (+) Babinski sign. (Note that infants will typically display a positive Babinski sign following this type of stimulus; this is normal.)

Challenge question: What would a "positive" Babinski sign in an adult tell you about the function of descending spinal cord tracts?

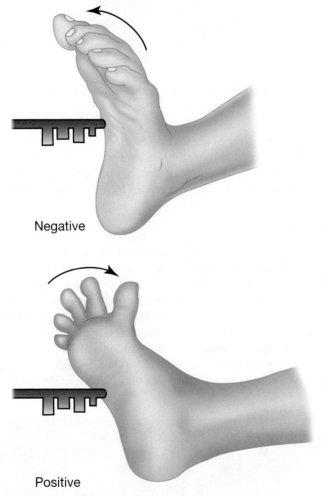

Negative

Positive

FIGURE 8-10 A "positive" Babinski sign indicates upper motor neuron damage. A positive Babinski is demonstrated by extension of the toes when the sole of the foot is stimulated.

Blood Supply

The spinal cord receives blood from three arteries that run vertically along its length: an anterior spinal artery and two posterior spinal arteries (see **Figure 8-11**). In addition, two small segmental arteries supply each spinal cord segment. The anterior spinal artery supplies the anterior two-thirds of the cord, and the posterior spinal artery supplies the posterior

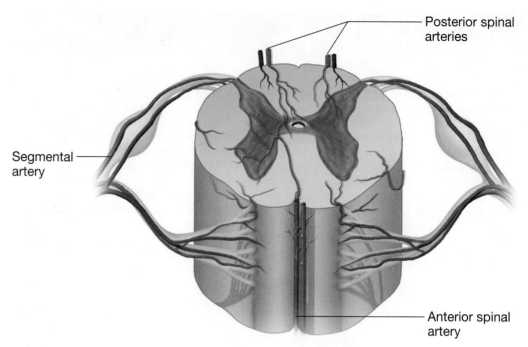

Posterior spinal arteries

Segmental artery

Anterior spinal artery

FIGURE 8-11 The vascular supply of the spinal cord consists of an anterior spinal artery, two posterior spinal arteries, and small segmental arteries.

third. All of the spinal cord arteries are interconnected, forming a network of small vessels that provides blood to the cord and to spinal nerves within the vertebral canal. The spinal cord is drained by small veins that empty into a venous plexus located outside the dura mater. From there, venous blood empties into larger veins located along the posterior body wall.

Spinal Cord Injury

Traumatic spinal cord injury can result from motor vehicle accidents, falls, sports injuries, and violence. In addition, diseases and disorders of the spine can produce the same symptoms as those from traumatic injury. Often, the spinal cord is injured because vertebrae have been fractured or dislocated. In some cases, the cord may experience traumatic bending (sometimes called subluxation). It can also be damaged directly (by a bullet or knife wound), or crushed by swelling or a tumor that kills neurons and compresses small blood vessels, causing ischemia. In addition, dead and dying neurons release large amounts of ATP (adenosine triphosphate), enzymes, and neurotransmitters that can be toxic to nearby cells. This results in secondary injury that can spread and enlarge the initial area of cell death caused by the traumatic event.

Clinical Box 8-2: Vascular Disorders of the Spinal Cord

Blood flow to the spinal cord can be interrupted by injury to the arteries that supply the cord, and by disease or trauma that causes swelling in the spinal column. This will compress the small vessels and cause an infarct (area of cell death) in the cord. An infarct of the anterior spinal artery produces anterior cord syndrome. This syndrome spares the dorsal columns, but damages axons in the anterior part of the cord. Usually, this causes paralysis and sensory loss, but proprioception is intact.

Challenge question: If a patient had a vascular infarct that damaged axons in the posterior portion of the spinal cord, but left the anterior and lateral parts intact, what signs and symptoms would you expect to see?

Classification of Spinal Cord Injury

Spinal cord injuries are classified in several different ways: according to the segmental level of injury, by the level of intact function, and by the number of limbs affected. If vertebrae have been fractured or dislocated, the orthopedic surgeon may describe a "bony" level of injury based on the affected bone(s). On the spinal cord itself, the physical site of the injury can be described as the lesion level. This may spread across several segments, and can be different on each side of the cord. Finally, rehabilitation professionals often describe the injury level by the lowest (most inferior) intact, functioning nerve roots (see Figure 8-12).

Spinal cord injury is also classified according to the number of limbs that have lost motor function. **Quadriplegia (tetraplegia)** is complete or partial paralysis (paresis) of all four limbs. **Paraplegia** refers to paralysis of the lower extremities only, and **hemiplegia** to paralysis of one side of the body. **Monoplegia** is paralysis of one limb.

Finally, spinal cord injury can be classified as either complete or incomplete. A **complete spinal cord injury** results in complete paralysis and a complete loss of sensation below the level of the injury. Spinal cord injuries where any motor function or sensation remains are considered **incomplete spinal cord injuries.** Patients are classified as complete or incomplete by testing the lowest nerve root level (S5). This is done by testing sensation and muscle function of the anal sphincter, which is innervated by S_5. A patient who has anal sensation or the ability to contract the sphincter (or both) has **sacral sparing,** and is considered to have an incomplete spinal cord injury. Sacral sparing is important because it indicates that some ascending and/or descending tracts are intact. It is also more likely that people with incomplete injuries will have some degree of motor and sensory return.

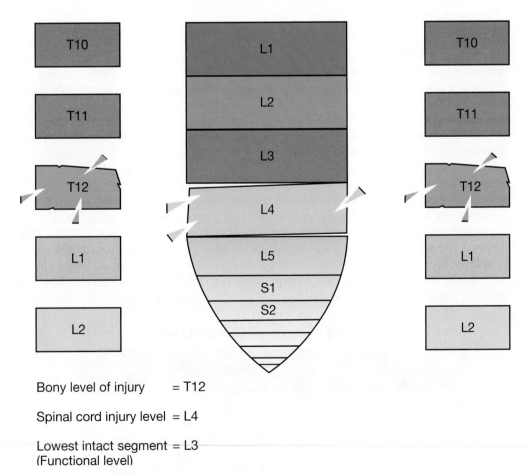

Bony level of injury = T12

Spinal cord injury level = L4

Lowest intact segment = L3
(Functional level)

FIGURE 8-12 Spinal cord injury: Methods of classification.

Neuroscience Notes Box 8-2: Reducing Swelling after Spinal Cord Injury

Because swelling within the spinal column is responsible for some of the damage caused by spinal cord injury, emergency room physicians attempt to reduce this swelling in order to prevent as much neurological damage as possible. Medications that reduce inflammation (for example, methylpredisone) have been shown to reduce swelling and improve patient outcomes. There are also some reports suggesting that therapeutic hypothermia (cooling the injured spinal region with a cold saline solution) can help prevent lasting neurological damage if used early enough, although more evidence is needed regarding this modality.

Progression of Spinal Cord Injury

The first several weeks after spinal cord injury are a period of **spinal shock.** During this time, there is no sensation or movement below the injured spinal cord segment. All reflexes below the lesion shut down, and usually bladder and bowel control are lost. Spinal shock is thought to result from swelling and trauma to the cord caused by the injury, as well as inflammation causing pressure within the vertebral canal.

Once the period of spinal shock is over, and the swelling goes down, some spinal reflexes may return. Usually flexor reflexes come back first, followed by extensor reflexes. Often, reflexes become exaggerated, so a deep tendon reflex test will produce a hyperactive response. Over time, patients may develop extensor spasms that are marked by overactivity of extensor muscles. Clinicians who work closely with this population do frequent sensory and motor assessments to monitor any changes in neural function.

Determining Injury Level

After the period of spinal shock has ended and the pattern of sensory and motor function has stabilized, it is possible to determine the specific segmental injury level. This is done by dermatome testing (for somatosensory levels) combined with deep tendon reflex testing (to determine motor function levels). Some patients will have slightly different results with these two tests but the definitive injury level is always defined by motor function. Spinal cord injuries are usually classified using the ASIA classification system (explained later in this chapter).

The two major symptoms of complete spinal cord injury are loss of sensation and paralysis (loss of voluntary motor function). The extent of functional loss is related to the segmental lesion level, the extent of damage in the spinal cord, and which specific tracts are affected (see **Table 8.3**).

Somatosensation is almost always changed after spinal cord injury (see **Figure 8-13**). All dermatomes *above* the physical lesion in the spinal cord will have normal function. *At* the physical lesion level, the entire dermatome will display loss of somatosensation. This is because the sensory neurons entering the **dorsal horn** have been destroyed. *Below* the lesion level, somatosensation is also lost; this is due to destruction of the ascending spinal cord tracts in the white matter. Thus, a dermatome test will show sensory loss both at and below the physical lesion level, and will exhibit normal sensation above.

Table 8.3 Determining Lesion Level (Complete Injury)

Physical Lesion Level	Sensation	Movement	Tone
Above	Normal	Normal	Normal
At	Lost	Paralyzed	Hypotonic
Below	Lost	Paralyzed	Hypertonic

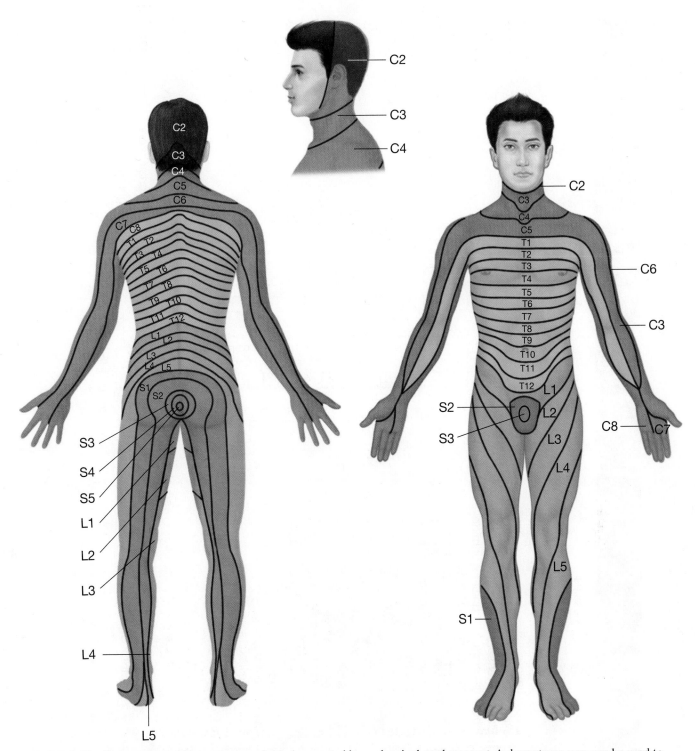

FIGURE 8-13 Dermatomes represent areas of skin innervated by each spinal cord segment. A dermatome map can be used to determine injury level after spinal cord injury.

Paralysis (loss of voluntary movement) is a major consequence of spinal cord injury. Paralysis results from an interruption in the pathway that connects the motor cortex to skeletal muscles. Injury to any of these components can produce paralyzed muscles (see **Figure 8-14**). At the physical injury level in the spinal cord, all muscles innervated by that spinal segment will be paralyzed due to destruction of spinal cord lower motor neurons. Muscles innervated below the spinal injury level will be paralyzed because the descending pathways cannot send action potentials past the level of the lesion. However, some patients have function for several segments below the injury site: This is called the zone of partial preservation.

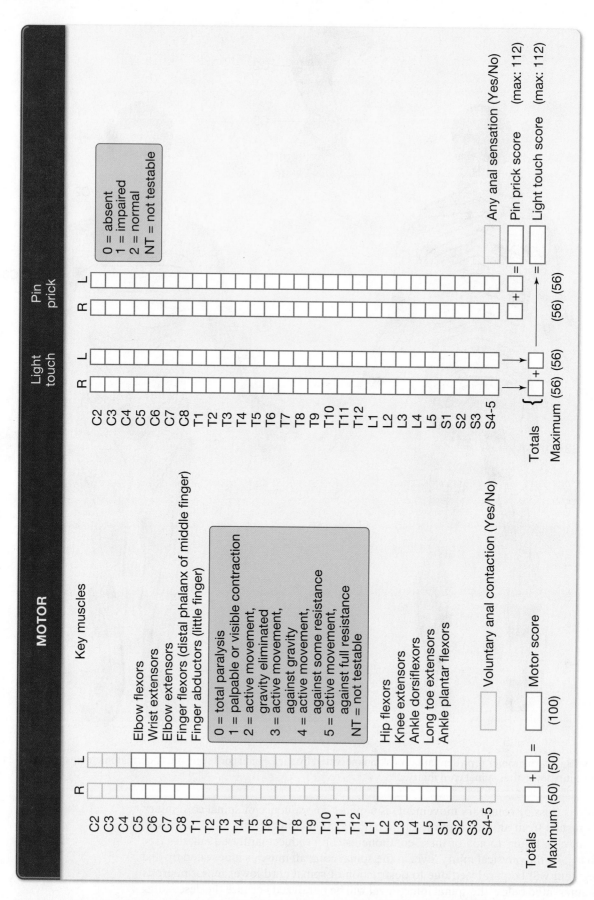

FIGURE 8-14 American Spinal Injury Association (ASIA) classification of spinal cord injury: Myotomes represent functional muscle groups innervated by each spinal cord segment, and dermatomes represent areas of the skin innervated by each segment.

Neuroscience Notes Box 8-3: Exercise and Spinal Cord Injury

Because the spinal cord is part of the central nervous system, damaged axons result in cell death and functional loss with no regeneration. Scientists are exploring ways to promote regeneration and restore function. In rats with incomplete spinal cord injuries, exercise increases chemicals called neurotrophins that promote regeneration of spinal cord axons (Vaynman and Gomez-Pinilla, 2005; Vavrek et al., 2006) and improve motor function (Vavrek et al., 2006; Kubasek et al., 2008). It is not yet known whether exercise promotes spinal cord regeneration in humans. However, exercise is beneficial for people with spinal cord injuries for the same reasons it is good for everyone: It promotes cardiovascular health, helps to maintain a healthy weight, and can improve mood.

Motor function level can be determined by deep tendon reflex testing. All muscles innervated by nerves *above* the physical lesion level will have normal function. Deep tendon reflex testing should produce normal reflex responses. *At* the lesion level, a DTR test will elicit no response; the muscles will be paralyzed and hypotonic. This condition is described as flaccid paralysis.

Muscles innervated *below* the physical lesion level will also be paralyzed, but will demonstrate hypertonicity and spasticity when tested. They are paralyzed because of damage to upper motor neurons. Deep tendon reflex tests produce an abnormally strong, intense muscle contraction.

Complications of Spinal Cord Injury

The primary signs of spinal cord injury are paralysis and sensory loss (see **Table 8.4**). Many secondary complications follow from these problems. They include pressure sores, heterotopic ossifications, autonomic dysreflexia, and spasticity. In addition, bladder and bowel control, as well as sexual functioning, are affected by most spinal injuries.

Pressure sores result from immobility, and often occur on parts of the body where a bony prominence puts pressure on skin and underlying tissues (for example, over the ischial tuberosities). Because many patients have sensory loss, they may be unaware that pressure sores are developing. If these sores are not carefully monitored, they can become infected and cause sepsis (a serious blood infection), which can be fatal.

Table 8.4 Spinal Cord Innervation

Spinal level	Structures innervated	Functional effect	Effect of injury
C1–C4	Neck muscles	Neck stability and mobility	Loss of neck stability
C3–C5	Diaphragm	Breathing	Ventilator dependent
C5–T1	Upper extremity	Upper extremity movement	Tetraplegia
T1–L5	Trunk muscles Intercostals Abdominal wall muscles	Trunk stability and movement Accessory respiratory muscles	Loss of trunk stability Decreased respiratory function
L2–S4	Lower extremity	Lower extremity movement	Paraplegia (diplegia)
S2–S4	Pelvic diaphragm Genitals	Sphincter control (bladder and bowel) Sexual function	Neurogenic bladder/bowel Loss of sexual function

Clinical Box 8-3: Autonomic Dysreflexia

Autonomic dysreflexia is a potentially life-threatening condition that can occur in people with spinal cord injuries above the T5 level. This condition results from a noxious stimulus, such as a kinked catheter, that sends pain signals toward the brain. However, because of the spinal cord injury, the signal cannot reach the brain. Instead, pain signals communicate with the sympathetic nervous system to produce an uncontrolled sympathetic response involving vasoconstriction and continually increasing blood pressure, along with a decreasing heart rate. Because this is a very serious condition, any clinician working with patients with spinal cord injuries should be aware of the signs and symptoms of autonomic dysreflexia as well as the immediate course of action. Some common signs and symptoms of autonomic dysreflexia include a pounding headache, a sudden increase in blood pressure (as high as 200/100), sweating and goose-bumps above the injury level, and a very flushed face. If a patient shows these symptoms, the blood pressure must be reduced immediately. The clinician should sit the patient upright, and find the cause (the noxious stimulus) as quickly as possible. Often, it is a kinked catheter or full bladder, but there are many other possible causes. If the cause cannot be found or resolved quickly, the nurse and/or MD should be called to help resolve the situation.

Challenge question: Which damaged spinal cord pathway prevents the pain stimulus from reaching the brain to alert the patient of a problem?

Heterotopic ossifications are small, calcified nodules found in muscles and joints after spinal cord injury. The exact cause of these is unknown, but it is thought that they may result from defects in bone and calcium metabolism due to trauma or immobility. Heterotopic ossifications that form inside joints can severely limit joint mobility.

Spinal cord injuries may produce clinically significant changes in muscle tone. Motor neurons in the spinal cord adjust tone for normal function. If these neurons are injured, muscles will display excessive tone and are described as spastic and hypertonic. A deep tendon reflex test of a hypertonic muscle produces an abnormally strong reflex contraction (spasticity). Over time, muscles below the injury level become supersensitive to sensory stimulation. This can cause extremely strong muscle contractions in response to a tendon tap or another sensory stimulus. It can also result in **clonus,** a series of rapid, rhythmic alternating movements.

Neuroscience Notes Box 8-4: Spasticity after Spinal Cord Injury

Spinal cord injury almost always affects tone in muscles innervated at and below the lesion level. At the level of the lesion, lower motor neurons to skeletal muscles are damaged. This results in loss of muscle tone (hypotonia or flaccidity). Below the lesion level, lower motor neurons are intact but the upper motor neurons controlling them are injured. Many of these upper motor neurons modify tone, so injury will often result in hypertonia and spasticity. This can be controlled with medications (such as Baclofen) that reduce the excess tone.

Clinical Box 8-4: Spinal Cord Syndromes

There are a number of spinal cord syndromes that can be identified based on the specific location of the damaged tissue. Four of these syndromes are described here (see **Figure 8-15**).

Brown-Sequard Syndrome
A lesion affecting exactly one-half (right or left) of the spinal cord is known as **Brown-Sequard syndrome.** Symptoms of Brown-Sequard syndrome include:

- Ipsilateral flaccid paralysis of muscle at the physical injury level
- Ipsilateral spastic paralysis of muscles below the lesion site
- Ipsilateral sensory loss at the lesion level
- Ipsilateral loss of proprioception, vibration, and two-point discrimination below the lesion level
- Contralateral loss of pain and temperature sensations below the level of the lesion

Central Cord Syndrome
Central cord syndrome is caused by damage to the center of the spinal cord. It usually occurs due to traumatic bending of the cord in the cervical region (from hyperextension or hyperflexion injuries). Central cord syndrome results in flaccid paralysis of upper extremity muscles along with upper extremity sensory loss. It is sometimes referred to as "reverse paralysis" because the upper extremities suffer more paralysis and sensory loss than do the lower extremities.

Anterior Cord Syndrome
Anterior cord syndrome results from damage to the anterior part of the spinal cord that spares the posterior white matter. Anterior cord syndrome can be caused by traumatic bending of the cord, or by conditions that narrow the vertebral canal (spinal stenosis). Because the posterior part of the cord is spared, the dorsal columns are usually not affected. Conscious proprioception, vibration, and two-point discriminative touch sensations remain intact, while other sensations and motor functions are lost. Although people with anterior cord syndrome appear completely paralyzed below the level of injury, they frequently display higher levels of functional balance than people with complete spinal cord injuries, due to the intact proprioceptive tracts.

Cauda Equina Syndrome In cauda equina syndrome, injury to the dorsal and ventral nerve roots in the cauda equina results in loss of sensation, flaccid paralysis, and loss of sympathetic and parasympathetic responses in the pelvis. Although the cauda equina is technically part of the peripheral nervous system, it seldom regenerates after injury because it lacks connective tissue pathways to guide regrowth. Because bladder and bowel function are controlled by sacral spinal levels S_2 through S_4, the most serious functional consequence of cauda equina syndrome is loss of bladder and bowel control.

Challenge question:
1. Which of the spinal cord syndromes described here is most likely to cause hemiplegia?
2. Which of the spinal cord syndromes described here would be considered incomplete?

The rectum and bowel are innervated by the same spinal cord segments as the bladder, and are controlled in a similar fashion. Spinal cord injury above S_2 cause a spastic neurogenic bowel, whereas injury at S_2 through S_4 produces a flaccid neurogenic bowel. In both cases, patients lose voluntary control of the anal sphincter. Constipation is a frequent consequence of SCI, partly due to decreased physical mobility.

Sexual function is often affected after spinal cord injury. Sexual function is a neurologically complex phenomenon that involves sensation, voluntary motor nerves, and autonomic

Clinical Box 8-5: Erection After Spinal Cord Injury

The sacral spinal cord (S_2 through S_4) houses neurons that cause reflex erections in males: These occur when there is physical stimulation of the penis. In contrast, psychogenic erections occur when a male thinks about sex and are facilitated by neurons connecting the brain with the sacral cord. If spinal cord injury damages these descending axons, psychogenic erections will be lost. However, if the sacral cord is intact, reflex erections will still occur.

Challenge question: Would a male with a complete spinal cord injury above S_2 be able to tell that he has an erection without looking?

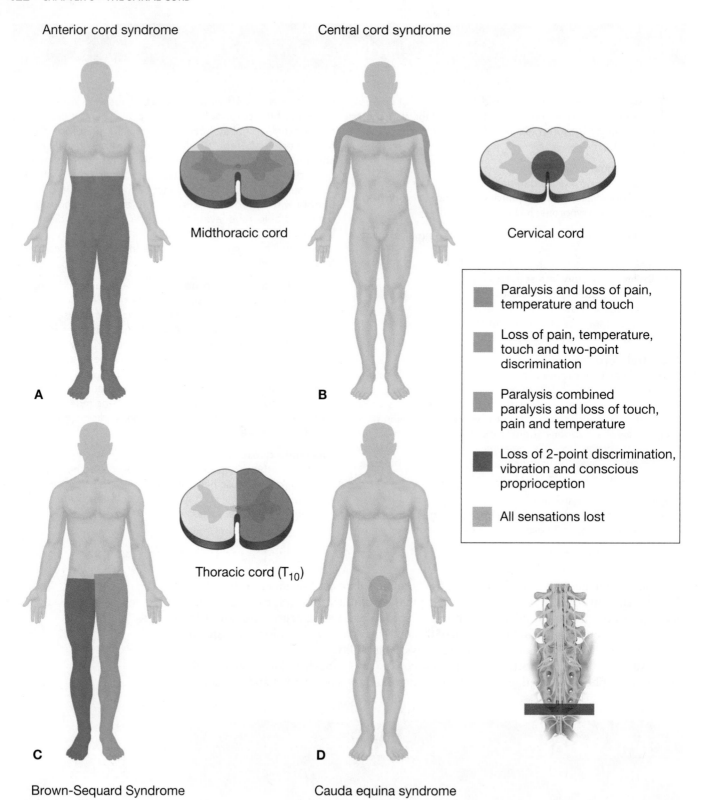

Anterior cord syndrome

Midthoracic cord

Central cord syndrome

Cervical cord

A

B

	Paralysis and loss of pain, temperature and touch
	Loss of pain, temperature, touch and two-point discrimination
	Paralysis combined paralysis and loss of touch, pain and temperature
	Loss of 2-point discrimination, vibration and conscious proprioception
	All sensations lost

Thoracic cord (T$_{10}$)

C

D

Brown-Sequard Syndrome

Cauda equina syndrome

FIGURE 8-15   Spinal cord syndromes (Brown-Sequard syndrome, anterior cord syndrome, central cord syndrome, cauda equina syndrome).

Neuroscience Notes Box 8-5: Bladder Function after Spinal Cord Injury

Normal urinary function requires intact sensory and motor connections between the bladder and the sacral spinal cord. Interruption of these connections at any point produces a neurogenic bladder (see **Figure 8-16**). Spinal cord lesions above S_2 through S_4 produce a reflex neurogenic (spastic) bladder. The bladder wall muscle maintains tone and can empty by reflex. When enough urine enters the bladder to stimulate stretch receptors in its wall, the muscular bladder wall will contract and the sphincters will relax. However, voluntary control is lost because patients are unaware of fullness and because control of voluntary sphincter muscles is lost.

Bilateral lesions involving spinal cord segments S_2 through S_4 result in a flaccid neurogenic bladder. Patients are not aware that the bladder is full and cannot voluntarily inhibit or initiate bladder emptying. Because lower motor neurons to the bladder wall and sphincters are lost, the bladder becomes flaccid and distended, until there is a continual dribbling incontinence. This creates urinary retention with a high risk of infection.

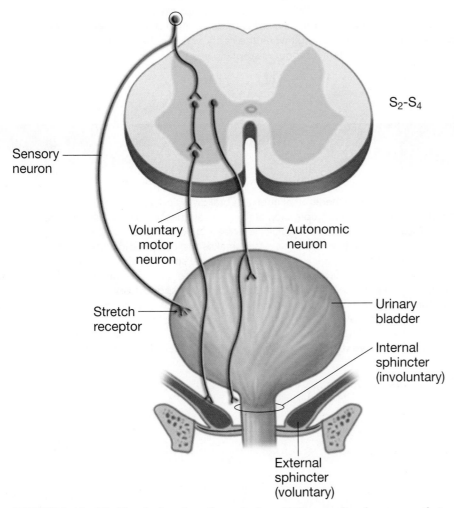

FIGURE 8-16 Bladder dysfunction after spinal cord injury results when nerves that control bladder sensation and emptying are damaged, causing loss of function.

neurons. It requires normal activity of spinal cord reflexes, as well as connections between the lumbosacral spinal cord and the brain. Erection (in males) and vaginal/clitoral swelling (in females) are controlled by sacral segments S_2 through S_4; damage to the cord at or above this level may affect these functions. In addition, injuries that disrupt sensation will cause patients to lose the ability to feel genital stimulation.

Neuroscience Notes Box 8-6:
Syringomyelia

Syringomyelia is a chronic degenerative disorder of the spinal cord. In syringomyelia, a fluid-filled cavity (syrinx) develops in the center of the cord. The cavity is usually found in the lower cervical and upper thoracic levels and extends through several segments. Occasionally the cavity extends into the brainstem or into lower thoracic segments. The cause of syringomyelia is unknown. The anterolateral spinothalamic tracts are affected first, so an early symptom is impairment of pain and temperature in the arms and hands. Since tactile and proprioceptive sensations are preserved, this selective loss of pain and temperature is referred to as a dissociated sensory loss. It may also cause weakness and atrophy of the hands and arms. These symptoms are due to destruction of ventral horn lower motor neurons. Autonomic disorders result when the cavity involves the lateral horn. Involvement of the lateral corticospinal tract produces spastic paresis and occasionally spastic paraplegia.

Clinical Box 8-6: Spinal Stenosis

In spinal stenosis, degeneration of intervertebral discs and bony outgrowths into the spinal canal can cause chronic compression of the cervical spinal cord. The disc becomes covered with fibrous tissue, and sometimes calcifies, creating bony ridges. This is often accompanied by enlargement of spinal ligaments, which makes the compression worse. When stenosis occurs in the cervical region, it may be called cervical **spondylosis.** The lower cervical spine is vulnerable to these degenerative changes because it is very mobile, and because the vertebral canal is narrow there. Signs and symptoms of spondylosis are a painful, stiff neck, arm pain along with numb hands, spastic leg weakness, and a positive Babinski sign. There may also be abnormal sensations of the limbs and trunk, often described as burning, pricking, tingling, or tickling sensations (parethesia).

   Challenge question: Why would cervical spondylosis cause pain, numbness, and weakness in the arms?

PATIENT SCENARIOS

Patient Case 8-1 (Jeremy)

Jeremy is a 20-year-old man who suffered a traumatic spinal cord injury in a motorcycle accident. He has been defined as an incomplete tetraplegic. Jeremy has spastic paralysis of both lower extremities and his trunk. In the upper limbs, Jeremy can flex both elbows and can extend his right wrist and right elbow, but cannot do either function on the left side. The right finger flexors are flaccid, as are his left wrist extensors. Jeremy does have some touch and pain sensation in his left lower extremity.

Questions

a) What is Jeremy's physical injury level? What is his functional level?
b) How would you test whether Jeremy's injury is complete or incomplete?
c) What will Jeremy's respiratory status be? What will his bladder and bowel function be?

Patient Case 8-2 (Annette)

Annette is a 60-year old woman with a medical diagnosis of spinal stenosis. She has hypertonic muscles in both lower extremities and a scissors gait. She also has marked ataxia in her legs, and decreased coordination is apparent in her upper limbs.

Questions

a) Which spinal cord tracts are most likely affected in this patient, based on her symptoms?
b) How do you think this patient's symptoms will progress, compared to a patient with a traumatic spinal cord injury? Would you expect Annette's symptoms to get worse over time, stay the same, or improve?

Patient Case 8-3 (Kathy)

Kathy has been diagnosed with Brown-Sequard syndrome due to a tumor that has degenerated the left half of her spinal cord at the T-4 level.

Questions

a) Which of Kathy's legs will display full motor function?
b) Would Kathy be able to feel a pin-prick sensation on her right medial malleolus?
c) Would Kathy display weakness or sensory loss of either upper extremity?

Review Questions

1. Describe the anatomy of the spinal cord, including its meningeal coverings.
2. For each afferent/sensory pathway in the spinal cord, name the type of sensation conveyed and its location in the spinal cord (dorsal, lateral, or ventral).
3. For each efferent/motor tract in the spinal cord, describe its location in the cord (dorsal, lateral, or ventral) and explain the role of each tract in producing movement.
4. Describe the blood supply to the spinal cord.
5. Explain the various ways that spinal cord injuries are classified.
6. Explain the motor and sensory signs that result from spinal cord injury. How could you distinguish flaccidity from spasticity in a clinical setting?
7. Describe the effects of spinal cord injury on respiratory function, bladder and bowel function, and sexual function.

References

1. Kubasak, M. D., Jindrich, D. L., Zhong, H., Takeoka, A., McFarland, C., Munoz-Quiles, C., Roy, R. R., Edgerton, V. R., Ramon-Cueto, A., & Phelps, P. E. (2008). OEG implantation and step training enhance hindlimb-stepping ability in adult spinal transected rats. *Brain, 131*, 264–276.
2. Vavrek, R. et al. (2006). BDNF promotes connections of corticospinal neurons onto spared descending interneurons in spinal cord injured rats. *Brain, 129*, 1534–1545.
3. Vaynman, S., & Gomez-Pinilla, F. (2005). License to run: Exercise impacts functional plasticity in the intact and injured central nervous system by using neurotrophins. Neurorehabil. *Neural Repair 19*, 283–295.

Further Reading

1. Boyd, J. G., Doucette, R., & Kawaja, M. D. (2005). Defining the role of olfactory ensheathing cells in facilitating axon remyelination following damage to the spinal cord. FASEB J. 19, 694–703.

2. Dunlop, S.A. (2008). Activity-dependent plasticity: implications for recovery after spinal cord injury. *Trends in Neurosciences, 31*(8), 410–418.

3. Feron, F., Perry, C., Cochrane, J., Licina, P., Nowitzke, A., Urquhart, S., Geraghty, T., & MacKay-Sim, A. (2005). Autologous olfactory ensheathing cell transplantation in human spinal cord injury. *Brain, 128,* 2951–2960.

4. FitzGerald, J., & Fawcett, J. (2007). Repair in the central nervous system. *J. Bone Joint Surg. Br., 89-B,* 1413–1420.

5. Harkema, A., Gerasimenko, Y., Hodes, J., Burdick, J., Angeli, C., Chen, Y., Ferreira, C., Willhite, A., Rejc, E., Grossman, R. G., & Edgerton, R. (2011). Effect of epidural stimulation of the lumbosacral spinal cord on voluntary movement, standing, and assisted stepping after motor complete paraplegia: A case study. *The Lancet.* doi:10.1016/S0140-6736(11)60547-3.

6. Kraft, U. (2005). Mending the spinal cord. *Scientific American, 16*(3), 68–73.

7. Pinter, M. M., & Dimitrijevic, M. R. (1999). Gait after spinal cord injury and the central pattern generator for locomotion. *Spinal Cord, 37,* 531–537.

8. Schwab, M. E. (2002). Repairing the injured spinal cord. *Science, 295,* 1029–1031.

PEARSON
myhealthprofessionskit™

Use this address to access the Companion Website created for this textbook. Simply select "Physical Therapy" from the choice of disciplines. Find this book and log in using your username and password to access self-assessment questions, a glossary and more.

Peripheral Nervous System

CHAPTER OBJECTIVES

After completing this chapter, the reader will be able to:

1 Discuss the structure and function of peripheral nerves.

2 Describe the anatomy and function of the cervical, brachial, lumbar, and sacral plexuses, and explain the anatomy and function of thoracic spinal nerves.

3 Explain how peripheral nerves can be damaged by injury or disease, and discuss the healing process.

KEY TERMS

alpha motor neurons
cervical plexus
dermatome
dorsal (posterior) ramus
endoneurium
epineurium
gamma motor neurons
growth cone
lumbar plexus
myotome
neuropathy
paresthesia
perineurium
peripheral nervous system (PNS)
plexus
sacral plexus
spinal cord segments
spinal nerves
ventral (anterior) ramus

Essential Facts··

▶ Peripheral nerves connect the spinal cord with body structures.

▶ Peripheral nerves contain motor, sensory, and autonomic nerve fibers, and are classified according to size, function, and conduction speed.

▶ Peripheral nerves form networks called plexuses.

▶ Peripheral nerves are protected by connective tissue coverings that assist with regeneration if the nerves are damaged by trauma or disease.

The **peripheral nervous system (PNS)** innervates the entire body. It connects the brain and spinal cord to body wall structures, including skin and subcutaneous tissue, skeletal muscle, tendons, bones, and joints. The PNS consists of 12 pairs of cranial nerves and 30 pairs of spinal nerves. This chapter will focus on the spinal nerves; cranial nerves were discussed in Chapter 7. Unlike the central nervous system, neurons in the PNS can heal (regenerate) if injured. A number of diseases and conditions affect peripheral nerves, including diabetes, Guillain Barre Syndrome (GBS), and carpal tunnel syndrome.

Nerve Composition

Peripheral nerves are composed of axons (nerve fibers). Most peripheral spinal nerves contain both motor and sensory axons, as well as some autonomic fibers. Motor neuron cell bodies are found in the ventral horn of the spinal cord (**Figure 9-1**). Motor nerve axons leave the central nervous system via ventral roots and innervate skeletal muscle. Because they directly innervate muscle, they are considered lower motor neurons.

Most peripheral nerves also contain somatosensory neurons. Their cell bodies are located in small ganglia adjacent to the spinal cord called dorsal root ganglia. Each sensory nerve axon carries sensation from the skin, subcutaneous tissue, muscle, bone, ligaments, and joints. They transmit sensations such as pain, temperature, touch, vibration, and proprioception.

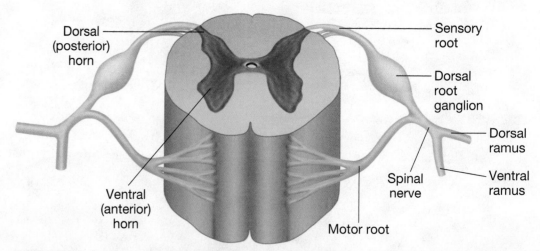

FIGURE 9-1 A spinal segment. The spinal cord is divided into 30 functional segments, each of which gives rise to a pair of spinal nerves. Each spinal nerve is formed by a sensory (dorsal) root and a motor (ventral) root.

Neuroscience Notes Box 9-1:
Local Anesthetic

Local anesthetics injected in the vicinity of peripheral nerves relieve or prevent pain by blocking the conduction of sensory action potentials. Local anesthetics bind to and block Na^+ channels in axons. This prevents Na^+ ions from flowing into the nerve fibers, thus impeding transmission of action potentials. Eventually the anesthetic agent diffuses away from the nerve fiber, and the anesthetic effect wears off. Because axons that carry pain signals are small and often unmyelinated, they are affected first when an anesthetic is applied, and are the last to recover function. This explains why people given local anesthetics may report feeling sensations of pressure or touch, but no pain (such as during dental procedures).

Many peripheral nerves contain autonomic nerve fibers. All 30 pairs of spinal nerves contain sympathetic autonomic neurons that innervate smooth muscle located in blood vessel walls and sweat glands. Spinal nerves in the pelvis also contain parasympathetic neurons. All autonomic neurons in the PNS have their cell bodies in the lateral horn of the spinal cord (spinal nerves) or in the autonomic motor nuclei of the brainstem (cranial nerves).

Spinal Nerves

The spinal cord is formed by 30 individual **spinal cord segments,** each of which gives rise to a pair of **spinal nerves** (right and left). Spinal nerves emerge from the vertebral column between the vertebrae, and innervate skin, subcutaneous tissue, muscle, tendons, bones, and joints. Spinal nerves are responsible for producing movement, and for conveying sensation from the body. They also contain sympathetic nerve fibers that primarily innervate sweat glands and blood vessels to control body temperature and blood pressure.

After emerging from the spinal column, the spinal nerves travel laterally to innervate body structures. Just lateral to the spine, each nerve divides into two branches called rami. The **dorsal (posterior) ramus** curves toward the back, where it innervates muscles, skin, and other structures on the back. The **ventral (anterior) ramus** curves anteriorly, and supplies structures of the anterior and lateral body regions, as well as the upper and lower extremities.

In some regions, the spinal nerves interweave to form a nerve network, or **plexus.** Four major plexuses have been identified: cervical, brachial, lumbar, and sacral.

Cervical Plexus

The **cervical plexus** (see **Figure 9-2**) consists of axons from spinal nerves C1-C5 that innervates structures in the neck. The two largest cervical plexus nerves are the ansa cervicalis and the phrenic nerve. The ansa cervicalis innervates many small muscles that are involved in swallowing and speech. The phrenic nerve travels down through the neck and thorax to innervate the thoracoabdominal diaphragm. The major spinal segment contributing to the phrenic nerve is C4, but it also contains fibers from C3 and C5. If the phrenic nerve is damaged bilaterally, or if the spinal cord is injured above C3, the diaphragm will be paralyzed and respiration will stop.

Neuroscience Notes Box 9-2: Hiccups

Hiccups are caused by spasms of the diaphragm, and usually result from irritation of the phrenic nerves. The sudden diaphragmatic contraction closes the vocal cords (glottis) very quickly, producing the characteristic "hic" sounds. The clinical term for hiccups is *singultus*. Usually hiccups go away on their own, but there are many home remedies that are thought to get rid of them faster; most of these involve raising the level of CO_2 in the blood (holding your breath, drinking a full glass of water).

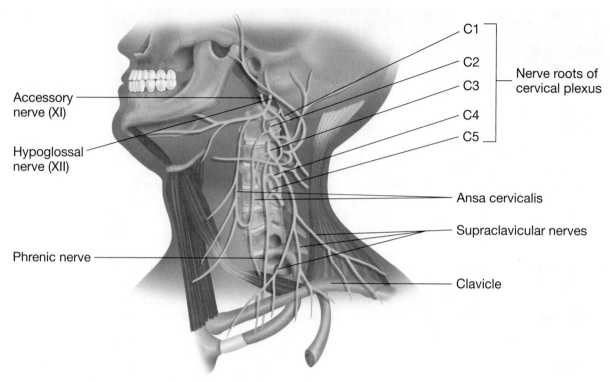

Accessory nerve (XI)

Hypoglossal nerve (XII)

Phrenic nerve

C1
C2
C3
C4
C5

Nerve roots of cervical plexus

Ansa cervicalis

Supraclavicular nerves

Clavicle

FIGURE 9-2 The cervical plexus is formed by spinal nerves C1-C5 and innervates structures in the neck, along with the diaphragm. The phrenic nerve is formed by C3-C5 and innervates the diaphragm.

Brachial Plexus

The brachial plexus innervates muscles of the upper extremity (see Figure 9-3). It is formed by spinal nerves C5 through T1. This complex network is located in the lower part of the neck and passes through the armpit (axillary region) on its way to the arm. It is organized into five separate regions: roots, trunks, divisions, cords, and branches. (A good way to remember these is the mnemonic "**R**eally **T**ired? **D**rink **C**offee **B**lack.")

The five ventral rami (C5, C6, C7, C8, and T1) are confusingly called the "roots" of the brachial plexus. (Remember that they are not really roots, but rami: They contain both motor and sensory nerve fibers as well as sympathetics.) In the neck, C5 and C6 combine

Clinical Box 9-1: Cervical Spinal Injury and Respiration

The phrenic nerves that innervate the diaphragm are part of the cervical plexus and emerge from spinal cord segments C3 through C5, with C4 as the primary segment. Other major muscles involved in respiration are the intercostals and abdominal wall muscles; these are innervated by thoracic and lumbar spinal nerves. A spinal cord injury at or above level C3 causes the phrenic nerves to be disconnected from respiratory centers in the brainstem that keep the diaphragm contracting automatically. This means that breathing can no longer occur spontaneously. People with high-level spinal cord injuries may require a mechanical ventilator to inflate their lungs, since they lack the ability to contract the respiratory muscles on their own.

Challenge question: Would a patient with an intact phrenic nerve but without innervation to the intercostal muscles have completely normal respiratory function?

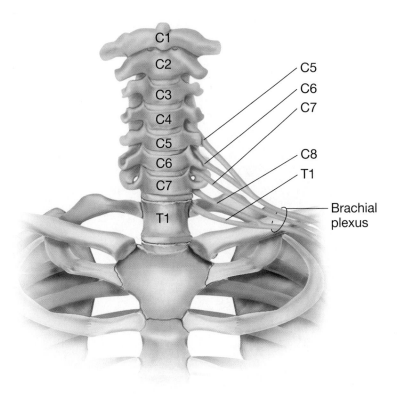

FIGURE 9-3 The brachial plexus is formed by spinal nerves C5-T1, and innervates the upper extremity.

to form the upper trunk, C7 alone forms the middle trunk, and C8 merges with T1 to form the lower trunk. Each trunk then splits into two divisions: anterior and posterior. The anterior division forms nerves that innervate muscles and skin found on the anterior aspect of the upper extremity; the posterior division forms nerves that supply posterior structures. Both divisions pass behind the clavicle and then give rise to the brachial plexus cords. The lateral cord is formed by nerve fibers from the upper and middle trunks, while the medial cord is composed of neurons derived from the lower trunk. The posterior cord contains nerve fibers from all three trunks.

In the armpit (axilla), the plexus gives rise to five major branches, or named nerves. In addition, numerous small branches sprout from the entire plexus. Together, the large and small branches supply most of the muscles and all of the sensation to the upper limb.

There are three large anterior division branches: musculocutaneous, median, and ulnar (see **Figure 9-4**). The musculocutaneous nerve supplies motor innervation to the

Clinical Box 9-2: Nerve Compression

Compression of a peripheral nerve preferentially affects large diameter sensory axons so that touch, pressure, and vibration sensations are reduced or lost first, while the function of small diameter pain, temperature, and autonomic fibers is preserved. For example, in carpal tunnel syndrome, compression of the median nerve at the wrist will usually cause decreased touch perception before it affects pain.

Challenge question: In which part of the hand would a patient with carpal tunnel syndrome experience sensory changes?

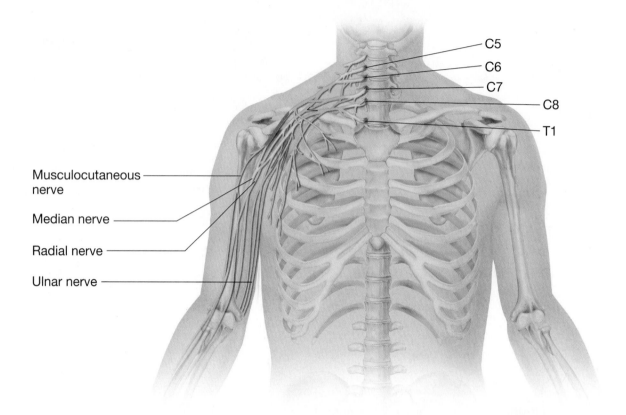

FIGURE 9-4 Major brachial plexus nerves include the musculocutaneous, median, ulnar, and radial nerves that innervate the upper extremity.

anterior arm muscles (biceps brachii, coracobrachialis, and brachialis). The nerve continues into the forearm where it becomes the lateral antebrachial cutaneous nerve that supplies sensation to the lateral forearm. The median nerve innervates muscles located in the anterior compartment of the forearm, and then passes through the carpal tunnel at the wrist to supply muscles of the thumb (thenar eminence) and sensory innervation to the lateral part of the hand. Finally, the ulnar nerve supplies a few muscles in the anterior forearm and most of the intrinsic hand muscles. It also provides sensation to the medial third of the hand.

Smaller anterior division nerves from the brachial plexus include the medial pectoral nerve and lateral pectoral nerve. The medial pectoral nerve branches from the medial cord and supplies the pectoralis minor and medial (sternal) part of the pectoralis major muscle. The lateral pectoral nerve sprouts from the lateral cord, and innervates the clavicular part of the pectoralis major.

Two large nerves are derived from the posterior cord of the brachial plexus: The axillary nerve supplies the deltoid and teres minor muscles, while the radial nerve innervates all posterior muscles of the arm and forearm, as well as sensory innervation to parts of the posterior arm, forearm, and hand. Smaller posterior division nerves include the dorsal scapular (rhomboid major and minor, levator scapulae), suprascapular (supraspinatus and infraspinatus), long thoracic (serratus anterior), thoracodorsal (latissimus dorsi), and subscapular nerves (subscapularis and teres major).

Two purely sensory nerves branch from the medial cord and supply sensation to the medial aspect of the arm and forearm: Respectively, these are the medial brachial and medial antebrachial cutaneous nerves (see **Figure 9-5**).

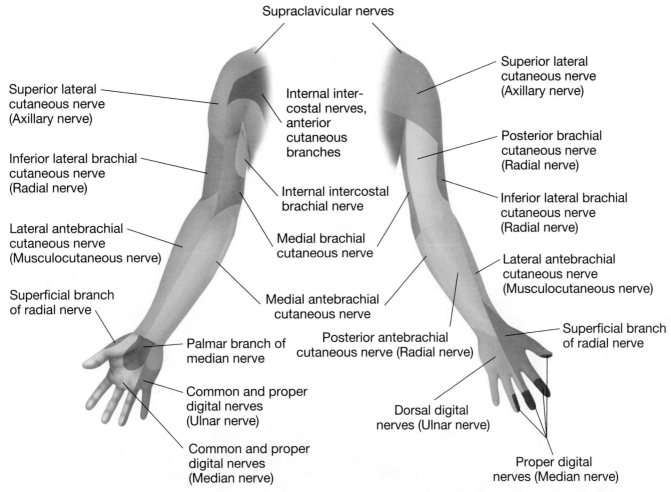

FIGURE 9-5 Sensory innervation of the upper extremity: Each brachial plexus nerve innervates a specific region of skin.

THORACIC SPINAL NERVES In the thorax, nerves do not form a plexus. Instead, they divide into dorsal and ventral rami; the dorsal rami innervate structures on the back, including the intrinsic back (paraspinal) muscles and overlying skin, whereas the ventral rami run laterally beneath the ribs to form intercostal nerves. These supply intercostal muscles and skin of the thoracic region (see **Figure 9-6**).

Neuroscience Notes Box 9-3: Brachial Plexus Injuries

Brachial plexus injuries include any injury that involves tearing, shearing, or overstretching of the nerves within the brachial plexus. Although this can occur in any population, most brachial plexus injuries affect newborns, most often due to the upper extremity becoming awkwardly stretched as the child is squeezed through the birth canal. The symptoms of a brachial plexus injury often include weakness, paresis, and impaired sensation of the upper extremity. The most severe form of injury is known as *avulsion*; this involves the nerve root being torn away from or severed from the spinal cord. This will typically be displayed as flaccid paralysis of the upper extremity. Therapists will often become involved after these injuries to help prevent stiffness and contractures, and to help retrain muscles as nerve function recovers.

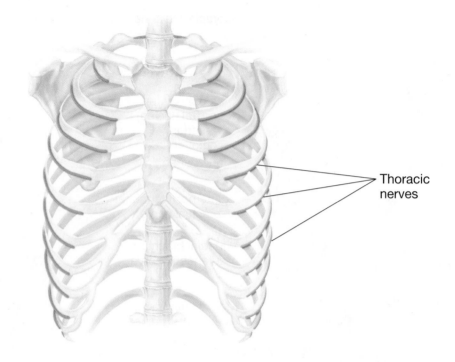

Thoracic nerves

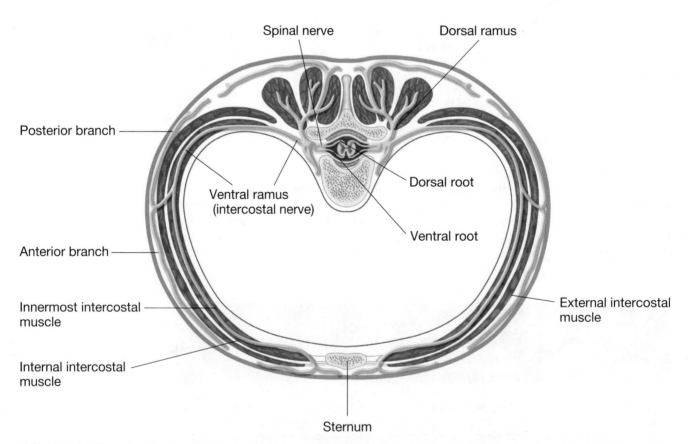

Spinal nerve

Dorsal ramus

Posterior branch

Ventral ramus (intercostal nerve)

Dorsal root

Anterior branch

Ventral root

Innermost intercostal muscle

External intercostal muscle

Internal intercostal muscle

Sternum

FIGURE 9-6 Thoracic spinal nerves innervate muscles and skin on the thorax. They divide into ventral rami (to the intercostal muscles) and dorsal rami (to the paraspinal muscles). The ventral rami divide into several additional branches.

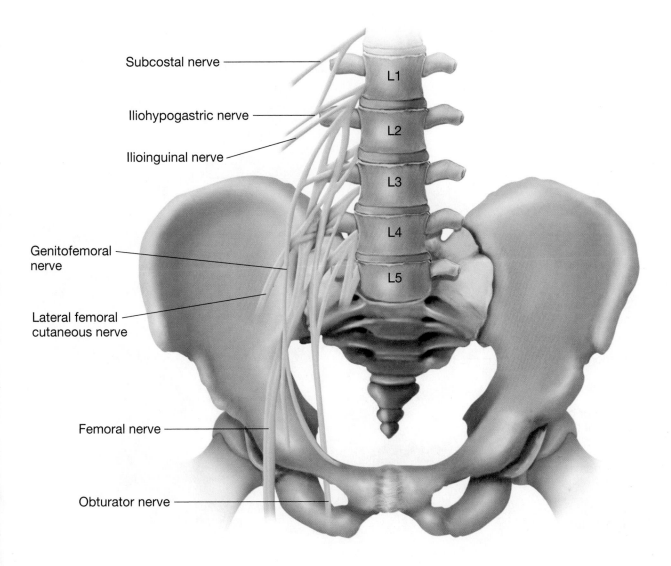

FIGURE 9-7   The lumbar plexus arises from the lumbar portion of the spinal cord and innervates muscles of the hip and thigh. The femoral and obturator nerves are the major nerves to the anterior and medial thigh.

Lumbar Plexus

The **lumbar plexus** is composed of nerve fibers from spinal segments L1 through L4 (see Figure 9-7). It gives rise to seven major nerves. Three of these are entirely sensory: the genitofemoral nerve supplies the scrotum (in males) and labia majora (in females), the lateral femoral cutaneous nerve supplies the lateral part of the thigh, and the saphenous nerve supplies the medial leg and foot as well as part of the knee joint. Four larger nerves contain both motor and sensory axons. The iliohypogastric nerve is sensory to the anterior abdominal wall, and provides motor innervation to the anterior abdominal wall muscles. The ilioinguinal nerves also supply anterior abdominal muscles and provide sensation to the groin. The obturator nerve (L2-L4) provides sensation to the medial thigh, and motor function to the hip adductor muscles.

The largest lumbar plexus branch is the femoral nerve. This nerve is derived from L2-L4 and passes from the pelvis to the thigh accompanied by the femoral artery and femoral vein. It innervates muscles of the anterior hip and thigh, including the iliacus, pectineus, sartorius, and all four heads of the quadriceps femoris. It also provides sensation to the anterior skin of the thigh and to both hip and knee joints.

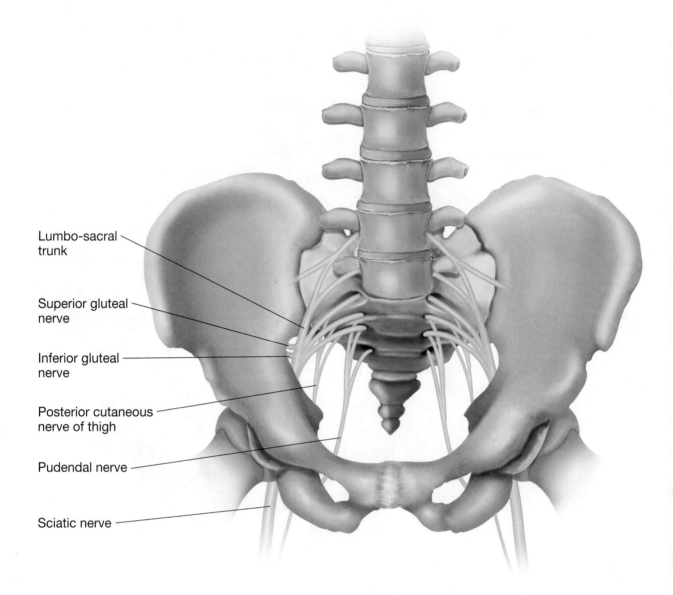

Lumbo-sacral trunk

Superior gluteal nerve

Inferior gluteal nerve

Posterior cutaneous nerve of thigh

Pudendal nerve

Sciatic nerve

FIGURE 9-8 The sacral plexus arises from the lower lumbar and sacral portions of the spinal cord, and innervates the lower extremity and pelvic regions. The sciatic nerve innervates muscles in the thigh, leg, and foot. The pudendal nerve innervates the pelvic floor muscles and the genitals.

Sacral Plexus

The **sacral plexus** contains nerve fibers from L4-L5, and the first four sacral segments (S1-S4) (see Figure 9-8). Six major nerves are derived from this plexus. The superior gluteal nerve (L4-S1) innervates three hip muscles: gluteus medius, gluteus minimus, and tensor fascia lata. The inferior gluteal nerve (L5-S2) innervates the gluteus maximus. The posterior cutaneous nerve is a purely sensory nerve that supplies sensation to the buttocks, posterior thigh, and anus.

The sciatic nerve is the largest nerve in the body. It is actually composed of the tibial nerve (L4-S3) and the common fibular (peroneal) nerve (L4-S2). The two nerves are wrapped together by a sheath of connective tissue. The sciatic nerve runs deep to gluteus maximus through the gluteal region, and then travels down the posterior thigh where it innervates the hamstring muscles. At the knee, the tibial and common fibular nerves separate. The tibial nerve continues down the posterior aspect of the lower leg, innervating posterior leg muscles. Just posterior to the medial malleolus, it branches into the medial plantar nerve and lateral plantar nerve. Together, the plantar nerves innervate all intrinsic foot muscles and the plantar surface of the foot.

Clinical Box 9-3: Piriformis Syndrome

Sciatica is a clinical condition that describes injury to or inflammation of the sciatic nerve. One cause of sciatica is *piriformis syndrome,* in which the sciatic nerve is compressed by the piriformis muscle. If the piriformis muscle becomes inflamed or excessively tight, the nerve will become pinched. This condition may cause radiating pain or numbness down the entire lower extremity. Luckily, piriformis syndrome may be treated quite effectively by stretches that help to elongate the piriformis muscle or by reducing the pressure generated by local swelling.

Challenge question: In what position could a therapist place the lower extremity in order to stretch the piriformis muscle? (Hint: piriformis performs external rotation of the hip, and can perform abduction when the hip is flexed.)

The common fibular nerve wraps around the head of the fibula and then splits into the superficial fibular nerve and the deep fibular nerve. The superficial fibular nerve innervates the lateral compartment muscles (fibularis longus and brevis), whereas the deep fibular nerve innervates the anterior compartment (dorsiflexor) muscles.

The pudendal nerve (S2-S4) is the most inferior branch of the sacral plexus. This nerve supplies muscles of the perineum and pelvic floor. Importantly, these muscles are responsible for voluntary control of the bladder and bowels, as well as for muscle contraction during orgasm and ejaculation. The pudendal nerve is also responsible for sensation to the penis and clitoris and to the skin of the scrotum, labia, and vagina.

Peripheral Nerve Coverings

Each peripheral nerve is covered by layers of connective tissue (see **Figure 9-9**). The **epineurium** is the outermost covering; it is continuous with the dura mater around the spinal cord. Epineurium is dense, fibrous, and tough. It provides a protective covering and is responsible for the tensile strength of peripheral nerves.

Internal to the epineurium, the **perineurium** groups individual nerve fibers into bundles called *fascicles.* Perineurial cells are joined by tight junctions that help to create the blood-nerve barrier. This barrier protects peripheral nerve axons from the blood, similar to the way that the blood-brain barrier separates the central nervous system from the blood. Some sensory receptors have connective tissue capsules that are continuous with perineurium (including Pacinian corpuscles, muscle spindles, and Golgi tendon organs).

Clinical Box 9-4: Dermatomes and Myotomes

A **dermatome** is a region of the body innervated by sensory nerves arising from one spinal cord segment. Similarly, a **myotome** describes a muscle or group of muscles innervated by motor neurons arising from a single spinal cord segment. Clinically, therapists use dermatomes and myotomes to check the function of specific nerve roots. For instance, spinal cord injuries are typically classified by the highest functioning dermatomes and myotomes a patient displays. The American Spinal Cord Injury Association (ASIA) has described the following dermatomes and myotomes to be used for spinal cord injury classification (see **Table 9.1**). (Also see chapter 8 for a more detailed description and figure regarding dermatomes and myotomes).

Challenge question: What muscle(s) would be innervated by myotome level C5? C7? L3?

Table 9.1 Spinal Level Innervation

Upper Extremity Dermatomes

Nerve Root	Area of Sensory Testing
C5	Lateral epicondyle of the humerus
C6	Proximal phalanx of the thumb
C7	Dorsum of the proximal phalanx of the middle finger
C8	Dorsum of the proximal phalanx of the fifth digit (little finger)
T1	Medical epicondyle of the humerus

Lower Extremity Dermatomes

Nerve Root	Area of Sensory Testing
L1	Midpoint between the ASIS and pubic crest
L2	Midpoint of the anterior thigh
L3	Medial epicondyle of the femur
L4	Medial malleolus
L5	Dorsum of the foot between the second and third toes
S1	Lateral malleolus
S2	Posterior knee (popliteal fossa)

Upper Extremity Myotomes

Nerve Root	Muscle Group Tested
C5	Elbow flexors
C6	Wrist extensors
C7	Elbow extensors
C8	Long finger flexors (distal phalanx of middle finger)
T1	Finger abductors (typically tested on fifth digit)

Lower Extremity Myotomes

Nerve Root	Muscle Group Tested
L2	Hip flexors
L3	Knee extensors
L4	Dorsiflexors
L5	Great toe extensors
S1	Plantar flexors

Neuroscience Notes Box 9-3: Herpes Zoster (Shingles)

Herpes zoster ("shingles") is a viral infection of the sensory ganglia of spinal and cranial nerves. Shingles and chickenpox are both caused by the varicella virus, which remains dormant in sensory ganglia for years after an initial chickenpox infection. In some people, the virus is reactivated; the specific reasons for reactivation are not clear but it is more common in people with decreased immune function. Following reactivation, the virus migrates back down the sensory axon to the skin where it causes the signs and symptoms of shingles. These include redness and small, painful blisters. The infection typically localizes to a single dermatome or cranial nerve. In most people the pain lasts for a few weeks, but in some cases the pain persists for months or years after the blisters have healed. About two-thirds of patients with shingles get it in one thoracic dermatome, and another 20% have it in their faces (usually in the distribution of a branch of the trigeminal nerve). When shingles infects the facial nerve, it is known as *Ramsay-Hunt syndrome*.

The innermost connective tissue sheath is the **endoneurium.** It wraps each individual nerve fiber (axon) with a coat of delicate, loose connective tissue. Internal to the endoneurium are bare (unmyelinated) axons, or Schwann cells that form the myelin sheath around myelinated axons.

When body parts move, peripheral nerves glide between other tissues. In addition, each fascicle within the peripheral nerve can glide somewhat independently. The movement of nerve fibers within their connective tissue sheaths is important for promoting blood flow to axons through small arterioles and capillaries, and also for the movement of axoplasm (the fluid inside axons). Axoplasmic flow helps promote movement of material inside neurons, which helps keep axons healthy.

Nerve Fiber Classification

There are two classification systems for peripheral nerve fibers (axons). Axons can be classified according to their size (diameter) and the amount of myelin covering them, or according to their conduction velocity. Because conduction velocity is correlated with axon diameter, the fastest-conducting nerve fibers are also the largest diameter axons with the thickest myelin sheaths. Sensory neurons are usually classified by size, and motor neurons by conduction velocity, but these classification systems are sometimes used interchangeably.

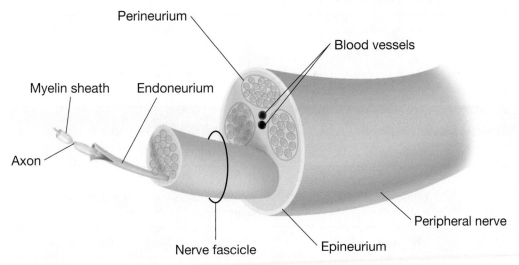

FIGURE 9-9 A peripheral nerve and its connective tissue coverings. Each axon is covered by endoneurium, each fascicle is covered by perineurium, and the entire nerve is wrapped with epineurium.

Sensory neurons can be classified according to the diameter of their axons. The largest-diameter axons are Type I, and are found in sensory nerves innervating muscle spindles (Type Ia) and Golgi tendon organs (Type Ib). Type II axons are smaller in diameter, with a thinner myelin sheath; they also innervate muscle spindles, as well as Merkel's discs (touch) and Pacinian corpuscles (vibration). Type III sensory axons innervate free nerve endings; they are smaller than type II axons and have a thin myelin sheath. Types I, II, and III fibers are all myelinated axons. Type IV nerve fibers are unmyelinated and are the smallest diameter fibers. They innervate free nerve endings for pain and temperature sensations.

Neurons that innervate muscles are called lower motor neurons. There are two types of lower motor neurons: alpha motor neurons and gamma motor neurons (see **Table 9.2**). **Alpha motor neurons** innervate muscle to create muscle tension and produce movement. Alpha motor neurons are about 12 to 20 μm in diameter, are fast-conducting, and have a thick myelin sheath. In contrast, **gamma motor neurons** are 6 to 12 μm in diameter, are slower-conducting, and innervate muscle spindles. They are involved in the maintenance and alteration of muscle tone, and do not produce movement.

The autonomic nervous system is formed by two kinds of involuntary motor neurons. β fibers are small and myelinated; C fibers are unmyelinated.

Table 9.2 Peripheral Nerve Fibers

Afferent Nerve Fibers

Name	Diameter (μm)	Modality	Receptor Type
Ia	12-20 (myelinated)	Quick stretch (muscle) Slow stretch (muscle)	Muscle spindle
Ib	12-20 (myelinated)	Muscle/tendon tension Ligament tension	Golgi tendon organ Ligament receptor (type III joint receptor)
II Aβ	8-12 (myelinated)	Slow stretch (muscle) Joint position, movement 2-point discriminative touch Vibration/deep pressure Skin stretch Pressure and texture Light touch	Muscle spindle Joint receptors (type I and type II) Meissner's corpuscle Pacinian corpuscle Ruffini ending Merkel's disk Hair follicle receptor
Aδ	1-6 (myelinated)	Sharp and burning pain Temperature (cold)	Free nerve ending
C (IV)	1-1.5 (unmyelinated)	Freezing and aching pain Temperature (hot) Itch	Free nerve ending

Efferent Nerve Fibers

Name	Diameter (μm)	Innervation	Function
α	7-22 (myelinated)	Extrafusal muscle fibers	Muscle contraction
γ	2-15 (myelinated)	Intrafusal muscle fibers (muscle spindles)	Adjusts sensitivity of muscle spindle to stretch (= spindle fibers = nuclear bag and nuclear chain fibers)
β	1-5 (myelinated)	Presynaptic autonomic	Stimulates postsynaptic autonomic neuron
C	0.2-0.5 (unmyelinated)	Postsynaptic autonomic	Contraction of cardiac and smooth muscle

Peripheral Nerve Injury and Healing

Peripheral nerves can be injured by trauma or disease. Common types of injury include excessive stretching, compression, and lacerations (cuts). Infections (for example, shingles and leprosy) can also injure nerve fibers. In addition, ischemia resulting from nerve compression, entrapment, or metabolic conditions such as diabetes mellitus can harm axons. Autoimmune disorders (e.g., Guillain-Barre syndrome) can damage peripheral nerves, often by targeting the myelin sheath that insulates axons.

Damage to peripheral nerves produces **neuropathy**. Most neuropathies cause impairment of both motor and sensory functions, although one may be affected more than the other. In most cases, sensation is decreased, lost, or abnormal. **Paresthesia** is an early symptom of peripheral nerve injury. It is an abnormal sensation described as a prickling, tingling, or "pins-and-needles" feeling. It may occur in one limb (such as in carpal tunnel syndrome), or bilaterally (in diabetes mellitus). Diabetic sensory loss is most severe in the hands and feet, so it is referred to as a "glove-and-stocking" sensory loss (see Figure 9-10).

Motor symptoms resulting from peripheral nerve injury are characterized by weakness (paresis) or paralysis and hypotonia. In many neuropathies, muscles of the feet and legs are affected first. Typically, tendon reflexes are either depressed or lost. Autonomic function may also be affected; this causes loss of sweating (anhydrosis) and orthostatic hypotension due to interruption of sympathetic neurons that regulate vasoconstriction and blood pressure. Bowel and bladder incontinence, sexual impotence, blurred vision, dry eyes and mouth, and vomiting may also occur.

Some peripheral nerve injuries are reversible, so function may be restored. When axons are damaged but their connective tissue sheaths are intact, healing is likely to occur since the connective tissue can guide axon regeneration. Recovery of function is slow

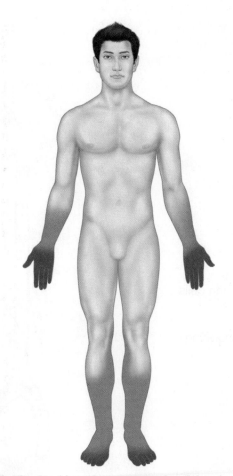

FIGURE 9-10 Stocking–glove pattern of peripheral neuropathy.

because the axon must re-grow and establish synaptic contact with its target structure, and then a new myelin sheath must be synthesized. A more severe injury, in which the axon, myelin sheath, and all connective tissue coverings are severed, is more difficult to recover from. However, axon regeneration does occur in the peripheral nervous system, and genes that are required for healing are beginning to be identified (Hammarlund, Nix, Hauth, Joregensen and Bastiani, 2009).

Following injury that cuts or crushes an axon, the axon degenerates. After this, a sprout called a **growth cone** begins to emerge from the neuron cell body (see Figure 9-11). Guided by chemical cues, the growth cone gradually elongates until it can reach a target tissue and establish a synapse. Many of the chemical cues that assist regeneration come from the Schwann cells that myelinate peripheral axons. In some cases, regeneration is impaired by excessive scar tissue that physically blocks elongation of the growing axon. Typically, neurons regenerate at about 1 mm/day, although they can grow as slowly as 0.5 mm/day or as fast as 9.0 mm/day. Some evidence suggests that exercise can improve recovery (Van Meeteren, Brakkee, Hamers, Helders and Gispen, 1997).

Recovery from peripheral nerve injury usually begins with fibers of the smallest diameter, followed gradually by larger fibers. Because pain and temperature are transmitted by small axons, these sensations usually return prior to touch and proprioception. Somatosensory receptors found in the skin and subcutaneous tissue can survive denervation for at least a year, so sensation can often be restored if axon regrowth takes place within that time frame.

Denervated skeletal muscle atrophies significantly, losing 70% of its cross-sectional area after 2 months. However, the motor end plates on muscle cells remain intact for about a year. If motor neurons can reconnect to muscle fibers within a year, motor function may be restored. Regenerated motor units are often larger than the originals, so muscle contraction will be less precise than before the injury.

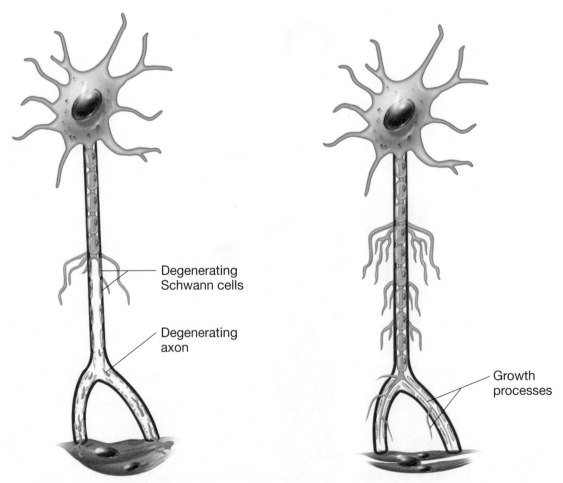

FIGURE 9-11 Axons in the peripheral nervous system degenerate following injury, and can often regenerate if guided by Schwann cells and connective tissue.

Clinical Box 9-5: Guillain-Barre Syndrome

The Guillain-Barre syndrome (GBS), also called acute inflammatory polyneuropathy, involves the demyelination of peripheral nerves. The syndrome is caused by an autoimmune reaction that targets the myelin sheath around peripheral nerve axons. In many cases, the onset of symptoms follows a respiratory or gastrointestinal infection. The major clinical manifestation of GBS is muscular weakness and fatigue. Usually the legs are affected first, and the weakness progresses to the trunk, arms, and head muscles. In a few patients, the weakness progresses to total motor paralysis, with death resulting from respiratory failure. Paresthesia and numbness are common early signs. Tendon reflexes are reduced and then lost. Nerve conduction testing demonstrates a reduction in the amplitude of muscle action potentials, slowed conduction velocity, or conduction block in motor nerves. Fortunately, most patients recover completely or nearly completely.

Challenge question: Since GBS often begins in the lower extremity, which dermatomes might be affected first?

Neuroscience Notes Box 9-4: Diabetic Neuropathy

Diabetes mellitus is a common cause of neuropathy. It is the most frequent long-term complication of diabetes, and can lead to limb amputations and sudden cardiac death from involvement of autonomic nerves. About 50% of people with diabetes have peripheral neuropathy. Once the condition begins, it cannot be reversed, so the best approach is prevention. People with diabetes who maintain good control of their blood sugar with diet, exercise, and medication can minimize the risk of acquiring neuropathy (Cade, 2008).

The symptoms of diabetic neuropathy are paresthesia (numbness, pain, and a pins-and-needles feeling) that often begins in the toes and feet. Small-diameter sensory axons are affected first, so pain and temperature sensations are affected before proprioception. As the disease progresses, these sensory symptoms gradually move proximally, and begin to affect the hands and fingers. Patients may become unaware of injuries to their feet, including routine blisters or sores. Coupled with the poor peripheral circulation, which is another common characteristic of diabetes, this can lead to infections that don't heal well and that can eventually affect muscle and bone. If these infections are untreated, the involved extremity may need to be amputated.

Diabetic neuropathy can also affect autonomic neurons, and eventually lower motor neurons. Autonomic symptoms include hypotension, tachycardia, digestive problems (constipation and diarrhea), and difficulty controlling bowel, bladder, and sexual functioning. When lower motor neurons are affected, patients will display paresis (weakness) and hypotonia (low muscle tone) that usually begins with intrinsic foot muscles and spreads proximally. Deep tendon reflexes will be weak or absent.

Nerve damage results from the direct effects of chronic high blood glucose (hyperglycemia) on peripheral axons. Excess glucose is converted to metabolites that damage axons. High glucose levels also cause thickening of blood vessel walls, resulting in ischemia (lack of oxygen) that decreases the oxygen supply to peripheral nerve fibers. Finally, people with diabetes often have elevated blood lipid levels that lead to arteriosclerosis, further reducing blood flow to axons.

PATIENT SCENARIOS

Patient Case 9-1 (Cindy)

Cindy is a 46-year-old woman who works as a cashier. She has recently been experiencing pain, numbness, and a "pins and needles" feeling in both hands, especially the right one. Her right hand also has some muscle atrophy, evident in the thenar muscles, and she is having trouble using her thumb. Cindy has been diagnosed with carpal tunnel syndrome.

Questions

a) Which peripheral nerve is compressed in patients with carpal tunnel syndrome?

b) Is it likely that the damaged nerve will recover its function? Why or why not?

Patient Case 9-2 (Rufus)

Rufus is 66 years old and has had Type II diabetes for about 9 years. He is experiencing a painful burning and "pins and needles" feeling in both feet that seems to be getting worse and that is keeping him awake at night. An examination of his feet reveals that there is a large blister on one heel (from a new pair of shoes) that he is not aware of, and an unhealed sore on the big toe of his other foot. His diagnosis is bilateral diabetic peripheral neuropathy.

Questions

a) Why are people with diabetes at high risk for serious foot problems?

b) What can he do to minimize these risks?

Review Questions

1. List the types of neurons found in peripheral nerves, and their connective tissue investments.

2. Name the four major nerve plexuses found in the human body and indicate the regions each plexus innervates.

3. Describe the healing process for peripheral nerves and list factors that help or hinder nerve regeneration.

References

1. Cade, W. T. (2008). Diabetes-related microvascular and macrovascular diseases in the physical therapy setting. *Physical Therapy, 88*(11), 1322–1335.

2. Hammarlund, M., Nix, P., Hauth, L., Jorgensen, E. M., & Bastiani, M. (2009) Axon regeneration requires a conserved MAP kinase pathway. *Science, 323,* 802–806.

3. Van Meeteren, N. L. U., Brakkee, J. H., Hamers, F. P. T., Helders, P. J. M., & Gispen, W. H. (1997). Exercise training improves functional recovery and motor nerve conduction velocity after sciatic nerve crush lesion in the rat. *Arch. Phys. Med. Rehabil., 78,* 70–77.

Further Reading

1. Greene, D. A., Sima, A. A. F., Pfeifer, M. A., & Albers, J. W. (1990). Diabetic neuropathy. *Annu. Rev. Med., 41,* 303–317.

2. Gulve, E. A. (2008). Exercise and glycemic control in diabetes: Benefits, challenges and adjustments to pharmacotherapy. *Physical Therapy, 88*(11), 1297–1321.

PEARSON
myhealthprofessionskit™

Use this address to access the Companion Website created for this textbook. Simply select "Physical Therapy" from the choice of disciplines. Find this book and log in using your username and password to access self-assessment questions, a glossary and more.

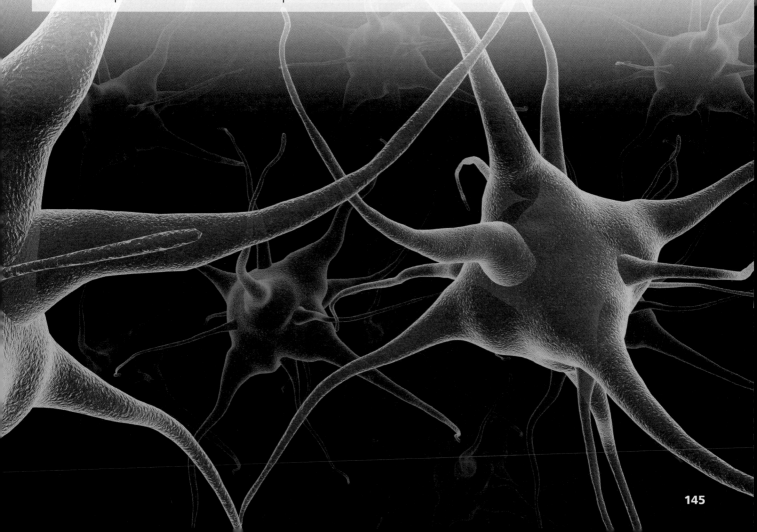

10

Autonomic Nervous System

CHAPTER OBJECTIVES

After completing this chapter, the reader will be able to:

1 Describe the structure of the sympathetic system, and explain the role of sympathetic neurotransmitters.

2 Discuss the function of the sympathetic system in regulating body functions, especially the function of the heart, respiratory system, sweat glands, and blood pressure.

3 Describe the structure of the parasympathetic system, and explain the role of parasympathetic neurotransmitters.

4 Explain the function of the parasympathetic system in regulating body functions, especially the function of the heart, the digestive system, the urinary bladder, and the reproductive system.

5 Discuss control of the autonomic nervous system, and the functional consequences that result from disruption of this control.

KEY TERMS

acetylcholine (Ach)

central autonomic fibers

homeostasis

hypothalamus

norepinephrine (NE)

parasympathetic system

splanchnic nerves

sympathetic system

sympathetic trunk

Essential Facts··

▶ The autonomic nervous system controls blood vessels and internal organs.

▶ The autonomic nervous system is divided into sympathetic and parasympathetic systems.

▶ The sympathetic system is activated during stress, during exercise, and in dangerous situations.

▶ The parasympathetic system maintains body systems in a resting state; it promotes digestion, slows the heart, and controls the urinary and reproductive systems.

The autonomic nervous system controls cardiac muscle and smooth muscle throughout the body. The autonomics affect activity of all organs and structures formed from cardiac or smooth muscle, including the heart, the respiratory system, the digestive tract, the urinary and reproductive systems, and the vascular system. The autonomic nerves also play a major role in controlling blood pressure.

The autonomic nervous system can be subdivided into **sympathetic** and **parasympathetic** parts. In general, the sympathetic system prepares the body to cope with emergency situations, and the parasympathetics are responsible for maintaining homeostasis (a balanced internal environment). The two subdivisions act in opposition to each other in some parts of the body, whereas other regions are controlled by only one subdivision. (For example, sweat glands are regulated only by sympathetic nerves.) In the heart and the digestive tract, the sympathetic and parasympathetic divisions have opposite effects; in the male reproductive system, the two divisions cooperate to fulfill a common function. Sympathetic and parasympathetic actions on the body are summarized in **Table 10.1**.

The Sympathetic System

The sympathetic part of the autonomic nervous system is designed for a fast response in case of threat or emergency. For this reason, the sympathetic system may be called the "fight-or-flight" system. An important function of the sympathetic nervous system is regulation of blood flow. This occurs by vasoconstriction (blood vessel narrowing) and vasodilation (blood vessel widening), targeted to control the amount of blood sent to organs and tissues. Increasing the blood supply to a region or organ (via vasodilation) will increase that organ's functional activity; decreasing blood flow (by vasoconstriction) diminishes action of the organ. In this way, the sympathetics can shunt blood around the body as needed to affect function.

Another major sympathetic function is to cause general vasoconstriction that increases systemic blood pressure. Overactivity of the sympathetics can cause hypertension (chronically high blood pressure).

Table 10.1 **Summary of Sympathetic and Parasympathetic Effects on Body Structures**

Organ	Sympathetic Action*	Parasympathetic Action
Systemic arterioles	Vasoconstriction (skin, skeletal muscles, GI tract) Vasodilation (skeletal muscles)	NONE
Systemic veins	Vasoconstriction	NONE
Heart	Stimulates SA node (increases heart rate and strength of contraction)	Decreases heart rate and strength of contraction
Bronchi	Dilates bronchial smooth muscle (airway dilation)	Constricts bronchial smooth muscle (airway constriction)
Digestive tract	Decreases motility; increases contraction of sphincters	Increases motility and relaxation of sphincters; stimulates digestive glands
Liver	Gluconeogenesis and glycogenolysis (increases blood sugar)	NONE
Pancreas	Inhibits secretion of digestive enzymes and insulin Promotes secretion of glucagon (increases blood sugar)	Increases secretion of digestive enzymes and insulin (decreases blood sugar)
Kidney	Produces renin (increases blood pressure)	NONE
Bladder	Sphincter contracts	Sphincter relaxes; smooth muscle of bladder contracts
Adrenal gland	Releases epinephrine and cortisol	NONE
Eye	Pupil dilates Ciliary muscle relaxes (far vision)	Pupil constricts Ciliary muscle contracts (near vision)
Reproductive organs	Constriction of ductus deferens, prostate, seminal vesicles (ejaculation)	Vasodilation of arterioles to erectile tissue (erection)
Sweat glands	Stimulation; sweating increased	NONE
Lacrimal gland	NONE	Increases tears produced
Salivary glands	Thick saliva	Copious, watery saliva

* Sympathetics may also act *indirectly* on organs by vasoconstriction, reducing their blood supply and thereby slowing down their function.

Sympathetic neurons have their cell bodies in the spinal cord at levels T1-L2. Sympathetic axons leave the spinal cord, exit the spinal column, and enter the **sympathetic trunk** (see **Figure 10-1**). There are two sympathetic trunks, one on each side of the vertebral column. Each sympathetic trunk is a series of 20 to 25 linked sympathetic ganglia that lie along the posterior body wall. After synapsing in the trunk, sympathetic axons join the spinal nerves. This means that every spinal nerve contains sympathetic axons.

Sympathetic axons innervate smooth muscle located in the skin, subcutaneous tissues, and muscles. The smooth muscle found in these tissues is located in blood vessel walls,

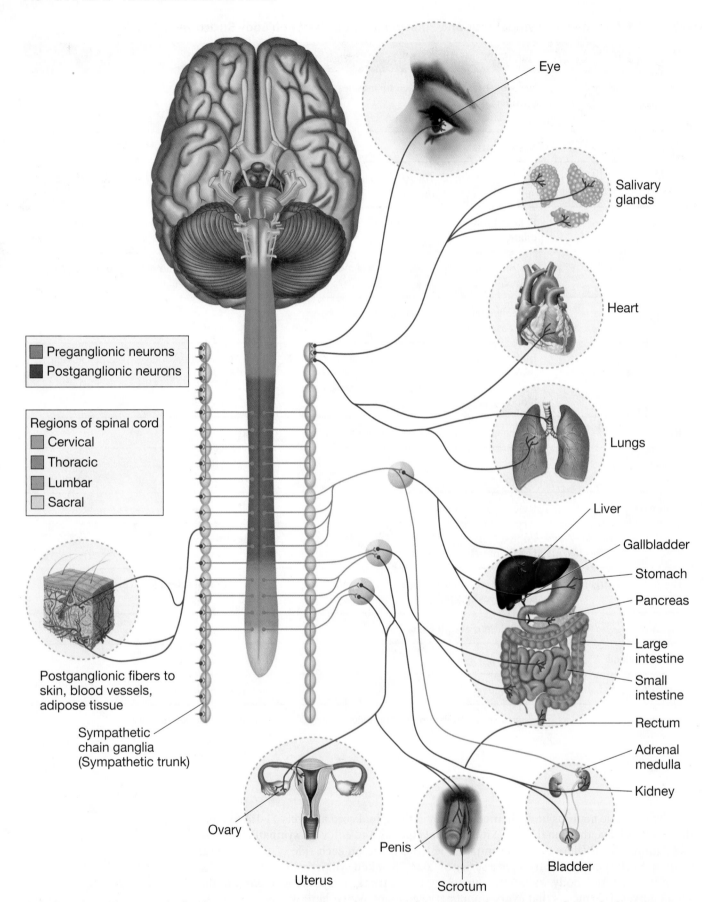

FIGURE 10-1 The sympathetic nervous system prepares the body to respond to emergencies or to stress. Sympathetic nerves go almost everywhere and innervate many body structures.

in the ducts of sweat glands, and in the piloerector muscles of the skin. Stimulation of these neurons causes sweating and the eruption of "goose bumps" on the skin (piloerector muscles). Sympathetic stimulation also regulates the flow of blood to the skin and skeletal muscles. For example, a person may turn pale if frightened because sympathetics cause vasoconstriction in the skin. The sympathetic system shunts blood to the organs most in need of energy and oxygen during an emergency situation, and away from areas where circulation is less important for immediate survival.

Sympathetic neurons also innervate smooth muscle located in the head. To reach the head, axons from the sympathetic trunk follow the common carotid artery (see **Figure 10-2**). In the head, sympathetic nerves innervate blood vessels, sweat glands, and piloerector muscles. They also innervate smooth muscle in the eyes and salivary gland ducts, resulting in dilation of the pupils and the production of thick saliva.

Finally, sympathetic neurons innervate important structures in the thorax and abdomen. In the thorax, smooth muscle wraps around the trachea and bronchi of the lungs. Sympathetics cause dilation of these structures, allowing more air to enter the lungs. Sympathetic nerves also innervate the heart, increasing both contraction strength and heart rate.

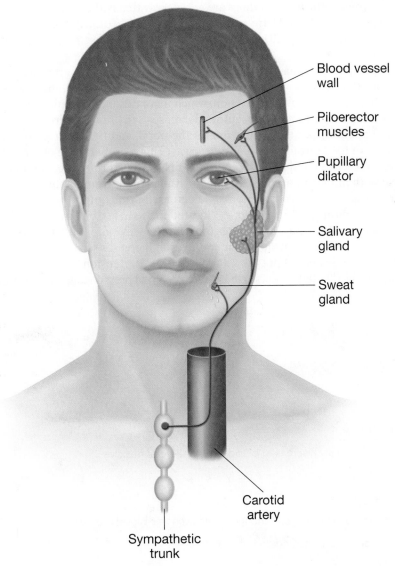

FIGURE 10-2 Sympathetic innervation of the head follows the carotid artery and its branches.

To reach abdominal and pelvic structures, sympathetic neurons follow blood vessels. Sympathetic axons form three **splanchnic nerves** that run medially and inferiorly from the sympathetic trunk to the abdominal aorta, and then follow the arteries to the abdominal organs. In the abdomen, smooth muscle is found in the walls of the digestive tract, and in pelvic organs, as well as in the walls of blood vessels supplying these organs. Sympathetic nerves generally decrease function of the digestive and urinary systems, and cause vasoconstriction that raises the systemic blood pressure.

One group of sympathetic axons from the splanchnic nerves innervates the adrenal gland. Sympathetic stimulation releases adrenalin (epinephrine) into the blood. This connection between the sympathetic and endocrine systems allows for a fast response (the adrenalin "rush").

The sympathetic nervous system uses two neurotransmitters: **acetylcholine (Ach)** and **norepinephrine (NE).** Synapses containing acetylcholine are called *cholinergic,* and synapses with norepinephrine are called *adrenergic.* Cholinergic synapses are found on sweat glands all over the body, and on arterioles that supply skeletal muscle. Stimulation of cholinergic neurons causes sweating. This may occur during exercise or in a stressful situation (resulting in a "cold sweat"). In addition, stimulation of cholinergic neurons produces vasodilation of the arterioles supplying skeletal muscle, thereby increasing blood flow to muscle.

Most sympathetic nerve endings are *adrenergic;* that is, they release the neurotransmitter norepinephrine (NE). There are three major NE receptor types, designated alpha (α), beta (β) –1 and beta (β) –2. The location and function of these receptors is summarized in **Table 10.2**.

Norepinephrine alpha (α) receptors are found in the walls of arterioles and small veins throughout the body. When the sympathetic system is activated, these vessels constrict. This results in general vasoconstriction, which increases the systemic blood pressure. Norepinephrine binding to alpha receptors decreases saliva production, (producing thicker saliva and a feeling of dry mouth), dilates the pupil, and tightens the sphincters, slowing the passage of food through the digestive tract. (This is probably the origin of the term *anal retentive* to refer to an uptight perfectionist.) Norepinephrine α receptors are also found in the smooth muscle of arterioles supplying the kidney; sympathetic stimulation of these receptors results in vasoconstriction and decreased urine output.

Norepinephrine β –1 receptors are located in the heart; binding of NE to these receptors increases the heart rate and causes the heart to beat more forcefully. β –1 receptors are also found in the kidney; sympathetic stimulation increases secretion of a hormone called renin that increases blood pressure. People with hypertension may be given drugs called β –1 antagonists ("beta-blockers") that decrease blood pressure and also slow the heart rate.

Review Concept 10-1: Sympathetic Neurotransmitter Function

Acetylcholine

- Vasodilation and increased blood flow to skeletal muscles
- Sweating and cooling of the body

Norepinephrine

- General vasoconstriction and increased systemic blood pressure
- Increased heart rate and contraction strength
- Relaxation of airways
- Decreased digestion and urinary function

Norepinephrine β –2 receptors are found in bronchial smooth muscle where they produce dilation (relaxation) of the airway when sympathetic activation occurs. People with asthma have excessive bronchial constriction, so people with asthma may be prescribed drugs called bronchodilators. These drugs are β –2 agonists that stimulate β –2 receptors and cause relaxation of bronchial smooth muscle to open the airways.

Table 10.2 Sympathetic Nervous System: Receptors

	Ach	NE α	NE β 1	NE β 2
Circulatory System				
Systemic arterioles		Vasoconstriction (general)	Vasoconstriction (indirect via renin/angiotensin II)	
Systemic veins		Vasoconstriction		
Heart			Increases rate and strength of contraction	
Kidney			Increases renin secretion	
Arterioles in skeletal muscle	Vasodilation	Vasoconstriction		
Blood pressure		Increases	Increases	
Digestive System				
G-I tract smooth muscle		Decreases motility; increases sphincter tone		
Liver		Increases blood glucose		Increases blood glucose
Pancreas		Decreases digestive enzymes; decreases insulin; increases blood glucose		Increases glucagon; increases blood glucose
Salivary glands		Thick saliva		
Genitourinary System				
Bladder wall		Decreases bladder wall tone; increases sphincter tone		
Reproductive system		Ejaculation		
Other				
Sweat glands	Increases sweat production			
Bronchial smooth muscle				Dilation (relaxation)
Eye (smooth muscle)		Pupil dilation		

Drugs of abuse, including cocaine and amphetamines ("speed"), increase the amount of norepinephrine, producing symptoms such as dry mouth, sweating, and a racing heart; an overdose can kill by pushing the heart beyond its capacity.

The Parasympathetic System

The parasympathetic portion of the autonomic nervous system maintains body **homeostasis.** (It is sometimes referred to as the system allowing us to "rest and digest.") Parasympathetics innervate internal organs, but do not innervate the skin, muscles, or blood vessels. Parasympathetic neurons have their cell bodies in the brainstem and in the sacral spinal cord (see **Figure 10-3**). Parasympathetic axons travel with cranial or spinal nerves to cardiac or smooth muscle cells. They regulate digestion, reproduction, urinary function, heart rate, and bronchial diameter. In general, the function of the parasympathetics is to keep the body in a quiet resting state.

Parasympathetic neurons innervate smooth muscle associated with the eye. They innervate the pupillary constrictor muscle of the eye, as well as the ciliary muscle that changes the shape of the lens. Parasympathetic activation will result in constriction of the pupil, and allows the lens to focus on close objects. It will also innervate the lacrimal (tear) and salivary glands to cause secretion of tears and saliva.

The vagus nerve (CN X) contains many parasympathetic neurons. The vagus nerves leave the head, pass through the neck, and innervate structures in the throat, thorax, and abdomen. Parasympathetic neurons slow the heartbeat, decrease the heart's contraction strength, and constrict the trachea and bronchi. Parasympathetics also innervate the digestive tract and stimulate activity of the liver, gall bladder, and pancreas. They increase peristalsis, promote relaxation of smooth muscle sphincters, and stimulate digestive enzyme release.

Parasympathetics from the sacral spinal cord form the pelvic splanchnic nerves. These nerves stimulate bladder emptying as well as vasodilation of erectile tissue in the penis and clitoris, producing erection. They also increase motility of the lower GI tract, and control defecation.

In the parasympathetic nervous system, all neurons release the neurotransmitter acetylcholine (Ach). Drugs that block Ach receptors (e.g., atropine) may be used to decrease parasympathetic function. Atropine causes dilation of the pupil and a decreased motility/contraction of the digestive tract.

The autonomic nervous system has a number of autonomic reflexes (see **Figure 10-4**) that control functions such as bladder emptying and defecation. In an autonomic reflex, a sensory neuron from an organ (bladder or rectum) enters the spinal cord and synapses onto an autonomic motor neuron. In this way, stretching of the bladder results in contraction of smooth muscle that allows the bladder to empty.

Autonomic Regulation

The autonomic nervous system is controlled by the **hypothalamus** in the brain. Neurons from the hypothalamus run inferiorly though the brainstem, traveling with the reticulospinal tracts. These axons are called the **central autonomic fibers** and they synapse onto autonomic neurons. This arrangement allows the hypothalamus to respond to body changes by increasing or decreasing autonomic activity. For example, when body temperature increases, the body's thermostat in the hypothalamus will send signals to the sweat glands via the central autonomic fibers and sympathetic nervous system to increase secretion (sweating). Sweating then cools the body, decreasing temperature.

The hypothalamus is influenced by numerous central nervous system structures and circuits that indirectly affect functioning of the autonomic nervous system. In particular, the limbic system is involved in regulation of the autonomics. Limbic areas regulate emotions (anger, fear), basic drives (sex, hunger), and memory. Connections between the limbic system and the hypothalamus account for the connection between emotional states and bodily responses; for example, most people blush when embarrassed (facial vasodilation), turn pale when afraid (facial vasoconstriction), and get sweaty palms when nervous (sympathetic activation of sweat glands).

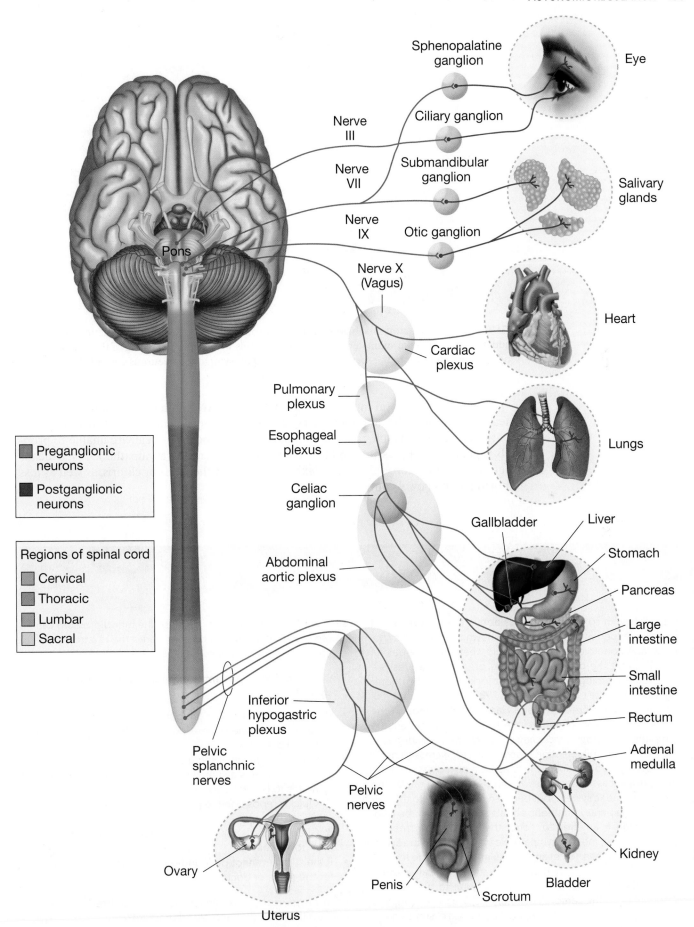

FIGURE 10-3 The parasympathetic system conserves energy, maintains homeostasis, and controls digestion and reproduction. Parasympathetic nerves arise from the brainstem and sacral spinal cord, and innervate selected body structures.

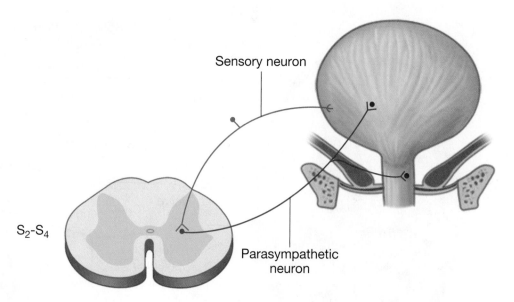

FIGURE 10-4 The autonomic bladder reflex controls urination by causing contraction of the bladder and relaxing the sphincter when the bladder fills with urine. Stretching of the bladder wall sends action potentials to the sacral spinal cord, and parasympathetic neurons control the bladder.

Injury to the central autonomic fibers (e.g., due to a spinal cord injury above T4) means that most of the autonomic nervous system is disconnected from its hypothalamic control center. As a result, patients cannot sweat in response to heat, are unable to properly regulate blood pressure, and lose control of the sacral parasympathetics. This means there is loss of psychogenic (nonreflexive) erection of the penis or clitoris, as well as loss of bladder and bowel control.

Clinical Box 10-1: Autonomic Dysreflexia

Patients with spinal cord injuries above the T6 level are at risk of experiencing a condition known as *autonomic dysreflexia*. Autonomic dysreflexia occurs when there is a painful stimulus that the patient is unaware of, such as a pressure sore, tight clothing or shoes, or a blocked/kinked catheter (McGarry, Woolsey, and Thompson, 1982; Kewalramani, 1980; Lindman, Joiner, Freehafer, and Hazel, 1980). Although the spinal cord patient cannot feel the stimulus, it causes a large sympathetic response, including constriction of the arteries in the extremities, piloerection (goose bumps), increased heart contractility, and continually increasing blood pressure. Normally, this excessive response would be balanced out by the parasympathetic system, but because of the injury to the spinal cord, the parasympathetic signals are blocked at the level of the lesion. In an effort to reduce the continually increasing blood pressure, the parasympathetic system causes bradycardia (decreased heart rate) and vasodilation above the level of injury. As a result of these measures, patients typically experience a distinct "pounding headache" (due to the massive vasodilation of the cerebral arteries), flushing of the skin, and sweating above the level of injury. Autonomic dysreflexia is a serious medical emergency, because the blood pressure can rise so high that it causes a cerebral hemorrhage (stroke) and can be fatal (Eltorai, Kim, Vulpe, Kasravi, and Ho, 1992).

What to do if your patient is experiencing autonomic dysreflexia

- Put the patient in an upright position.
  1. Do NOT lay the patient down, this will only increase blood pressure.
- Check for the noxious stimuli.
  1. Most often it is a kinked catheter or a full bladder that needs to be emptied.
  2. Quickly reposition the patient if he or she is sitting in a wheelchair.
  3. Check for potential pressure areas caused by clothing or footwear.
- If the stimuli cannot be found quickly, immediately call for the nurse or doctor.

Challenge question: Which neurotransmitter is mainly responsible for controlling blood pressure?

Neuroscience Notes Box 10-1: Complex Regional Pain Syndrome

Complex regional pain syndrome (CRPS) is an abnormal response of the sympathetic nervous system to injury. Following damage to a part of the body (frequently a limb), the affected part will remain exquisitely painful even after the initial injury appears to have healed. Symptoms include intense, burning pain in the affected area, sweating, edema, and red, shiny skin. Some evidence suggests that norepinephrine released by sympathetic nerve endings in the affected region causes touch and pressure receptors to become abnormally sensitized, so that touch and other stimuli cause excruciating pain. Patients often avoid touching or moving the affected body part, causing stiffness and eventual disuse atrophy.

PATIENT SCENARIOS

Patient Case 10-1 (Jerry)

Jerry, a 29-year-old man, suffered a complete spinal cord injury 5 weeks ago. His cord was injured at spinal level C8. Jerry uses an indwelling (Foley) catheter for urinary function. While participating in physical therapy, his catheter was "kinked" and urine began to collect until the bladder was very full. Jerry's face turned red, and he complained of a very severe headache. His blood pressure was 220/110. The therapist recognized that Jerry was experiencing autonomic dysreflexia and immediately checked his catheter. Once the catheter was readjusted, Jerry's symptoms subsided.

Questions

a) Which part of the autonomic nervous system is responsible for the sudden and dramatic increase in Jerry's blood pressure?

b) Why does a high-level spinal cord injury predispose a patient to autonomic dysreflexia (which neurons are damaged, and what is their function)?

c) Explain what could happen if this situation is not resolved quickly.

Patient Case 10-2 (Eduardo)

Eduardo is a 42-year old man who injured his right arm in a construction accident. Although the arm injury has healed, Eduardo continues to experience significant pain and disability in the arm. He keeps it cradled against his chest, and does not like to have anyone touch it. Examination of the arm reveals that the skin is red, shiny, and swollen. Eduardo indicates that he tries not to use the arm because it hurts so much. The diagnosis is CRPS.

Questions

a) Why might Eduardo's arm be so painful?

b) Do you think that the swelling is caused by the sympathetic system, or by lack of use of the arm? Why?

Review Questions

1. Compare the functional effects of sympathetic and parasympathetic (if any) stimulation on the following structures:

- Heart
- Bronchial smooth muscle
- Adrenal gland
- Arterioles supplying skeletal muscles
- Digestive tract
- Arterioles supplying skin
- Sweat glands
- Salivary glands
- Urinary bladder
- Penis/Clitoris
- Liver
- Pancreas
- Pupil of the eye

2. Describe the location and function of α and β –1 and β –2 adrenergic nerve endings. How do beta-blockers affect the heart? To which receptors do asthma medications bind? How do cocaine and amphetamines affect sympathetic function?

3. Explain the role of central autonomic fibers.

4. Describe the causes and symptoms of autonomic dysreflexia.

References

1. Eltorai, I., Kim, R., Vulpe, M., Kasravi, H., & Ho, W. (1992). Fatal cerebral hemorrhage due to autonomic dysreflexia in a tetraplegia patient: case study and review. *Paraplegia, 30*(5), 355–360.

2. Kewalramani, L.S. (1980). Autonomic dysreflexia in traumatic myelopathy. *Am. J. Phys Med., 59*(1), 1–21.

3. Lindman, R., Joiner, E., Freehafer, A. A., & Hazel, C. (1980). Incidence and clinical features of autonomic dysreflexia in patients with spinal cord injury. *Paraplegia, 18*(5), 285–292.

4. McGarry, J., Woolsey, R. M., & Thompson, C. W. (1982). Autonomic hyperreflexia following passive stretching to the hip joint. *Phys. Ther.*, 62 (1), 30–31.

Further Reading

1. Bycroft, J., Rizwan, H., Shah, J., & Craggs, M. (2003). Management of the neuropathic bladder. *Hosp. Med.*, 64(8), 468–472.

2. Bycroft, J., Shergill, I., Choong, E., Arya, N., & Shah, P. (2005). Autonomic dysreflexia: A medical emergency. *Postgrad. Med. Journal*, 81(954), 232–235.

3. Carnethon, M. R., Prineas, R. J., Temprosa, M., Zhang, Z. M., Uwaifo, G., & Molitch, M. (2006). The association among autonomic system function, incident diabetes, and intervention arm in the diabetes prevention program. *Diabetes Care, 29,* 914–919.

PEARSON
myhealthprofessionskit™

Use this address to access the Companion Website created for this textbook. Simply select "Physical Therapy" from the choice of disciplines. Find this book and log in using your username and password to access self-assessment questions, a glossary and more.

Somatosensation

CHAPTER OBJECTIVES

After completing this chapter, the reader will be able to:

1 Describe the structure, function, and location of all somatosensory receptors and sensory nerve fibers.

2 List the major spinal cord pathways that convey somatosensation to the brain.

3 Discuss how the brain uses and interprets somatosensory information.

4 Explain the protective function of pain and distinguish among different types of pain.

KEY TERMS

acute pain
afferent neuron
ascending (somatosensory) tract
chronic pain
gamma motor neuron
Golgi tendon organ (GTO)
hair follicle receptors
Meissner's corpuscle
Merkel's disc
muscle spindle
neuropathic pain
nociceptive pain
nociceptor
Pacinian corpuscle
primary somatosensory cortex
proprioceptor
receptor
Ruffini corpuscle
sensitization
somatosensory system
special sensory system
stereognosis
thermal receptor

Essential Facts··

▸ Somatosensation includes pain, temperature, touch, pressure, vibration, and proprioception (position and movement).

▸ Somatosensory receptors are located everywhere in the body, except for the brain.

▸ Sensation is perceived in the brain's primary somatosensory cortex.

The nervous system can be divided into motor and sensory portions. The sensory nervous system detects and responds to information about the body's external environment (What is the temperature like? Are there any dangerous predators around? Did I just step on something sharp?) as well as the body's internal environment (Am I hungry? Thirsty? Anxious? Ill?). The brain uses this information to respond to changes, threats, and other challenges. Without sensation, life would be both brief and dull.

The sensory system can be subdivided into two parts: a **somatosensory (general sensory)** portion, and a **special sensory** portion. The term *somatosensory* refers to sensations experienced by the skin and subcutaneous tissue as well as by muscles, tendons, bones, and joints. These senses include pain, temperature, pressure, touch, vibration, and position sense (proprioception). Special sensations are vision, hearing, smell, taste, and balance; these are described in chapter 12. This chapter will describe how the nervous system detects, transmits, and interprets somatosensation.

Somatosensory Receptors

Receptors are tiny structures located all over the body that convert stimuli into action potentials (nerve impulses). They are classified according to their structure, location, or function. Here, they are organized by function.

Touch Receptors

Touch (tactile) receptors are located in the skin and subcutaneous tissue all over the body. Each touch receptor consists of a small connective tissue capsule that contains a specialized nerve ending (sensory dendrite). When stimulated by touch, Na⁺ channels in the receptor open, triggering an action potential. Thus, all touch receptors convert a mechanical stimulus (touch) into a nerve impulse (see Figure 11-1).

Touch sensation is sometimes divided into "crude touch" and "fine touch," or "light touch" and "deep pressure." Several different kinds of touch receptors are usually activated at the same time, so touch sensations are very complex.

Pacinian corpuscles detect vibration and deep pressure. They are located in the dermis and subcutaneous tissues, in the periosteum around bones, and in ligaments and intramuscular connective tissue. **Meissner's corpuscles** detect two-point discriminative touch,

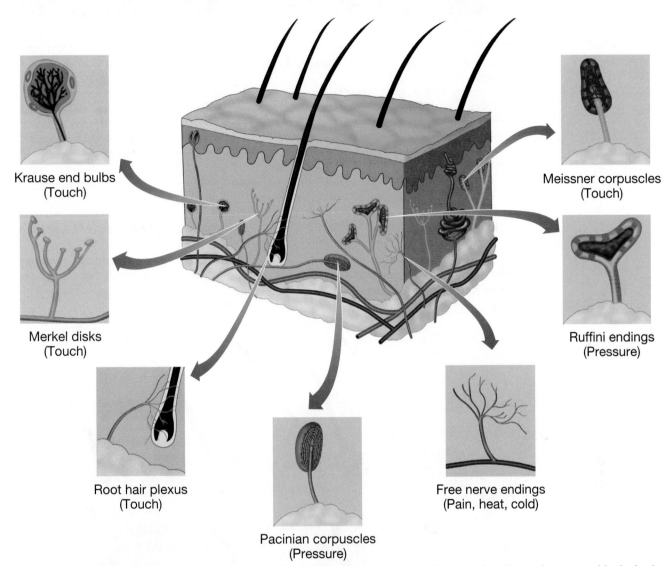

Krause end bulbs
(Touch)

Merkel disks
(Touch)

Root hair plexus
(Touch)

Pacinian corpuscles
(Pressure)

Free nerve endings
(Pain, heat, cold)

Ruffini endings
(Pressure)

Meissner corpuscles
(Touch)

FIGURE 11-1 Tactile (touch) receptors are located in the skin and subcutaneous tissue, and work together to provide the brain with tactile information.

or what is sometimes referred to as "fine touch." They allow specific, precise location of stimuli on the body surface, and are located in the skin; they are especially dense on the fingertips. **Merkel's cells (discs)** detect texture; some people use the term "crude touch" to distinguish this from two-point discrimination. They are found in large numbers on the fingertips, lips, and external genitalia.

Hair follicle receptors detect "light touch." They are composed of small nerve fibers that wrap around the roots of hairs. Bending of the hair stimulates the receptors and generates action potentials. Hair follicle receptors are found all over hairy skin (everywhere except the palms of the hands and soles of the feet). A good way to stimulate these is to blow gently across the back of your hand. **Ruffini corpuscles (endings)** detect stretching of the skin. They are found near folds of skin at joints, and beneath fingernails and toenails. Ruffini corpuscles are made of collagen fiber bundles that are connected to the collagen fibers in the dermis. **Table 11.1** briefly summarizes the various types of touch receptors.

Working together, the touch receptors allow us to determine the qualities of touch and texture. **Stereognosis** is the ability to determine the identity or meaning of an object by touch. This requires integration of different kinds of somatosensation, most of which is

Table 11.1 Touch Receptors

Type of Stimulus	Receptor	Spinal Cord Pathway
Vibration and deep pressure	Pacinian corpuscle	Dorsal column
Two-point discrimination (Fine touch)	Meissner's corpuscle	Dorsal column
Light touch	Hair follicle receptor	Anterior spinothalamic tract
Stretching of the skin	Ruffini ending	Anterior spinothalamic tract
Pressure texture	Merkel's disc	Anterior spinothalamic tract

facilitated by the touch receptors. If you have ever rummaged in the bottom of a bag for a pen or keys, you have used stereognosis to identify the object you want.

Pain and temperature are detected by receptors called "free nerve endings" because they do not have a connective tissue capsule. Some free nerve endings detect changes in temperature (thermal receptors); others detect pain (nociceptors) (see Figure 11-2).

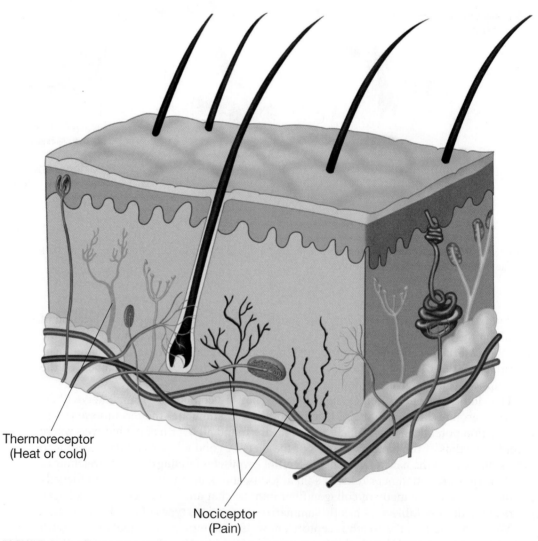

Thermoreceptor
(Heat or cold)

Nociceptor
(Pain)

FIGURE 11-2 Free nerve endings detect pain (nociceptors) and temperature (thermoreceptors: there are different thermoreceptors for hot and for cold).

Thermal Receptors

Thermal receptors respond to changes in temperature. At a constant temperature, the receptors send action potentials at a slow steady rate; they fire faster when there is a change in temperature. Hot thermal receptors detect increasing temperature, whereas cold thermal receptors detect decreasing temperature. Thermal receptors are inactive at absolute temperatures above 50°C or below 5°C; these extreme temperatures are felt as pain rather than hot or cold. Thermal receptors are located in the subcutaneous tissue all over the body.

Nociceptors

Nociceptors detect pain. They are free nerve endings located throughout the body (although they are not found in the brain itself). Nociceptors respond to stimuli that either *do* damage tissue or that *could* damage tissue. This means that they can signal potential damage to cells before it actually occurs.

Four different types of nociceptors have been identified. Each kind responds to a different type of painful stimulus and each sends signals that determine the quantity and quality of pain we experience.

The first type of pain receptor is a mechanical nociceptor. These respond to cutting or pinching; they produce a feeling of sharp, intense pain. A second type is called a thermal hot nociceptor; these respond to extremely high temperatures (over 50°C) and create a feeling of burning pain. A third kind of pain receptor is a thermal cold nociceptor that responds to temperatures below 5°C, giving a sensation of freezing pain. Finally, polymodal pain receptors are activated by mechanical stimuli and also by the chemicals released when there is inflammation. These produce a sensation of aching pain.

Another group of free nerve endings respond specifically to chemicals such as histamine, producing the sensation of itch. Itchy sensations have their own free nerve ending receptors that are located in the skin.

When a tissue or body part is chronically inflamed, pain receptors can become sensitized. This means that they are easily activated, even by stimuli that do not normally cause pain. For example, lightly stroking skin that has been burned will be painful, even though gentle touching usually does not hurt. This probably serves to protect injured tissues from further damage by causing us to protect the painful areas. See **Table 11.2** for a short summary.

Proprioceptors

Proprioceptors detect body position and movement. The brain uses this information to accurately control and guide motion. Proprioception can be conscious (sent to a conscious level in the brain), or unconscious (subconscious). Unconscious proprioception is processed in the brain, but is not available to the mind at a conscious level. This allows us to move without thinking about it; if you can walk and carry on a conversation at the same time, you are using your unconscious proprioception. Both conscious and unconscious proprioception are important for normal movement.

Proprioceptors are located in muscles, tendons, ligaments, and joint capsules. They detect muscle length (stretch), muscle tension, and the position and movement of joints.

Muscle spindles are stretch receptors that detect changes in muscle length (see **Figure 11-3**). They are found in most skeletal muscles, and appear in large numbers in muscles used for posture, in the extraocular (eye) muscles, and in the intrinsic muscles of

Table 11.2 Pain Receptors (Nociceptors)

Type of Pain Receptor	Modality
Mechanical	Cutting, pinching
Thermal hot	Temperature over 50°C
Thermal cold	Temperature below 5°C
Polymodal	Mechanical stimuli and inflammation

the hand. Muscle spindles are connected to the connective tissue inside the skeletal muscle (the perimysium), and stretch or shorten along with the muscle. They send the central nervous system information concerning two different aspects of muscle length: (1) whether the muscle's length is changing and (2) how quickly the muscle's length is changing.

Muscle spindles are innervated by specialized motor neurons called **gamma motor neurons.** Gamma motor neurons synapse onto spindle muscle fibers and can cause a very small contraction of each spindle muscle fiber. This pulls on (lengthens) the central part of the spindle fiber and makes it stiffer. When spindles are stiffer, they become more sensitive to stretching of the entire muscle. So, gamma motor neurons control how sensitive the muscle spindles are to muscle stretch. This is important because the more sensitive the spindles are, the more action potentials they will send to the brain. When the brain processes information about muscle length from all of the muscles acting at a joint, it can determine the angle of the joint as well as whether the joint is moving and in what direction.

Gamma motor neurons are controlled by motor centers in the spinal cord and brain. This means that the brain can regulate how sensitive muscles are to being stretched. It also means that brain injury or disease can affect the muscle's sensitivity to stretch. People with damage to the brain or spinal cord may display either increased or decreased sensitivity to muscle

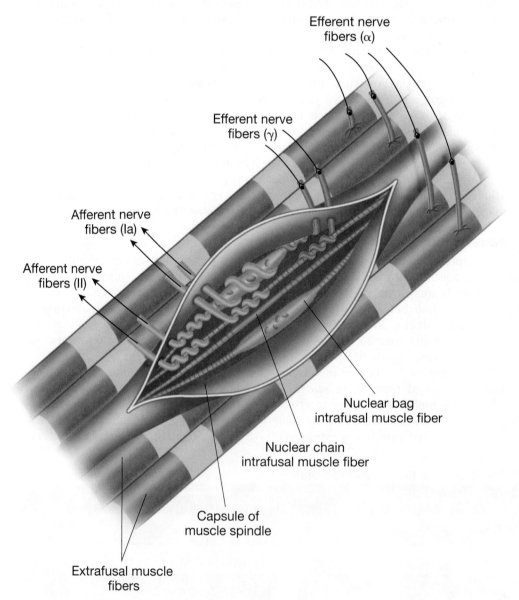

Efferent nerve
fibers (α)

Efferent nerve
fibers (γ)

Afferent nerve
fibers (Ia)

Afferent nerve
fibers (II)

Nuclear bag
intrafusal muscle fiber

Nuclear chain
intrafusal muscle fiber

Capsule of
muscle spindle

Extrafusal muscle
fibers

FIGURE 11-3 Muscle spindles are sensory structures located within skeletal muscles. They detect muscle stretch and convey this to the brain via the afferent nerve fibers. Their sensitivity to stretch is modified by gamma motor neurons.

stretching. For example, many people with traumatic spinal cord injuries have an abnormally strong reaction to muscle stretch that causes the muscles to become tight and spastic.

Golgi tendon organs (GTOs) are located in the tendons of most skeletal muscles, usually near the junction between the muscle and its tendon (see **Figure 11-4**). Their primary function is to detect muscle and tendon tension. When a muscle contracts, it pulls on its tendon, creating tension that stimulates an action potential in the neuron. The action potential is sent to the central nervous system.

Somatosensory receptors located in and around the joints respond to mechanical stress placed on the joint capsules and ligaments. They send the brain and spinal cord signals about the position and movement of joints. There are four types of joint receptors (see **Figure 11-5** and **Table 11.3**):

- Type I joint receptors are located in joint capsules and are stimulated when the joint capsules are stretched. They signal joint position.
- Type II joint receptors are also located in joint capsules and are activated by stretching of the joint capsule. They respond to joint movement.
- Type III joint receptors are located inside ligaments, and are also known as ligament receptors. They detect ligament stretching and signal that stress is being placed on a joint.
- Type IV joint receptors are pain receptors that function just like nociceptors located elsewhere in the body. They respond to stimuli that can damage joint tissues and are especially active when inflammatory reactions occur in and around joints (e.g., in arthritis).

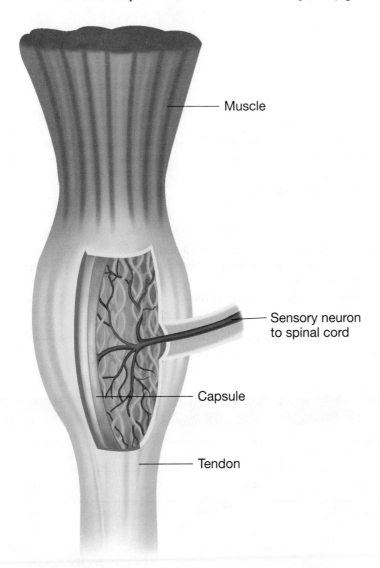

Muscle

Sensory neuron to spinal cord

Capsule

Tendon

FIGURE 11-4   Golgi tendon organs are located inside tendons and detect muscle tension and contraction.

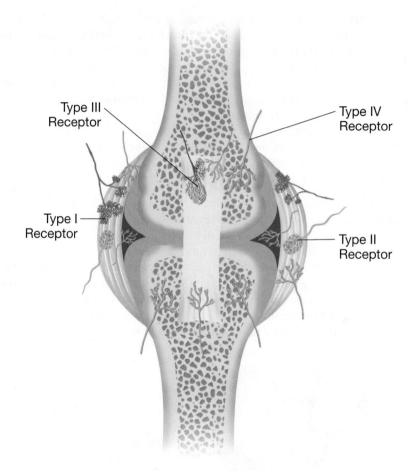

FIGURE 11-5 Joint receptors are located within joint capsules and ligaments, and detect joint position, movement, and pain and inflammation within the joint.

Somatosensory Pathways

Transmission of somatosensory information from the body to the brain requires a complete somatosensory pathway (see Figure 11-6). A pathway consists of:

1. A somatosensory receptor that converts a stimulus into an action potential
2. An afferent (sensory) neuron in a peripheral nerve that carries the action potential to the central nervous system
3. A neuron that sends the action potential up through the spinal cord to the brain

Some sensory pathways also have:

4. A neuron that conveys the sensation to the **primary somatosensory cortex** where conscious awareness of the sensation occurs

Table 11.3 Proprioceptors

Proprioceptor	Location	Stimulus
Golgi tendon organ	Tendons, near myotendinous junction	Muscle tension/contraction; tendon stretch
Muscle spindle	Most skeletal muscle	Muscle stretch/length
Joint receptors Type I Type II Type III Type IV	 Joint capsules Joint capsules Ligaments Joint capsules and ligaments	 Joint position Joint movement and velocity Ligament tension Pain (and inflammation)

LESION IN :

EFFECT ON DISCRIMINATIVE
TOUCH AND CONSCIOUS
PROPRIOCEPTIVE INFORMATION :

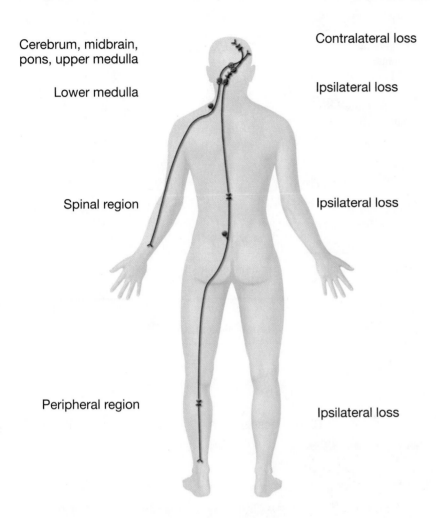

Cerebrum, midbrain,
pons, upper medulla

Contralateral loss

Lower medulla

Ipsilateral loss

Spinal region

Ipsilateral loss

Peripheral region

Ipsilateral loss

FIGURE 11-6 Somatosensory pathways convey sensations to the brain via peripheral nerves and the spinal cord. The pathway shown here is the dorsal column pathway that detects vibration, discriminative touch, and conscious proprioception.

Afferent Fibers (Sensory Axons)

Every somatosensory receptor in skin, muscles, or joints is connected to an afferent (sensory) neuron. After the receptor converts a sensory stimulus into an action potential, the afferent nerve fiber sends the action potential into the central nervous system. Somatosensory neurons form part of all spinal nerves (except for C1) and several cranial nerves. In spinal nerves, sensory axons make up about 60% of the nerve fibers (see **Table 11.4**).

Sensory axons that are found in peripheral nerves range in diameter from 1 μm to 20 μm (see **Figure 11-7**). The larger the fiber (axon) diameter, the thicker its myelin sheath, and the faster action potentials are transmitted. Axons that transmit proprioception are the largest and fastest, whereas axons that transmit aching pain, freezing pain, and heat are small, slow, and unmyelinated.

When somatosensory action potentials reach the central nervous system, the sensory information can be used in several ways. First, it can be sent directly to motor neurons to form a reflex. Second, it can be sent to the brain for higher-order processing, forming an emotional response, or for conscious awareness of the stimulus. To reach the brain, the action potentials must travel up the spinal cord in a sensory (ascending) tract.

Table 11.4 Afferent Nerve Fibers

Classification	Sensory Modality	Receptor Type	Diameter (µm)	Transmission Speed
Ia	Quick stretch (muscle)	Muscle spindle	12–20 (myelinated)	Fast
Ib	Muscle/tendon tension Ligament tension	Golgi tendon organ Ligament receptor (type 3 joint receptor)	12–20 (myelinated)	Fast
II (Aβ)	Slow stretch (muscle) Joint position and movement; 2-point discriminative touch, Vibration, and deep pressure; Skin stretch Pressure, texture (light touch)	Muscle spindle Joint receptors (type 1 and type 2) Meissner's corpuscle Pacinian corpuscle Ruffini ending Merkel disk	8–12 (myelinated)	Moderate
III (Aδ)	Sharp and burning pain; temperature (cold)	Free nerve ending	1–6 (myelinated)	Slow
IV (C)	Freezing and aching pain; temperature (hot)	Free nerve ending	1–1.5 (unmyelinated)	Very slow

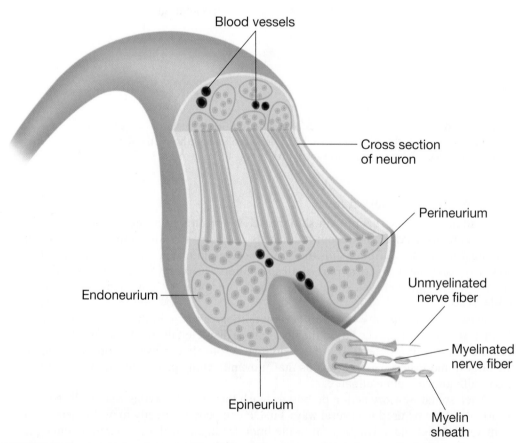

FIGURE 11-7 A peripheral nerve with myelinated and unmyelinated axons. Both kinds of axons are wrapped with endoneurium (connective tissue).

Clinical Box 11-1: Local Anesthetics and Nerve Fiber Regeneration

Local anesthetics relieve pain by blocking transmission of action potentials in sensory axons. They do this by preventing Na^+ channels from opening, so Na^+ ions cannot flow into the nerve cell (Tsang, Tsushima, Tomaselli et al., 2005). When peripheral nerves are anesthetized, the smallest axons are blocked first, followed by larger fibers according to their diameter. This means that pain sensations will be numbed initially, and proprioception is the last sensation lost (Sakai, Tomiyasu, Yamada et al., 2004). Local anesthetics are used for minor surgical procedures (such as dental work or suturing a cut).

When peripheral nerves regenerate after an injury, sensations return in the same order that they are lost following local anesthesia: Slow aching pain is first, then temperature and fast, sharp pain, followed by touch, and culminating finally by proprioception. Smaller neurons regenerate and begin to function sooner than large-diameter axons. Thus, the return of pain following a peripheral nerve injury means that nerve regrowth is taking place.

Challenge question: Why would a local anesthetic block pain signals while allowing touch or pressure to be perceived?

In the spinal cord, neurons with similar functions cluster together to form axon bundles known as columns or tracts. The spinal cord contains three types of tracts:

- Ascending (action potentials travel up from the body to the brain)
- Descending (action potentials travel down from the brain to the body)
- Intersegmental (short tracts that connect spinal cord segments)

In this chapter, the focus will be on the ascending tracts. The term *ascending* means that the action potentials flow upward from the body to the brain. There are four major **ascending (somatosensory) tracts,** and each conveys a different kind of sensation to the brain. The ascending tracts are summarized in **Table 11.5.**

Anterior and Lateral Spinothalamic Tracts

The anterior spinothalamic tract (pathway) conveys sensations of pressure and texture, light touch, and stretching of the skin (see **Figure 11-8**). Combined, these sensations comprise what might be called "light touch" or "crude touch." This system provides information

Table 11.5 Somatosensory Tracts

Ascending (Sensory) Tract	Sensation(s)	Destination
Anterior spinothalamic	Pressure, texture, light touch, stretching of the skin	Sensory cortex, opposite side
Lateral spinothalamic	Pain, temperature	Sensory cortex, opposite side
Dorsal columns	Vibration, two-point discriminative touch, conscious proprioception	Sensory cortex, opposite side
Spinocerebellar	Unconscious proprioception	Cerebellum, same side

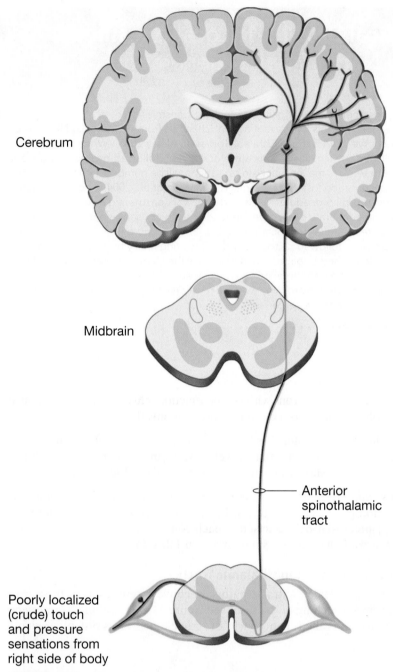

Cerebrum

Midbrain

Anterior spinothalamic tract

Poorly localized (crude) touch and pressure sensations from right side of body

FIGURE 11-8 The anterior spinothalamic tract conveys touch and pressure sensations to the contralateral sensory cortex. The tract is located in the anterior white matter of the spinal cord.

about the texture, consistency, and shape of objects, as well as information about superficial sensory stimuli that affect the skin (light stroking, air blowing across the surface, etc.). The anterior spinothalamic tract terminates in the brain in the primary somatosensory cortex, located in the parietal lobe. The sensation is perceived once the action potential reaches somatosensory cortex on the contralateral side of the brain.

The lateral spinothalamic tract conveys sensations of pain and temperature (see Figure 11-9). These sensations travel through the spinal cord and brainstem, and are perceived in the primary somatosensory cortex on the contralateral side of the brain. Action potentials in the pain system also connect with emotional centers throughout the CNS, as well as with autonomic nerves. These connections are responsible for emotional and physiological reactions to pain (e.g., crying, sweating, and nausea).

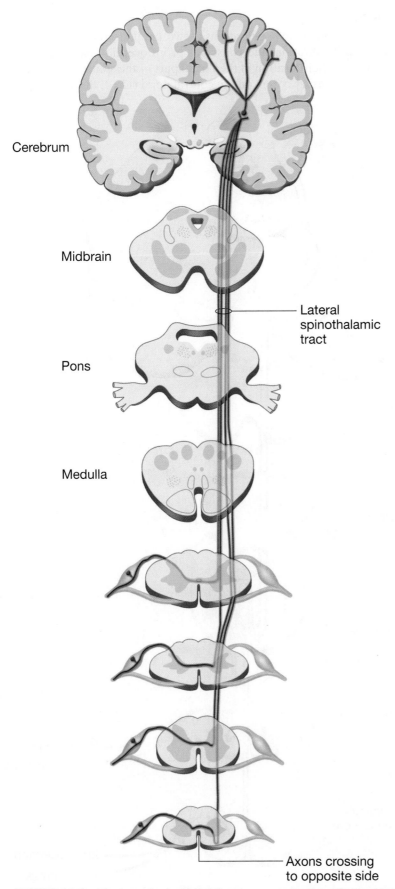

Cerebrum

Midbrain

Lateral
spinothalamic
tract

Pons

Medulla

Axons crossing
to opposite side

FIGURE 11-9   The lateral spinothalamic tract conveys pain and temperature to the contralateral sensory cortex. This tract travels to the brain in the lateral white matter of the spinal cord.

Dorsal Columns

The dorsal column tracts convey sensations of two-point discriminative touch (sometimes called "fine touch"), vibration, and conscious proprioception (see **Figure 11-10**). These tracts are named for their location in the dorsal part of the spinal cord. They terminate in the primary somatosensory cortex on the contralateral side of the brain.

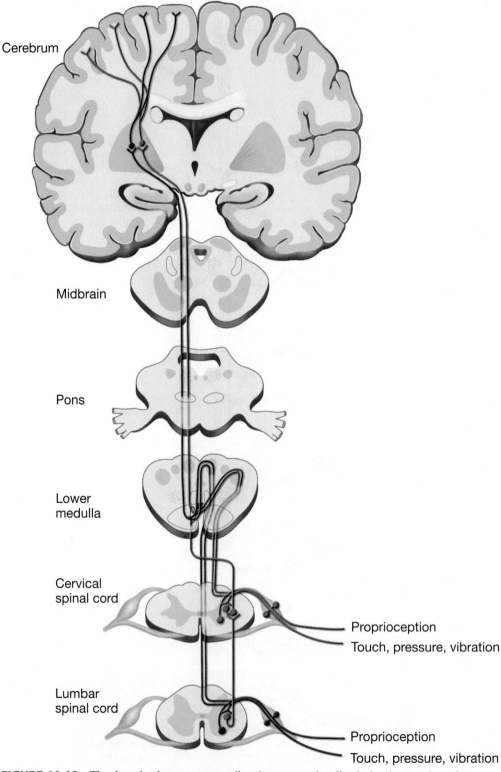

FIGURE 11-10 The dorsal columns convey vibration, two-point discriminative touch, and conscious proprioception to the contralateral sensory cortex. These tracts travel in the dorsal (posterior) white matter of the spinal cord.

Spinocerebellar Tracts

There are four spinocerebellar tracts that carry unconscious proprioception regarding muscle length and tension from muscle spindles and Golgi tendon organs (see **Figure 11-11** and **Table 11.6**). Most neurons in these tracts terminate in the ipsilateral cerebellum, which is responsible for coordinating unconscious (subconscious) balance, posture, and movement. A few end in the contralateral cerebellum, so the spinocerebellar tracts are usually described as bilateral.

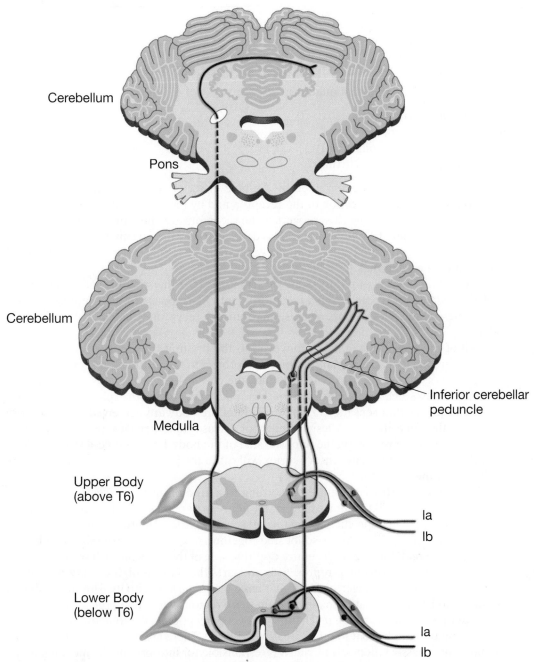

Cerebellum

Pons

Cerebellum

Inferior cerebellar peduncle

Medulla

Upper Body (above T6)

Ia

Ib

Lower Body (below T6)

Ia

Ib

FIGURE 11-11 The spinocerebellar tracts all convey unconscious proprioception to the cerebellum. They travel in the lateral white matter of the spinal cord.

Table 11.6 Spinocerebellar Tracts

Spinocerebellar Tract	Body Region
Anterior spinocerebellar	Lower extremities
Posterior spinocerebellar	Lower extremities
Cuneocerebellar	Upper extremities
Rostrospinocerebellar	Upper extremities and neck

Somatosensory Perception and Processing

Sensation has four important qualities:

1. Modality (What is it?)
2. Location (Where is it?)
3. Intensity (How strong is it?)
4. Timing (When is it occurring)?

Stimulus modality is determined by the type of receptor that is activated. Stimulus location is based on the location of the receptor, and by the density of receptors in a particular part of the body; the closer together the receptors are, the more precisely stimulus location is determined. Stimulus intensity is determined by the sensitivity of each receptor and by the frequency of action potentials generated; the stronger the stimulus, the more frequent the nerve impulses.

Eventually, all receptors stop sending signals, even if the stimulus continues. This is called *receptor adaptation*. When a receptor adapts, its response to the stimulus declines over time. All receptors adapt; some somatosensory receptors adapt slowly and others adapt rapidly.

All of the sensations that are conveyed to the brain in the anterior spinothalamic, lateral spinothalamic, and dorsal column tracts project to the contralateral (opposite side) somatosensory cortex. Because they all reach the cortex, these sensations reach the level of conscious awareness. In addition, all of these pathways cross in the spinal cord or brainstem. This means that sensations from one side of the body are perceived in the sensory cortex on the opposite side. A lesion (injury or disease) that damages the sensory cortex will cause loss of sensation on the opposite side of the body. For example, a stroke (CVA) that destroys the left somatosensory cortex will cause the patient to lose sensation on the right side of the body (see **Figure 11-12**).

The sensory cortex is organized according to a kind of map representing each body region (see **Figure 11-13**). For example, all neurons carrying sensation from the right thumb are located in a specific spot on the left sensory cortex. Neurons carrying sensation from the right index finger are also located together, next to those from the thumb. This arrangement creates a map of the entire opposite side of the body on each sensory cortex. The largest areas of this map represent body parts that have a high density of sensory receptors (lips, tongue, fingertips) and that have the highest sensitivity. This arrangement allows us to localize sensations coming from these regions with great precision.

After the somatosensation reaches the level of perception in the somatosensory cortex, the information can be sent to other areas of the brain. There are many connections to the somatosensory association cortex, which is responsible for interpreting the meaning of the sensation, for stereognosis, and for a kind of "touch" memory. Other connections go to motor areas of the cortex, so that sensations can be used to guide movement. Finally, the somatosensory cortex sends signals to cognitive and emotional centers.

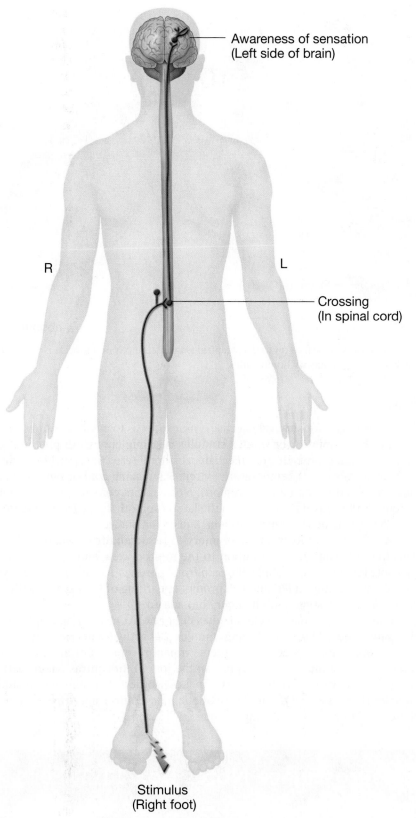

FIGURE 11-12 Most kinds of somatosensation project to the contralateral (opposite) side of the brain and cross in either the spinal cord or in the brainstem.

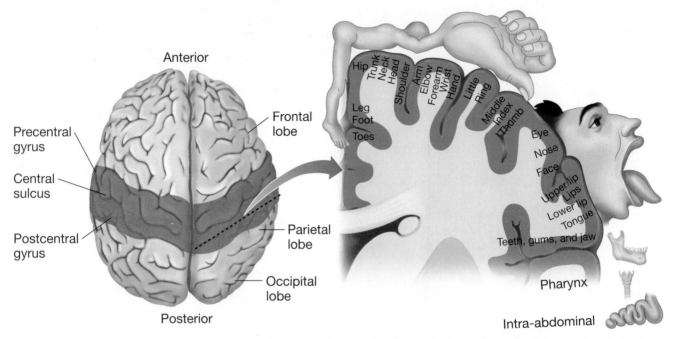

FIGURE 11-13 Primary somatosensory cortex is located on the postcentral gyrus in the parietal lobe. It is organized by body region to form a sensory map that is known as the sensory homunculus.

Pain

Pain is necessary for survival because it motivates us to avoid harmful stimuli. Pain begins when cells are injured, or when a stimulus is strong enough to potentially damage cells. Painful stimuli can result from mechanical stimuli (crushing, pinching, squeezing, stretching), chemicals (acid), temperature extremes (freezing cold or burning hot), or ischemia (lack of blood flow to a body region). Nociceptors convert painful stimuli into action potentials that travel to the brain in the lateral spinothalamic tract. Perception of pain can vary depending on thoughts, emotions, and circumstances.

Acute pain results from direct injury to tissue and from the resulting inflammation. This kind of pain directs attention to the injured area, and encourages behaviors that promote healing. For example, the pain from a broken femur will prevent you from trying to walk on the injured leg, and will promote guarding of the limb. Usually acute pain is of short duration, lasting until the injury has healed.

Long-term pain can be classified as either nociceptive or neuropathic pain. **Nociceptive pain** is caused by a long-lasting stimulus that activates nociceptors. For example, it can result from cancer (when tumors press on pain receptors) or arthritis (when continuous inflammation stimulates nociceptors in the joints). In contrast, **neuropathic pain** results from direct injury to peripheral nerve fibers. Disorders that cause neuropathic pain include shingles (herpes zoster), diabetes (diabetic neuropathy), and trigeminal neuralgia. All of these conditions involve damage to sensory neurons.

Neuroscience Notes Box 11-1: Sensitization

Tissue injury and inflammation not only cause pain but also temporarily increase the sensitivity of the entire pain perception system. This is called **sensitization.** Sensitization results from the release of chemicals by damaged cells. Some of these chemicals directly activate nearby nociceptors, whereas others make the nociceptors more easily stimulated. Anti-inflammatory analgesics (aspirin, ibuprofen) inhibit some of these chemicals and thus reduce pain.

Neuroscience Notes Box 11-2: Chronic Pain

When peripheral nerves are damaged by disease or injury, the sensory pathway that conveys pain into the spinal cord is affected. Instead of reducing painful sensations, it often causes increased, long-term, chronic pain. **Chronic pain** persists even when the initial injury has healed. The pain occurs because injured axons become overexcited and generate action potentials spontaneously. For example, people with diabetic neuropathy feel a constant "pins and needles" type of pain, usually in their feet. It begins in the small-diameter nerve fibers that transmit pain, and gradually spreads to affect larger axons in the peripheral nerves (Greene, Simal, Pfeifer et al., 1990). Changes in the spinal cord that affect the ascending pain pathways can also cause chronic pain. Inflammation can cause more synapses to develop between pain fibers (Type C afferents) and the spinal cord neurons in the lateral spinothalamic tract (Ikeda, Stark, Fischer, Wagener, Drdla, Jager and Sandkulher, 2006).

Acute and nociceptive pain can be divided into two subtypes: "fast" pain and "slow" pain. Fast pain has a rapid onset, is usually sharp and intense, and can be localized very accurately. Slow pain has a slower onset, is more prolonged and achy, and is less precisely localized. Imagine stubbing your toe: Initially you feel an intense, "fast" pain that is followed by a longer-lasting achy "slow" pain. Both kinds of pain travel in the lateral spinothalamic tract; about 25% of the nerve fibers in the tract transmit fast pain, and the remaining 75% carry slow pain. Slow pain neurons have many connections in the thalamus and hypothalamus. These synapses are responsible for autonomic responses to pain such as nausea, sweating, fainting, and increased heart rate. They are also the reason for our emotional reaction to pain as being unpleasant or unbearable.

Pain perception can be decreased by some forms of touch that activate neurotransmitters in the spinal cord that slow or stop transmission of pain signals. This may explain why many people gently rub the skin near the injury to diminish pain, and why massage often has therapeutic benefits. The cerebral cortex, hypothalamus, and limbic (emotional) regions of the brain can also affect perception of pain. For example, the placebo effect shows that an expectation of pain relief actually does decrease pain perception. On the other hand, anxiety can cause pain perception to increase.

PATIENT SCENARIOS

Patient Case 11-1 (Wilma)

Wilma, age 82, suffered a stroke (CVA) that damaged the primary somatosensory cortex. Sensory tests for pain, light touch, and conscious proprioception show that Wilma has lost these sensations on the left side of her body (her left shoulder, arm, forearm, and hand).

Questions

a) Since Wilma's sensory loss is evident on her left side, which side of the cerebral cortex has been injured by the stroke?

b) Which ascending sensory pathways carry each of the three sensations mentioned above?

Patient Case 11-2 (Paul)

Paul is a 58-year-old man who has Type II diabetes. He has had the disease for about 7 years, and admits he does not always take his medication. Also, he does not exercise regularly even though he knows he should. Now Paul is experiencing a painful, tingly, "pins and needles" feeling in both of his feet. He says that he feels it all the time, no matter which shoes he wears.

Questions

a) What do you think might be causing Paul's foot pain? How would you classify this type of pain?

b) If Paul continues to undertreat his diabetes, which type of nerve fibers in his peripheral nerves may be affected next?

c) If Paul were given a local anesthetic, which sensation(s) would he lose first? Which would he lose last?

Review Questions

1. Name each type of somatosensation, and name the receptors that detect the sensation as well as the pathway that conveys each sensation to the brain. Where does conscious perception of sensations occur?

2. Explain why injury to somatosensory cortex on one side of the brain can cause sensory loss on the opposite (contralateral) side of the body.

3. Distinguish between acute, nociceptive, and neuropathic pain.

References

1. Greene, D. A., Simal, A. A. F., Pfeifer, M. A., et al. (1990). Diabetic neuropathy. *Annual Review of Medicine, 41,* 303–317.

2. Ikeda, H., et al. (2006). Synaptic amplifier of inflammatory pain in the spinal dorsal horn. *Science, 312,* 1659–1662.

3. Sakai, T., Tomiyasu, S., Yamada, H., et al. (2004). Quantitative and selective evaluation of differential sensory nerve block after transdermal lidocaine. *Anesth. Analg., 98,* 248–251.

4. Tsang, S. Y., Tsushima, R. G., Tomaselli, G. F. et al. (2005). A multifunctional aromatic residue in the external pore vestibule of Na⁺ channels contributes to the local anesthetic receptor. *Mol. Pharmacol., 67,* 424–434.

Further Reading

1. Eide, P. K. (1998). Pathophysiological mechanisms of central neuropathic pain after spinal cord injury. *Spinal Cord, 36,* 601–612.

2. Miller, G. (2007). Grasping for clues to the biology of itch. *Science, 318,* 188–189.

3. Robinson, A. J. (1997). Central nervous system pathways for pain transmission and pain control: issues relevant for the practicing clinician. *J. Hand Therapy, 10,* 64–77.

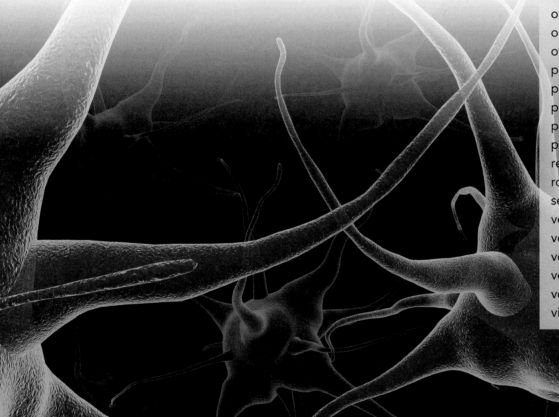

12

Special Sensory Systems

CHAPTER OBJECTIVES

After completing this chapter, the reader will be able to:

1 Describe the sensory receptors and pathways responsible for vision, hearing, and balance.

2 Explain common clinical conditions involving the visual, auditory, and vestibular systems.

3 Discuss the structure and function of the neural systems for smell and taste, and list several clinical conditions involving these systems.

KEY TERMS

anosmia
auditory ossicles
cochlea
cones
cortical blindness
extraocular muscles
hemianopsia
macula
Meniere's disease
olfactory receptors
olfactory nerve (tract)
optic chiasm
optic nerve
optic tract
organ of Corti
otolithic organs
photoreceptors
primary auditory cortex
primary olfactory cortex
primary visual cortex
proprioceptors
retina
rods
semicircular canals
vertigo
vestibular apparatus
vestibular nuclei
vestibulocerebellum
vestibulocochlear nerve
visual cortex

Essential Facts··

▶ The special senses include vision, hearing, balance, taste, and smell.

▶ Vision is detected in the eye, and transmitted by the optic nerves to the visual cortex.

▶ Each visual cortex perceives visual stimuli from the opposite visual field.

▶ Hearing and balance (head movement) are detected in the inner ear and transmitted by the vestibulocochlear nerve to the brain.

▶ Olfactory receptors located in the nose detect odors and transmit them via the olfactory nerve to the olfactory cortex.

▶ Taste receptors on the tongue detect taste; the sense of smell is an important component of taste.

The special sensations are vision, hearing, balance, taste, and smell. All of these senses are detected by sensory receptors located in the head, and all are transmitted to the brain by cranial nerves. Special senses undergo processing within the brain and are essential for normal function. Pathologies involving the special senses include blindness and visual deficits, deafness and tinnitus (a constant ringing in the ears), and disorders of balance, smell, and taste.

The Visual System

Vision is our most prominent sense. Human beings have millions of sensory receptors, and about 70% of them are visual receptors. Visual receptors convert light into action potentials that are transmitted from the eyes to the brain, where we perceive and interpret the world.

The Eye and Retina

The eye (eyeball) is about 1 inch in diameter and is located inside a skull cavity called the orbit (see Figure 12-1). Each eyeball is surrounded by fat, and is protected by the eyelids. Eyelids are formed of connective tissue covered by muscle and skin. The lacrimal gland, located at the superior and lateral corner of the eye, produces tears that help to keep the eyeball moist and wash away dirt.

The eyeball's external surface (except for the front) is made of a thick, white connective tissue (the sclera). In the front of the eye, the outer surface is formed by the clear cornea, which is very sensitive to touch and contains many pain receptors. This serves an important protective function. Six small **extraocular muscles** attach to the sclera and move the eyeball (see **Table 12.1**). All of the extraocular muscles are innervated by cranial nerves.

Just behind the cornea, smooth muscle forms the colored iris. The iris surrounds the pupil, an opening that admits light into the eye. The iris changes the diameter of the pupils to control how much light gets into the eye. In bright light, the pupil constricts so less light gets in; in dim light, the muscle relaxes so pupils are dilated and more light can enter the eye.

The eye's visual receptors are all located on the **retina,** which is found at the back of the eyeball inside the sclera. Light comes into the eye though the clear cornea in front, passes through the clear lens, and strikes the retina (see Figure 12-2). The lens focuses the light, so that it strikes the retina precisely. If the eyeball is not perfectly spherical, light cannot

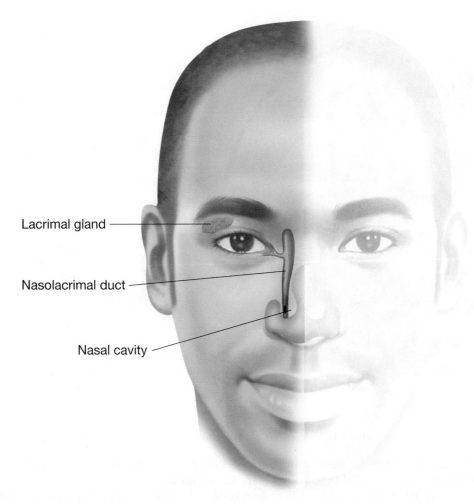

FIGURE 12-1 The eye is located within the orbit, and kept moist by tears that are produced in the lacrimal gland. Tears drain into the nasal cavity via the nasolacrimal duct.

hit the retina accurately, and vision will be blurry. This is one reason that many people must wear glasses or contact lenses in order to improve visual clarity. In many people, the lens becomes cloudy with age and must be replaced; this is called a cataract. The shape of the lens can be adjusted to allow focusing on objects that are far away, or close up. This adjustment of the lens is called accommodation; it is controlled by smooth muscle fibers that pull on the lens to change its shape.

Table 12.1 **Extraocular muscles**

Muscle	Function
Medial rectus	Moves eyeball medially
Lateral rectus	Moves eyeball laterally
Inferior rectus	Moves eyeball inferiorly
Superior rectus	Moves eyeball superiorly
Superior oblique	Moves eyeball inferiorly and laterally
Inferior oblique	Moves eyeball superiorly and laterally

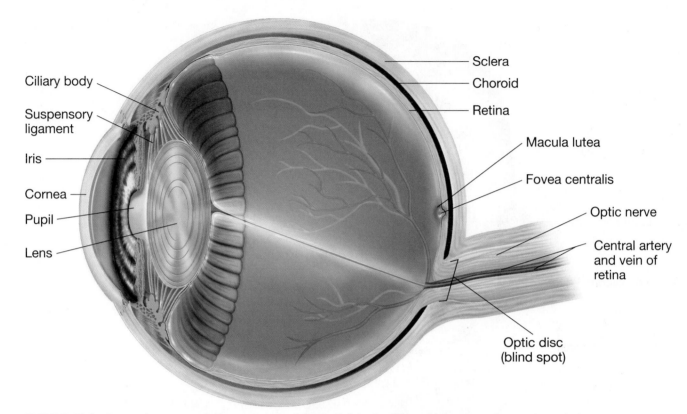

Ciliary body

Suspensory ligament

Iris

Cornea

Pupil

Lens

Sclera

Choroid

Retina

Macula lutea

Fovea centralis

Optic nerve

Central artery and vein of retina

Optic disc (blind spot)

FIGURE 12-2 Internal anatomy of the eye; anterior is to the left in the figure. Light enters the eye through the cornea, passes through the lens, and strikes the retina where it is converted into action potentials by photoreceptor cells (rods and cones).

When light strikes the retina, it stimulates cells called **photoreceptors** that convert the light into action potentials. Photoreceptors are named for their shapes: rods and cones (see Figure 12-3). Each eye has about 125 million rods and 7 million cones. **Rods** are located all over the retina. They work in dim light and they are responsible for black and white vision. **Cones** are concentrated in the middle of the retina, at a spot called the **macula.** Cones are important for clear, sharp visual perception, and need bright light to work. They are responsible for color vision. Three kinds of cones are found in most people: one reacts to blue light, another to green light, and the third to red. People who are color-blind are missing one or more of these types of cones.

Neuroscience Notes Box 12-1:
Eye Diseases

Detached Retina   A detached retina can occur when the retina comes loose and pulls away from the back of the eyeball. Sometimes, a detached retina results from a blow to the head, but it can also occur for no clear reason. The retina must be surgically reattached quickly so that rods and cones do not die. If it is not reattached, vision will be permanently lost in that eye.

Macular Degeneration   Macular degeneration causes death of photoreceptors (mainly cones) in the macula and can cause decreased vision or blindness. It usually occurs in older people (age-related macular degeneration), but can sometimes occur in young people. Macular degeneration appears to be an inherited condition; in older people it is also linked to high levels of blood cholesterol.

Retinopathy of Prematurity   Retinopathy of prematurity results from supplemental oxygen given to babies born too early. Once the oxygen is removed, many small blood vessels grow inside the eyes. The vessels have thin walls and often leak, producing bleeding inside the eye that can cause the retina to detach. Because the retina and optic nerve cannot regenerate, the blindness is permanent.

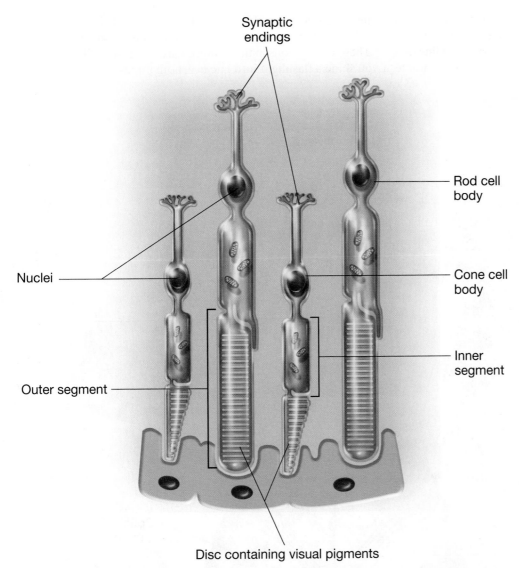

Synaptic
endings

Rod cell
body

Cone cell
body

Nuclei

Inner
segment

Outer segment

Disc containing visual pigments

FIGURE 12-3 Photoreceptor cells in the retina convert light into action potentials. Rods work
in dim light and are responsible for black and white vision, whereas cones need bright light to
function and are responsible for color vision.

All photoreceptor cells (rods and cones) contain special visual pigments that can absorb
light. When light strikes a rod or cone, the light is absorbed by the visual pigment inside the
cell. Absorption of light triggers a series of chemical reactions that result in an action potential. The action potential is then transmitted to the optic nerve and conveyed to the brain.

The Optic Nerves

Each eyeball is connected to a large **optic nerve** (cranial nerve II; see **Figure 12-4**). The
optic nerve contains about 1 million neurons. It runs from the back of each eyeball into the
skull through the optic canal. Inside the skull, the two optic nerves meet on the undersur-
face of the brain and form an "X" that is called the **optic chiasm.** Here, about half of the
axons in each optic nerve (the axons in the medial part of the nerve) cross the midline and
join with axons from the other eyeball. Posterior to the chiasm, the axons form the optic
tract. Within each optic tract, about 50% of the axons come from the ipsilateral eye (on the
same side), and about 50% come from the opposite (contralateral) eye. All axons in each
optic tract carry visual information from the opposite visual field.

Each optic tract sends axons to three major locations in the brain: the hypothalamus,
the midbrain, and the **primary visual cortex** (with a synapse in the thalamus on the way).
Axons going to the hypothalamus are used to establish circadian rhythms and sleep/wake
cycles. Axons projecting to the midbrain form connections with cranial nerves that control

the extraocular muscles. This allows visual tracking, so that the eye muscles can coordinate the eye with visual stimuli. (Without moving your head, try watching a game of ping-pong or scanning a line of text). These connections in the midbrain are also responsible for visual reflexes. For example, if you shine a flashlight into one eye, both pupils will automatically constrict.

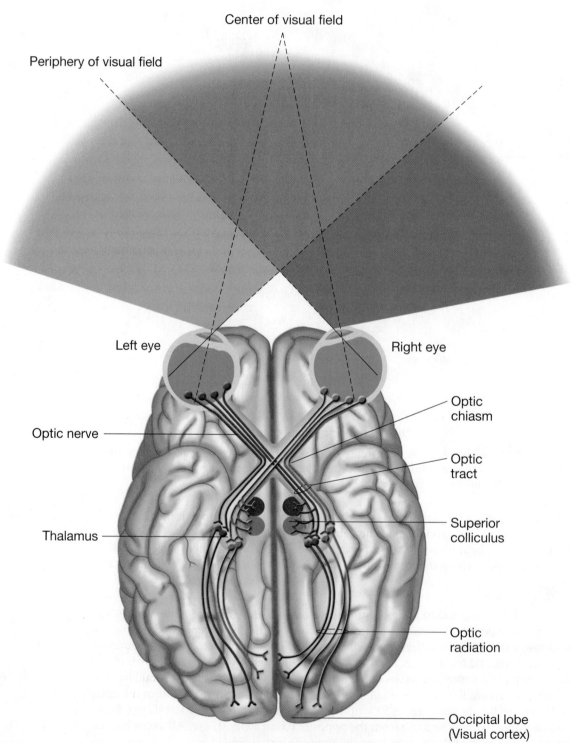

FIGURE 12-4 Each visual field is projected to the contralateral visual cortex in the occipital lobe of the cortex. The visual signals from each eye project to visual cortex in both cerebral hemispheres.

Clinical Box 12-1: Pupillary Constriction

Doctors treating a patient with head trauma often shine a small flashlight into the patient's eye to see if the pupil constricts appropriately. Interestingly, the doctor often pays equal—if not more attention—to the opposite eye. If one pupil constricts, and the other does not, it may be a sign of a concussion or bleeding affecting the midbrain.

Challenge question: What should a clinician do if he or she notices that a patient's pupils are unequal?

Most axons in the optic tracts project to the thalamus, where they synapse onto neurons that carry action potentials to the primary visual cortex. This pathway allows perception of visual stimuli. Primary visual cortex is located in the occipital lobe at the back of the brain. When action potentials reach the primary visual cortex, we are able to consciously perceive the visual information.

Visual Perception and Processing

Visual perception takes place in the primary visual cortex. From there, axons project to other areas of the brain that allow us to interpret and understand what we are seeing, and to determine its meaning (see **Figure 12-5**). Some neurons travel to the visual association cortex, which allows visual recognition of objects. Other neurons project to the parietal lobe, where they connect to neurons concerned with locating objects in space and

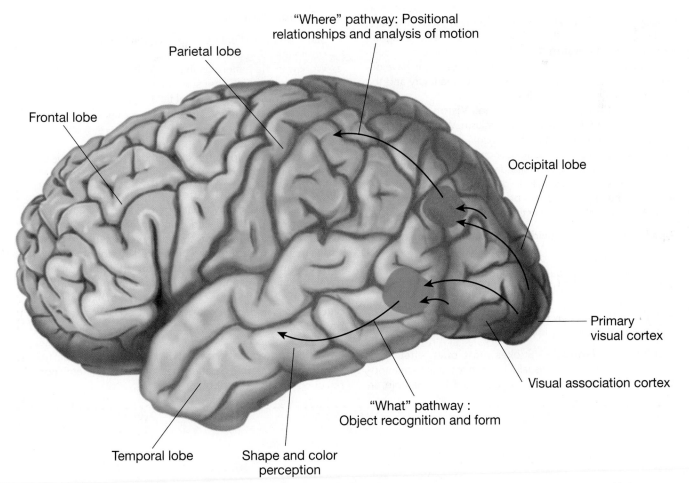

FIGURE 12-5 The primary visual cortex projects to visual association cortex, to the parietal lobe, and to the temporal lobe. These connections allow interpretation and functional use of visual information.

perceiving spatial relationships. (This is sometimes referred to as the "where" pathway.) Finally, a third group of neurons from the primary visual cortex projects to the temporal lobe. Here, a region called inferotemporal cortex allows us to determine the size, color, shape, and texture of what we are seeing. (This might be called the "what" pathway.) Parts of inferotemporal cortex are devoted only to visual recognition of faces; they are sometimes called the "grandmother cells." Damage to these cells causes a clinical condition called prosopagnosia, in which people cannot identify faces of famous or familiar people.

Damage to one optic tract, or to primary visual cortex on one side of the brain causes loss of vision in the opposite visual field; this is called **hemianopsia.** Hemianopsia is common after CVA (stroke). If the primary visual cortex is injured on both sides, the patient will have **cortical blindness.** People with cortical blindness cannot perceive (see) anything, even though their eyes and optic nerves are intact. This is because visual perception actually takes place in the visual cortex.

Clinical Box 12-2: Three Different Lesions—Three Different Results

A properly functioning visual system provides a wide visual field. With the use of "peripheral vision" an individual is able to visually detect objects and motion to a nearly 180-degree field. As discussed earlier in the chapter, information in the left visual field is sent to the right hemisphere, and information from the right visual field is sent to the left hemisphere (see **Figure 12-6A**). Injuries to the brain—such as tumors, traumatic brain injuries, and strokes—can have different outcomes based on the location of the injury and the neuroanatomical structures involved.

Optic Chiasm Lesion—Tunnel Vision Tumors or even strokes can damage the optic chiasm. When this occurs, visual information from the outer visual fields is prevented from crossing the optic chiasm. As shown in **Figure 12-6B**, this results in a very narrow, centralized visual field and is clinically referred to as *tunnel vision*. Individuals who suffer from tunnel vision have a high risk of falls because they do not perceive objects (potential fall risks) in the outer half of the visual field.

Tips for treating an individual with tunnel vision

- Stand directly in front of the patient when communicating or demonstrating.
- Remove rugs and objects from the floor as they may pose a fall risk.
- Balance training may be appropriate, as the lack of peripheral vision may impair balance.

Stroke—Hemianopsia Strokes most often affect one hemisphere of the brain. Visually, this can result in hemianopsia—loss of vision to the opposite visual field. For example, an individual who suffers a stroke affecting the left hemisphere or left optic tract is unable to receive information from the right visual field (see **Figure 12-6C**).

Tips for treating an individual with hemianopsia

- Stand on the patient's unaffected side when communicating or demonstrating.
- Work with the patient on improving his or her visual field and assessing his or her surroundings by rotating the head to scan the entire visual field.
- Promote the use of the affected extremities—prevent neglect.
- Balance training.
- Reduce household clutter and remove throw-rugs to help prevent falls.

Optic Nerve or Eye Damage Individuals who suffer damage to a single optic nerve, damage one eye, or are required to wear an eye patch will all display similar deficits. Although loss of an eye is significant, this injury results in a relatively small visual field loss (this can be verified by closing one eye, and looking around the room). Because information from both visual fields can be gathered from just one eye, there is minimal visual field loss (see **Figure 12-6D**). The loss of one eye does impact depth perception, so clinicians should be cautious when performing activities involving throwing or catching an object.

Challenge question: What might be a good clinical test to distinguish whether a patient has tunnel vision, hemianopsia, or optic nerve damage?

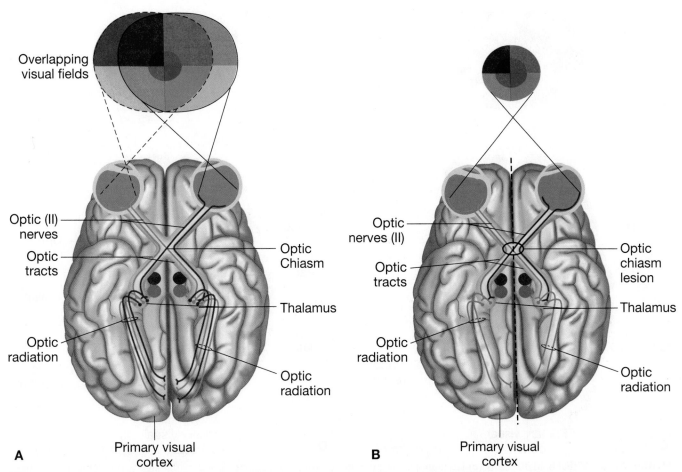

FIGURE 12-6   Visual field diagrams. (a) In a normally functioning visual system, information from each visual field projects to the contralateral visual cortex. (b) Tunnel vision results when there is damage to the optic chiasm that causes patients to lose peripheral vision.

The Auditory System

The auditory system allows us to perceive sound, to locate it in space, and to understand its meaning. For most people, it is important for understanding language and has many connections to language centers in the brain.

The Ear

The ear has three parts: an external, middle, and inner ear (see **Figure 12-7**). The external ear collects sound waves and funnels them to the middle ear. In between the external and middle ears is a thin sheet of tissue called the eardrum (tympanic membrane). When sound waves strike the eardrum, it vibrates, and transmits the vibrations into the middle ear.

The middle ear is a small space (cavity) inside the temporal bone of the skull. It contains three tiny bones called the **auditory ossicles** (the hammer, the anvil, and the stirrup) that are the smallest bones in the human body. The hammer (malleus) rests on the inner surface of the eardrum. When the eardrum vibrates, the malleus moves in response, and transmits the vibration to the anvil (incus), which sends it to the stirrup (stapes). The stapes is attached to another membrane called the oval window, which separates the middle ear from the inner ear. Thus, the auditory ossicles transmit the vibration caused by sound waves through the middle ear cavity into the inner ear.

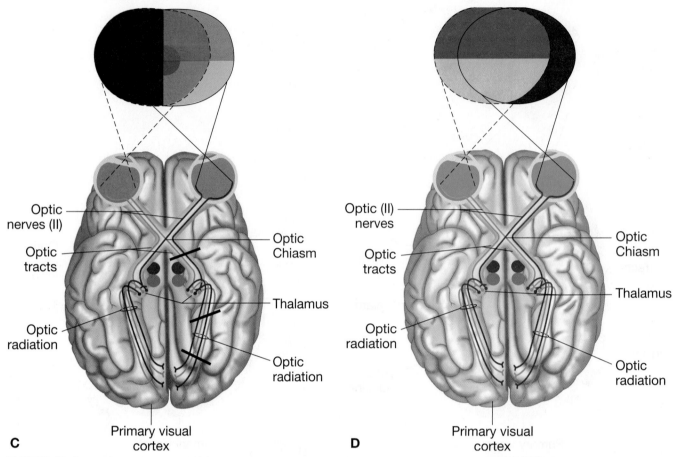

C **D**

FIGURE 12-6 Visual field diagrams. (c) Hemianopsia is a unilateral visual field deficit caused by damage to one optic tract, optic radiation, or to the primary visual cortex on one side. Patients lose vision in the visual field contralateral to the lesion. (d) Loss of vision in one eye results from damage to the ipsilateral optic nerve.

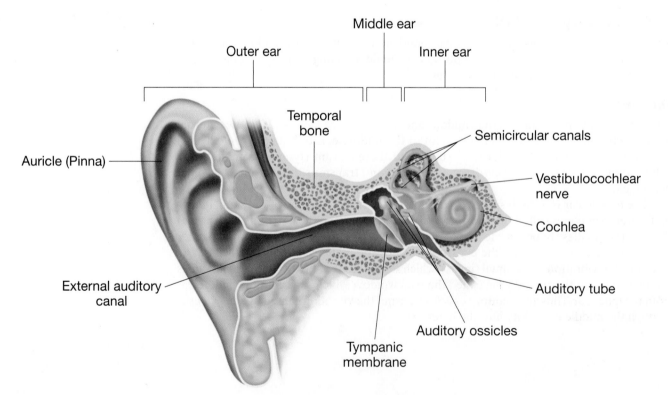

FIGURE 12-7 • The ear consists of three parts: the external ear channels sound waves, the middle ear transmits sound waves to the inner ear, and the inner ear contains sensory receptors for both hearing and head movement (used to maintain balance).

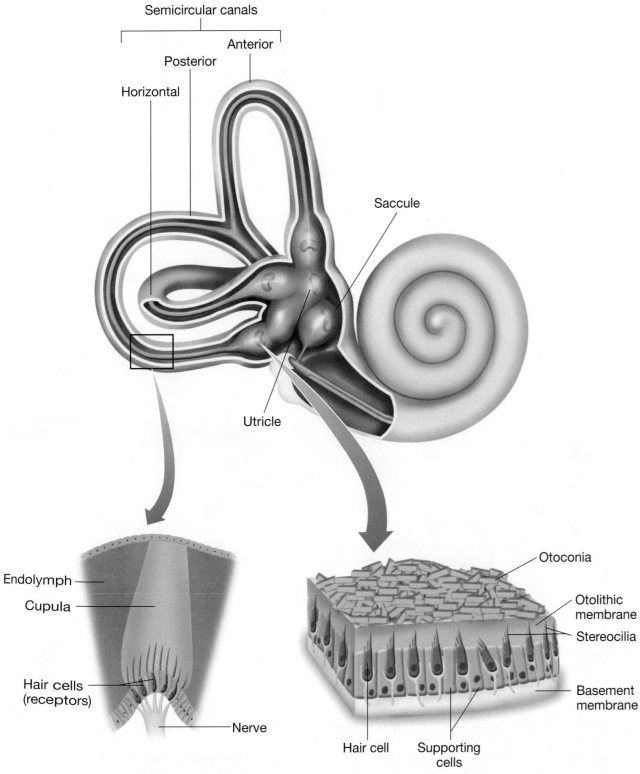

FIGURE 12-10 The vestibular apparatus consists of the semicircular canals and the otolithic organs (utricle and saccule); together, these detect head position and movement.

Neuroscience Notes Box 12-2:
Osteogenesis Imperfecta

O steogenesis imperfecta, sometimes referred to as "brittle bone disease," is an inherited condition that causes bones to form poorly and break very easily. People with osteogenesis imperfecta may display hearing loss or become deaf because the small middle ear bones are malformed or become fractured, so sounds are not transmitted through the middle ear cavity.

There are two parts to the inner ear: the **cochlea** (for hearing) and the **vestibular apparatus** (for balance). The cochlea is a spiral-shaped hollow space located deep inside the temporal bone. It is lined with a membrane (the basilar membrane) and contains fluid (endolymph). The fluid is secreted by cells in the basilar membrane, and it fills both the cochlea and the vestibular part of the inner ear.

The sensory receptors for sound are located in the inner ear. Inside the cochlea, the receptor cells responsible for hearing are found within the **organ of Corti** (see **Figure 12-8**).

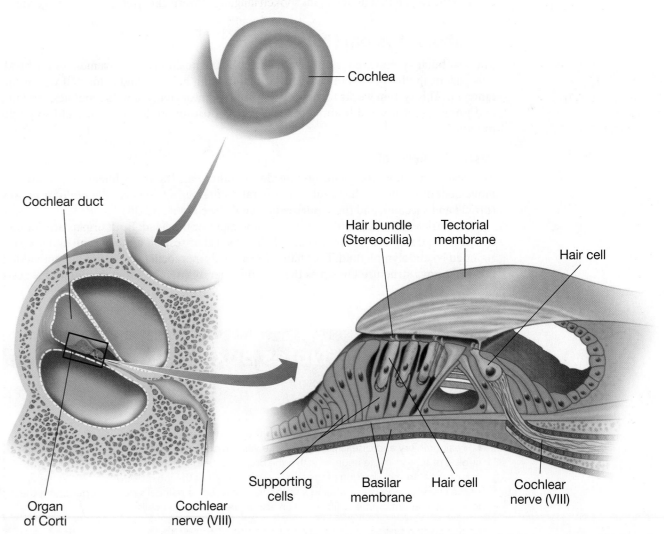

FIGURE 12-8 The cochlea is part of the inner ear and contains auditory receptors called "hair cells" that convert sound into action potentials. The hair cells are stimulated by movement of the tectorial membrane in the organ of Corti.

The organ of Corti consists of about 18,000 auditory receptor cells called "hair cells." These cells look hairy because each has many long projections called stereocilia on its surface. The tips of the "hairs" are embedded in a goo-like substance called the tectorial membrane.

When sound waves are transmitted through the middle ear by the auditory ossicles, they cause movement of the oval window. When the oval window moves, endolymph fluid inside the cochlea also moves, as does the gooey tectorial membrane. Movement of the tectorial membrane pulls on the tips of the hair cells embedded in it, causing them to bend. This opens ion channels in the hair cell membranes, and releases a neurotransmitter that activates the vestibulocochlear nerve (CN VIII). So, bending of the hair cell stereocilia triggers the nerve impulse that allows hearing.

Vestibulocochlear Nerve (CN VIII) and Auditory Processing

Cochlear hair cells in the inner ear form synapses with neurons in the cochlear part of the **vestibulocochlear nerve** (see Figure 12-9). The cochlear portion of the nerve joins with the vestibular portion and together they enter the skull.

Neurons conveying hearing project to neurons located on both sides of the brainstem. From the brainstem, they connect to the thalamus, and from there, neurons project to the **primary auditory cortex** in the temporal lobe where perception of the sound takes place. Each primary auditory cortex receives input from both ears, and each ear sends signals to both sides of the brain. This is important for locating sounds in space. From primary auditory cortex, projections travel to the auditory association area where sounds are interpreted. There are also many neurons connecting auditory cortex to the language areas of the brain, especially to the region that understands spoken language (Wernicke's receptive language area).

Vestibular System (Balance)

The vestibular system is concerned with detecting the position and movement of the head. It is part of the body's overall system for maintaining balance, and is located within the inner ear. This system works together with proprioceptors located in the muscles, tendons, and joints to inform the brain about the body's position and movement, and to guide motion.

Vestibular Apparatus

The vestibular apparatus is located inside the inner ear. It detects linear and rotational movement of the head. The vestibular apparatus consists of two parts: the **otolithic organs** (utricle and saccule), and the **semicircular canals** (see Figure 12-10).

The utricle and saccule detect linear movement of the head. Both organs are formed by specialized sensory receptor cells ("hair cells") that rest on a membrane and are surrounded by endolymph fluid. The "hairs" are actually stereocilia whose tips are embedded in a gelatinous structure known as the otolithic membrane. The otolithic membrane rests

Neuroscience Notes Box 12-3:
Hearing Loss

Hearing loss can result from damage to the middle ear bones, the hair cells in the inner ear, or injury and diseases affecting the vestibulocochlear nerve. It can also occur when strokes or tumors injure neurons within the brain that help process these signals. Loud noises can cause extreme vibration of the tectorial membrane in the inner ear, which causes the tips of the stereocilia to break off and kills the hair cells. Since hair cells do not regenerate, this loss is permanent. Some antibiotics can also injure and kill hair cells.

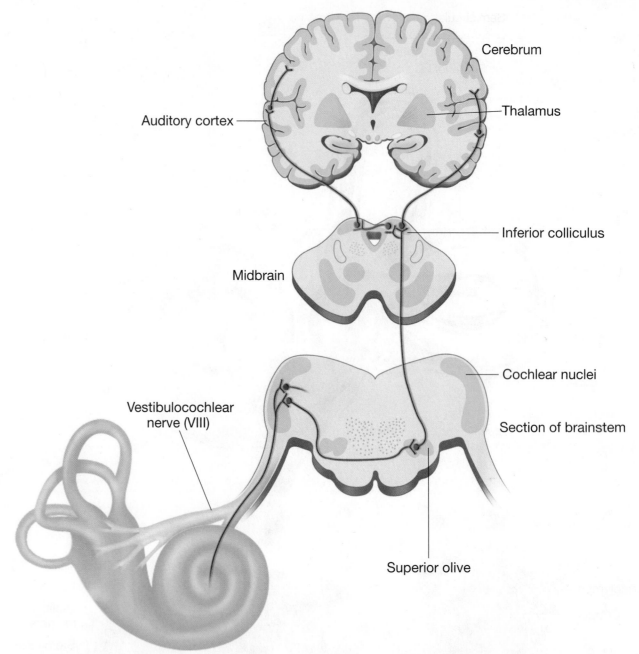

FIGURE 12-9 The auditory pathway begins in the cochlea, and conveys auditory information to the auditory cortex on both sides of the brain.

on top of the hair cells. It is covered with small calcium carbonate crystals called otoliths or otoconia (they are also called "ear stones" or "ear sand").

When the head moves, the otoliths, otolithic membrane, and endolymph all move along with it. Because the otolithic membrane and the tiny crystals embedded in it are much denser and heavier than the endolymph, the membrane moves at a much slower rate than does the fluid. This difference results in displacement (bending) of the stereocilia. When the tips of the hair cells bend one way, the hair cell is depolarized and releases a neurotransmitter. When they bend the other way, the cell is hyperpolarized and stops releasing the neurotransmitter.

The utricle detects horizontal plane motion, such as when accelerating forward in a car or in an airplane that is accelerating down a runway for takeoff. The saccule is responsible

for detecting vertical (up and down) movement such as when jumping up and down or when traveling in a fast-moving elevator.

The semicircular canals are also located inside the inner ear. There are three pairs of semicircular canals; each pair is responsible for detecting a different direction of head movement. Each semicircular canal contains specialized "hair cells" with stereocilia on their surface. The stereocilia are embedded in a gelatinous membrane known as the cupula. (It is similar to the otolithic membrane found in the utricle and saccule, but it lacks the tiny otoconia.) Movement of the head causes the endolymph and the cupula to move, which causes the stereocilia to bend. As in the otolithic organs, movement in one direction depolarizes the hair cells, whereas movement in the other direction hyperpolarizes and therefore inhibits them.

When hair cells in the utricle, saccule, or semicircular canals are depolarized, they stimulate the vestibular portion of the vestibulocochlear nerve (CN VIII). This signal travels along the nerve, eventually synapsing in the brainstem **vestibular nuclei.** From there, axons project to the motor cortex, the cerebellum, and the spinal cord. The brain uses this information to coordinate balance and guide movement (see **Figure 12-11**).

Proprioceptors

Normal balance and movement requires input from three sources: the inner ear vestibular apparatus, the visual system, and peripheral structures including muscles, tendons, and joints. The sensory receptors responsible for detecting the state of these structures

Neuroscience Notes Box 12-4: Vertigo

Vertigo is a sensation of extreme dizziness; it feels as though you are spinning even when you are stationary. It can be caused by injury or disease that affects the vestibular apparatus, cerebellum, or vestibulocochlear nerve. Some causes of vertigo include Meniere's disease, migraine, multiple sclerosis, vestibular neuritis (inflammation of the vestibulocochlear nerve), and benign paroxysmal positional vertigo (BPPV). Regardless of the cause, vertigo results from conflicting information sent to the vestibular cortex from the inner ear, the visual system, and the proprioceptors located in muscles and joints.

The two parts of the inner ear are connected by a small duct through which fluid (endolymph) flows; thus, diseases of, or injuries to, one part of the inner ear can affect both parts. **Meniere's disease** is a condition in which excess endolymph causes swelling inside the vestibular apparatus and cochlea. This inflammation can cause debilitating vertigo as well as hearing loss. Meniere's disease is usually treated with medication to decrease the amount of fluid in the inner ear.

A common cause of vertigo is benign paroxysmal positional vertigo (BPPV). People who suffer from BPPV have episodes of dizziness or vertigo that last from 5 to 30 seconds, most often resulting from a rapid change in head position such as rolling over in bed or tipping the head back to look upward. BPPV is caused by otoconia (the "ear rocks") that have become dislodged from the utricle, and fall into the posterior semicircular canal, where they bend the hair cells. Bending of the hair cells sends a message to the brain that the head is rotating or moving—even though it is not. This message is in direct conflict with the positional messages sent to the brain from the eyes that "the head is *not* moving." The inability of the brain to determine which signal is correct results in vertigo. A clinical sign of vertigo is nystagmus, characterized by "jumping" of the eyes. Therapists often confirm a diagnosis of BPPV by performing a Dix-Hallpike test that involves moving a person from sitting to supine while rotating and extending the head. If person displays nystagmus after this test, it is likely they have BPPV.

Trained clinicians commonly treat BPPV by performing either the Epley or Semont maneuvers (see **Figure 12-12**). Both of these treatments involve a sequence of head movements that help to re-position the dislodged otoconia back into the utricle (or to a less sensitive part of the semicircular canal).

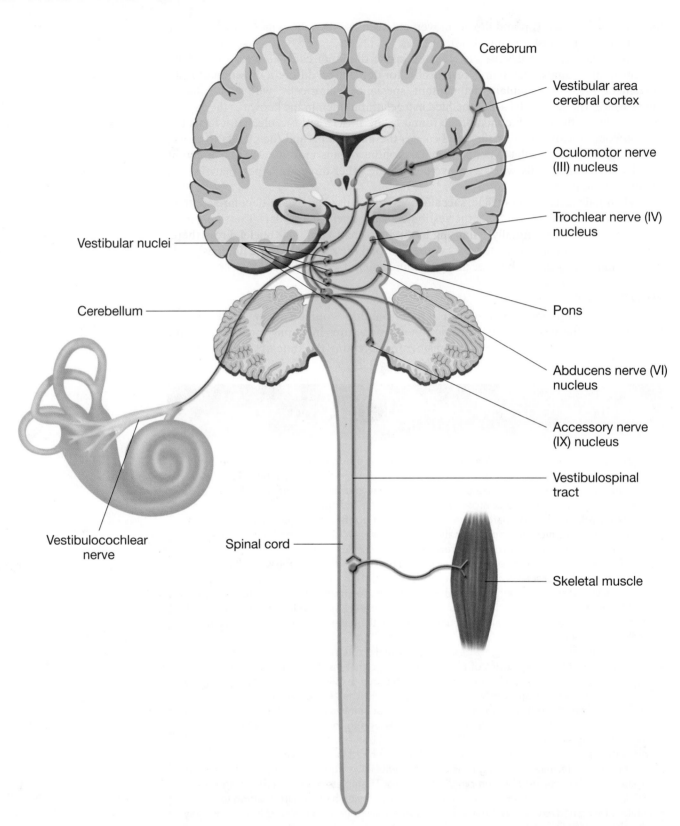

FIGURE 12-11 The vestibular apparatus sends action potentials into the brainstem vestibular nuclei where they project to the sensory cortex, cerebellum, cranial nerves that control eye and neck movement, and spinal nerves that control skeletal mucles.

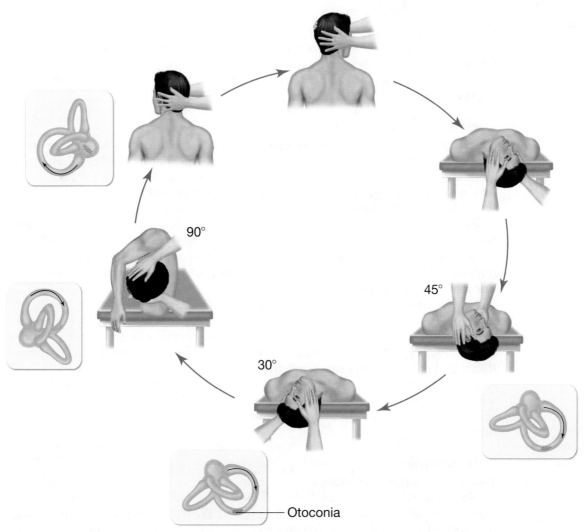

90°

45°

30°

Otoconia

FIGURE 12-12   The Epley maneuver places the patient's head in a sequence of positions in order to move otoconia out of the semicircular canal.

are called **proprioceptors.** Proprioceptors include muscle spindles (to detect muscle stretch), Golgi tendon organs (to detect muscle tension), and joint receptors (to detect position and motion of joints; these are found in joint capsules and ligaments). Information gathered from the proprioceptors is processed in the brain along with information from the visual and vestibular systems to provide proper control of balance and movement.

The most important brain structure for controlling balance is the cerebellum. The cerebellum receives input from the vestibular nuclei, from visual cortex, and from muscles, joints, and tendons. It has many connections to motor centers in the brain. A very important connection is to the ipsilateral (same side) vestibular nuclei in the brainstem. From these nuclei, the vestibulospinal tracts descend in the spinal cord to control motor neurons. The vestibulospinal tracts primarily control muscles used to maintain balance, including hip and knee extensors, as well as ankle plantarflexors and dorsiflexors.

Smell and Taste

The senses of smell and taste are essential for making sure that we do not eat spoiled food and that we avoid substances that could be harmful (e.g., feces, rotten meat, anything potentially diseased). These senses also add pleasure to life; people who lose one or both of them report that many experiences seem dull and bland. Smell and taste work together to provide a rich sensory experience.

Smell (Olfaction)

The receptors for smell **(olfactory receptors)** are located in the top of the nasal cavity (see Figure 12-13). The receptor cells are shaped like bowling pins. Part of each cell projects down into the nose, and a thin layer of mucus covers them. When air flows across these cells, molecules to be smelled are dissolved in the mucus and bind to the receptor cells. When the odor molecule binds to a receptor cell, the receptor cell is activated and an action potential results. The axons of each receptor cell poke up through tiny holes in the ethmoid bone to the base of the brain. There, they synapse onto neurons in the olfactory bulb, which sends axons through the **olfactory tract** to two main areas of the brain: the limbic system (for emotional responses to odors) and the **primary olfactory cortex** in the temporal lobe (for conscious awareness of the odor).

Loss of one's sense of smell is called **anosmia.** This can be temporary if the olfactory receptors in the nose are blocked by mucus (such as from a head cold or influenza). The receptor cells can also be damaged by head trauma, especially to the ethmoid bone. Olfactory cells can regenerate, so the sense of smell usually returns (Barber and Raisman, 1982). Anosmia can result from trauma to the temporal lobes of the brain, and is also common in people with Parkinson Disease and some forms of dementia. Sometimes a brain tumor or epileptic seizure can stimulate the primary olfactory cortex and produce olfactory hallucinations. These are usually unpleasant odors (like burning rubber).

Taste (Gustation)

Taste receptors (taste buds) are located on the tongue. They are found along the sides of the lingual papillae (the bumps visible on the tongue; see Figure 12-14). We have about 10,000 taste buds, and they are constantly replaced. Food molecules are dissolved in saliva (or another liquid) and bind to receptor molecules located on the taste bud cells. Without the fluid, taste cannot be perceived. (If you dry your tongue and put some salt or sugar on it, you will not be able to taste it.)

Taste buds respond to five different kinds of tastes: (1) salty, (2) sweet, (3) sour, (4) bitter, and (5) umami, which conveys a sense of "flavorfullness." Chemicals in food either release ions that enter taste bud cells, or they bind to proteins on the taste bud cell surface. Either way, taste bud cells generate action potentials that are conveyed to the brain through several cranial nerves (VII, IX, and X). Interestingly, ATP is the neurotransmitter that connects the taste bud cells to the cranial nerves (Finger et al., 2005). In the brain, taste is perceived in a small gustatory (taste) region of the sensory cortex. Recent evidence suggests that different kinds of tastes (bitter, sweet, etc.) have separate neural pathways and circuits (Sugita and Shiba, 2005). However, a great deal of the flavor of food is conveyed by its smell. Without the sense of smell to accompany taste, food loses much of its flavor.

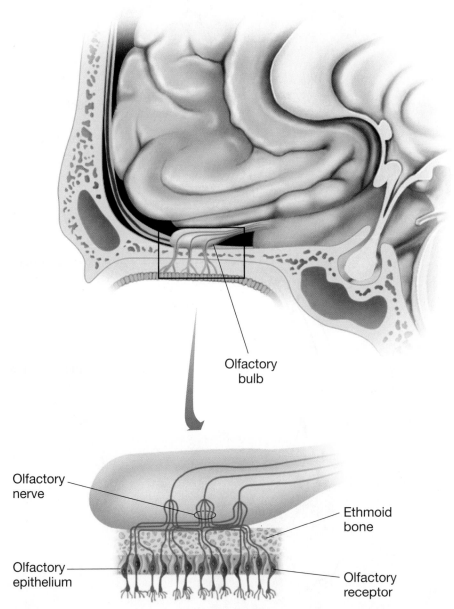

Olfactory
bulb

Olfactory
nerve

Ethmoid
bone

Olfactory
epithelium

Olfactory
receptor

FIGURE 12-13 The olfactory system converts odors into action potentials and sends them to the brain where they are perceived. Olfactory receptors are located in the olfactory epithelium in the nasal cavity and connect to the olfactory nerve (Cranial nerve I).

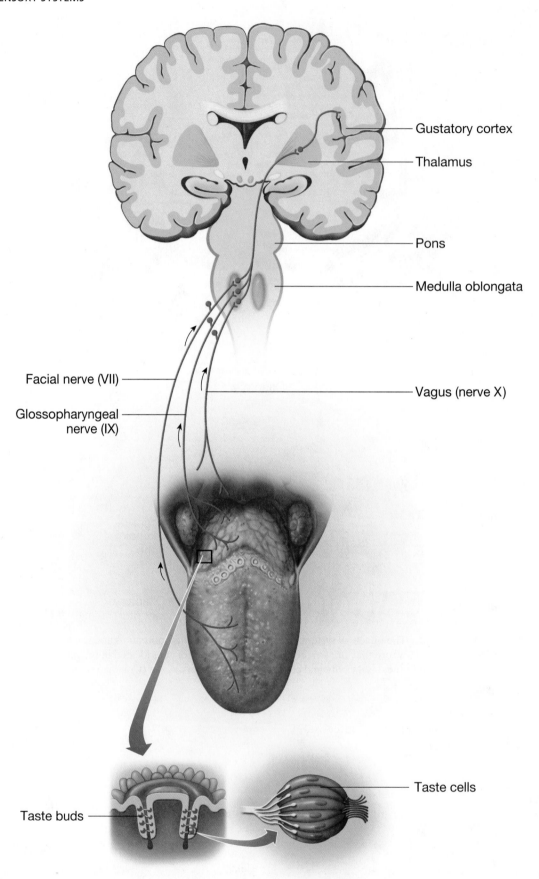

FIGURE 12-14 The gustatory (taste) system converts molecules dissolved in salvia into action potentials that are conveyed to the brain by several cranial nerves.

PATIENT SCENARIOS

Patient Case 12-1 (Jennie)

Jennie is a 21-year-old college student who hit her head in a bicycle accident one month ago and has subsequently experienced bouts of vertigo that last for several seconds or minutes at a time. The vertigo tends to begin when she moves her head suddenly or changes her position quickly. Jennie's diagnosis is benign paroxysmal positional vertigo (BPPV). She is referred to physical therapy and her physical therapist performs a series of specific motions to her head. This procedure is known as the Epley maneuver. After the treatment, Jennie's dizziness disappears.

Questions

a) What structures were probably dislodged in the bike accident, causing vertigo?
b) How did the displacement of the structures produce the symptoms of vertigo?
c) Besides BPPV, what are some other common causes of vertigo?

Patient Case 12-2 (Hazel)

Hazel, age 77, suffered a stroke that affected the right side of her brain, including the right occipital lobe. Hazel is having difficulty seeing anything in her left visual field. For example, she is unaware of someone seated on her left side, and she combs only the hair on the right side of her head. She tends to look toward the right and it is easiest to get her attention by standing on her right side.

Questions

a) What is this type of visual deficit called?
b) Why is Hazel able to see what is on her right side, but not what is on her left?
c) If Hazel is your patient, how might you modify your treatment approach in view of this visual field deficit?

Review Questions

1. Describe the structure and function of the eyeball, including the function of photoreceptors.

2. Explain the connections between the optic nerve and major regions of the brain involved in perceiving and processing visual information. How are the "what" and "where" visual pathways different?

3. Predict the functional consequences of damage to the eye, retina, optic nerve, optic tract, and primary visual cortex. What would happen if the primary visual cortex on both sides of the brain were destroyed?

4. Describe how sound waves reach the sensory receptors for hearing inside the inner ear. How are sound waves converted into action potentials? Which cranial nerve transmits signals from the cochlea to the brain? Where is hearing perceived?

5. Describe the structure and function of the vestibular system. Which cranial nerve sends signals from the vestibular apparatus to the brain?

6. Describe symptoms associated with vestibular system pathologies, including Meniere's disease and benign paroxysmal positional vertigo (BPPV).

7. Where are sensory receptors for smell and taste located? Which cranial nerves transmit these sensations to the brain? Where are smell and taste perceived?

References

1. Barber, P. C., & Raisman, G. (1982). Cell division in the vomeronasal organ of the adult mouse. *Brain Res.*, *141*, 57–66.

2. Finger, T. E., Danilova, V., Barrows, J., Bartel, D. L., Vigers, A. J., Stone, L., Hellekant, G., & Kinnamon, S. C. (2005). ATP signaling is crucial for communication from taste buds to gustatory nerves. *Science, 310*, 1495–1499.

3. Sugita, M., & Shiba, Y. (2005). Genetic tracing shows segregation of taste neuronal circuitries for bitter and sweet. *Science, 309*, 781–785.

Further Reading

1. Bhandawat, V., Reisert, J., & Yau, K-W. (2005). Elementary response of olfactory receptor neurons to odorants. *Science, 308,* 1931–1934.

2. Grueter, T. (2006, February/March). Picture this: How does the brain create images in our minds? *Scientific American Mind,* 18–23.

3. Kim, J., Wu, H.-H., Lander, A. D., Lyons, K. M., Matzuk, M. M., & Calof, A. L. (2005). GDF11 controls the timing of progenitor cell competence in developing retina. *Science, 308,* 1927–1930.

PEARSON

myhealthprofessionskit™

Use this address to access the Companion Website created for this textbook. Simply select "Physical Therapy" from the choice of disciplines. Find this book and log in using your username and password to access self-assessment questions, a glossary and more.

Motor Systems and Movement

CHAPTER OBJECTIVES

After completing this chapter, the reader will be able to:

1. Describe how lower motor neurons produce muscle contraction, and the effects of lower motor neuron injury on function and muscle tone.

2. Explain how upper motor neurons control lower motor neuron function, describe the spinal cord pathways that contain upper motor neurons, and discuss the effects of upper motor neuron injury on function and muscle tone.

3. List the functions of the cerebellum, and discuss the effects of cerebellar injury.

4. Explain how the basal ganglia are involved in movement, and how basal ganglia pathologies affect movement, thought, and mood.

5. Discuss the role of the motor planning areas of the brain and describe the effects of injury to these regions.

KEY TERMS

apraxia
ataxia
basal ganglia (nuclei)
bradykinesia
cerebellum
corticobulbar tract
corticospinal tract
disequilibrium
dysdiadochokinesis
dyskinesia
lower motor neuron
motor end plate
motor homunculus
motor neuron
motor point
motor unit
muscle fiber (myofiber)
muscle tone
neuromuscular junction
paralysis
paresis
primary motor cortex
reticulospinal tract
supplementary motor area (SMA)
tectospinal tract
upper motor neuron (UMN)
vestibulospinal tract

Essential Facts···

▶ Motor neurons are required for skeletal muscle function.

▶ Lower motor neurons directly innervate skeletal muscles and form synapses with muscle cells.

▶ Upper motor neurons from the brain control activity of lower motor neurons through descending tracts in the spinal cord.

▶ The cerebellum directs function of the upper motor neurons and controls coordination, muscle tone, balance and gait.

▶ The basal ganglia control upper motor neuron activity and are responsible for movement initiation and inhibition.

▶ The supplementary motor area stores motor memories.

This chapter describes the nerves and brain regions that produce normal body movement. Movement requires integration of many parts of the nervous system, including the cerebral cortex, cerebellum, basal ganglia, brainstem, spinal cord, and the peripheral nerves. Injury to any of these can alter or even eliminate the ability to move normally.

Motor Neurons

Motor neurons are nerve cells that cause muscles to contract. Three kinds of muscle tissue are found in the human body: skeletal muscle, cardiac muscle, and smooth muscle; this chapter will focus on the nervous system's control of skeletal muscle. Skeletal muscle tissue forms the body's voluntary muscles. The regulation of cardiac and smooth muscle (involuntary muscle) is performed by the autonomic nervous system, and is discussed in chapter 10.

Lower Motor Neurons and Muscle Contraction

Skeletal (voluntary) muscle is made up of cells known as **muscle fibers;** these are also called *myofibers* or *myocytes*. The motor neurons that innervate skeletal muscle are known as **lower motor neurons.** Lower motor neurons synapse directly into skeletal muscle fibers. Their cell bodies are located in either the brainstem or the spinal cord, and their axons form part of many spinal nerves and cranial nerves.

Every peripheral (motor) nerve enters the belly of a skeletal muscle at a **motor point.** From there, each lower motor neuron divides into numerous branches. Each branch ends in an axon terminal, and each axon terminal forms a synapse with one skeletal muscle cell (fiber). The synapse between a lower motor neuron and a muscle fiber is called the **neuromuscular junction** (see Figure 13-1). Each neuromuscular junction is enclosed by a connective tissue sheath that protects the synapse and separates it from the surrounding tissue.

At the neuromuscular junction, each axon terminal releases the neurotransmitter acetylcholine (Ach). The muscle cell membrane at neuromuscular junctions is called the **motor end plate.** It is extensively folded, and it contains membrane proteins that are receptors for acetylcholine. When acetylcholine is released from the axon terminals, it binds to its receptors on the motor end plate and Na^+ ions flow into the muscle cell. The Na^+ influx moves along the muscle cell membrane, causing the muscle cell to depolarize.

Inside the muscle cell, Ca^{+2} ions are stored inside small chambers that are connected to the muscle cell membrane. The chambers are called the *sarcoplasmic reticulum (SR)*, and have many voltage-gated Ca^{+2} channels in their membranes. When the muscle cell

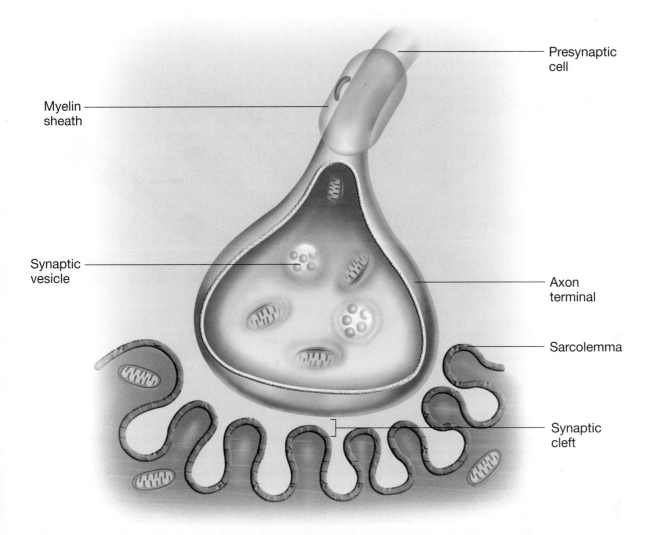

Myelin
sheath

Synaptic
vesicle

Presynaptic
cell

Axon
terminal

Sarcolemma

Synaptic
cleft

FIGURE 13-1   The neuromuscular junction is a synapse between a motor neuron and a skeletal muscle cell. The neuron releases the neurotransmitter acetylcholine, which diffuses across the synaptic cleft and stimulates skeletal muscle contraction.

depolarizes, Ca^{+2} ions are released from the sarcoplasmic reticulum and enter the muscle cell cytoplasm. The Ca^{+2} ions trigger contraction of the muscle, producing tension and movement. After muscle contraction begins, the Ca^{+2} ions are pumped back into the sarcoplasmic reticulum where they are stored until the next contraction of that muscle fiber.

In order to inactivate the neuromuscular junction, acetylcholine must be removed from its receptor. An enzyme (acetylcholinesterase) degrades acetylcholine within the synaptic cleft. This frees the receptor so that another molecule of acetylcholine can bind to it, and muscular contraction may continue. Clinically, drugs that inhibit acetylcholinesterase can be used to improve muscle function (e.g., in people with myasthenia gravis where the immune system destroys some of the acetylcholine receptors).

Skeletal muscle activation can occur only when lower motor neurons stimulate the muscle. Similarly, relaxation of a voluntary muscle can occur only when the lower motor neurons to that muscle are inhibited. Thus, the lower motor neuron is the only means by which the rest of the nervous system can communicate with skeletal muscles. The lower motor neuron is sometimes referred to as the "final common pathway" to a muscle, because all other parts of the nervous system control muscles through interaction with lower motor neurons.

Lower motor neurons that activate skeletal muscles can become damaged from disease or injury. Without stimulation, a muscle fiber will be unable to contract. If enough muscle cells lose their motor neurons, the muscle as a whole will be denervated and the result is **paresis** (weakness) or **paralysis** (loss of function).

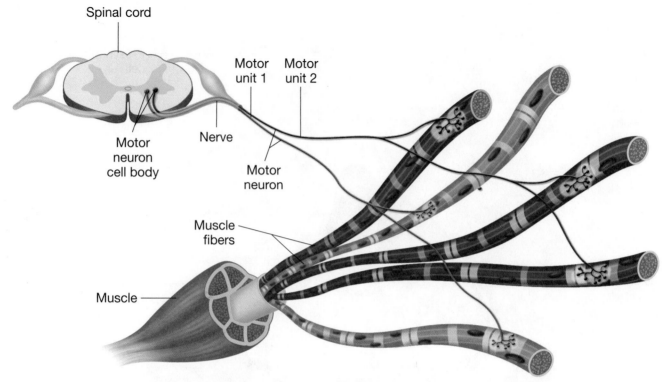

FIGURE 13-2   A motor unit consists of one lower motor neuron and all muscle fibers it innervates.

A single lower motor neuron and all of the muscle fibers it innervates form a **motor unit** (see Figure 13-2). Motor units range in size from small (1 lower motor neuron innervating about 20 muscle fibers) to very large (1 lower motor neuron innervating about 2,000 muscle fibers). The nervous system can control muscles that have small motor units very precisely. Thus, small motor units are found in muscles that move the eyes (extraocular muscles), the vocal cords (laryngeal muscles), the face (muscles of facial expression), and the fingers (intrinsic hand muscles). In contrast, muscles with large motor units—such as the intrinsic back muscles, the gluteus maximus, and the quadriceps femoris—generate strong, powerful contractions, and contract to maintain posture.

Muscle force is controlled by activating (recruiting) individual motor units until the desired amount of force is achieved. Usually, small motor units are recruited first, and gradually larger motor units are added to generate increased tension in the muscle. This is known as the size principle, and it allows the gradual development and control of muscle tension and force.

Upper Motor Neurons and Motor Tracts

Upper motor neurons (UMNs) connect the brain with lower motor neurons. The cell bodies of UMNs are located in the cerebral cortex and brainstem (see Figure 13-3). All other brain structures that influence movement, such as the cerebellum, basal ganglia, and the supplementary motor area act via these upper motor neuron systems.

Cortical upper motor neurons have their cell bodies in the frontal lobe. In humans, most (60%) of these neurons are located in the **primary motor cortex** (see Figure 13-4). Other cortical upper motor neurons are located in the premotor cortex, the supplementary motor area, and the primary somatosensory cortex on the postcentral gyrus.

Cortical upper motor neurons are organized in a specific pattern that creates a detailed map of the body (a **motor homunculus;** see Figure 13-5). The motor homunculus is organized so that areas of the body used for executing precise movements (e.g., fingers, lips, tongue) take up a large amount of space on the motor cortex, whereas areas with less precise movements use less space. This is known as proportional representation. The motor homunculus is "plastic" or flexible, and can be altered by increased or decreased use of a body part. For example, violin players have a larger part of the motor cortex for digits 2 through 5 on the left hand (which plays the notes) compared to the right hand (which holds the bow). Removal of a digit reduces the size of that body part on the motor homunculus.

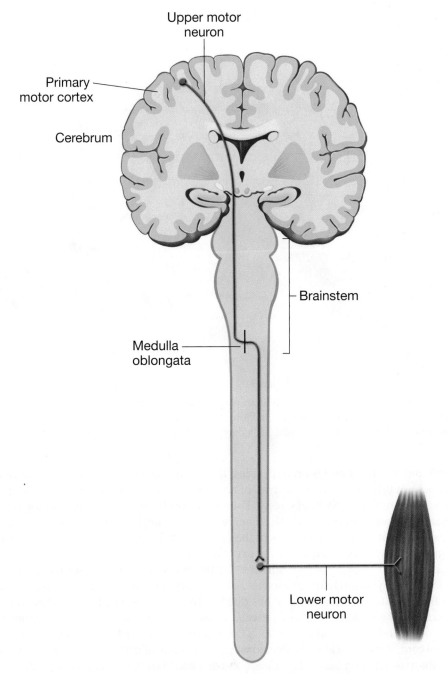

FIGURE 13-3 Upper motor neurons originate in the brain and control activity of lower motor neurons, which stimulate skeletal muscle contraction. Upper motor neurons that originate in the primary motor cortex usually control skeletal muscles on the contralateral (opposite) side of the body, as shown here.

Upper motor neurons that begin in the cerebral cortex form several descending (motor) tracts. *Tracts* are bundles of upper motor neuron axons that travel together in the white matter of the brainstem and spinal cord. The axons that connect the cortex to spinal cord lower motor neurons form the **corticospinal** (pyramidal) **tracts** (see Figure 13-6). Axons that connect the cortex to lower motor neurons located in cranial nerves form the **corticobulbar tracts.** Together, the corticospinal and corticobulbar tracts are responsible for generating complex, precise movements. They innervate all skeletal muscles, but most of them control lower motor neurons to distal limb muscles, as well as muscles used in speech production, eye movements, and facial expressions.

Fibers in the corticospinal tracts cross in the brainstem, so the right motor cortex controls muscles on the left side of the body (and vice versa). Most corticobulbar tracts are

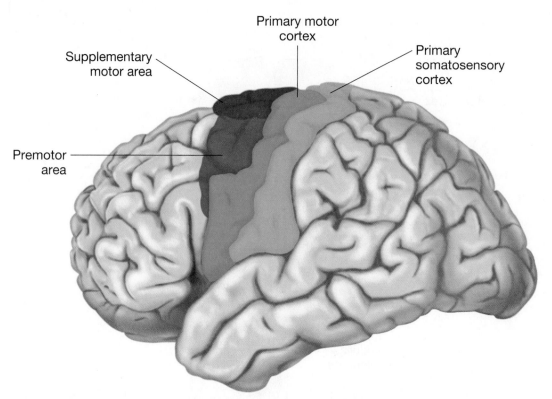

FIGURE 13-4 Motor areas of the cortex include primary motor cortex, premotor cortex, and the supplementary motor area, all located in the frontal lobe. Some upper motor neurons originate in the primary somatosensory cortex in the parietal lobe, providing a connection between sensation and movement.

bilateral, and control muscles on both sides. Thus, a unilateral lesion to the corticobulbar fibers does not usually result in paralysis of muscles innervated by cranial nerves, although there may be mild paresis (weakness). The exception to bilateral upper motor neuron innervation of cranial nerves is the facial nerve (CN VII); upper motor neurons that supply muscles located in the bottom portion of the face have only contralateral upper motor neuron control. Sometimes voluntary facial expression may be lost after upper motor neuron injury, but emotional expression is still present; this is because some upper motor neurons to the facial nerve originate in emotional areas of the brain (e.g., anterior cingulate cortex).

In the brainstem, corticospinal axons divide into two tracts. The majority (90%) of the axons cross to the opposite side and descend in the lateral white matter of the spinal cord, forming the lateral corticospinal tract (LCST; see Figure 13-7). The LCST is the largest tract in the spinal cord. It is almost always affected when there is any injury to the cord. The remaining 10% of the axons stay on the ipsilateral side and descend in the ventral part of the spinal cord to form the anterior corticospinal tract (ACST). The ACST contains upper motor neurons that synapse only onto lower motor neurons innervating muscles of the neck, trunk, and proximal upper extremity. This tract extends as far as the lower thoracic level of the spinal cord.

Upper motor neurons in the lateral corticospinal tract synapse directly into lower motor neurons in the ventral horn of the spinal cord, and also form synapses with interneurons in the grey matter. *Interneurons* are small nerve cells located in the spinal cord that connect other neurons together into networks or circuits. They also synapse onto lower motor neurons. Thus, lateral corticospinal tract upper motor neurons control lower motor neurons both directly and indirectly. Most of the direct connections control distal limb muscles and allow the motor cortex to generate independent movements of the fingers at individual joints. The indirect connections synapse onto interneurons that either activate or inhibit lower motor neurons. These allow the motor cortex to influence reflex activity and control complex patterns of muscle contraction that are "hard-wired" in the spinal cord.

A second group of upper motor neurons called the extrapyramidal tracts originate in four brainstem nuclei: the reticular formation, the vestibular nuclei, the superior colliculus, and the red nucleus (see Figure 13-8). Together, these upper motor neurons are responsible

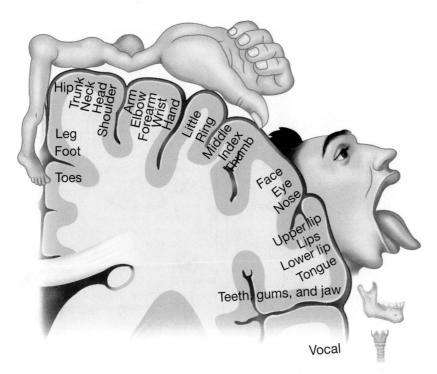

FIGURE 13-5 The motor homunculus is a representation of the body on the primary motor cortex.

for controlling movement of the trunk and proximal extremities, for postural reflexes, and for maintaining and modifying muscle tone.

Upper motor neurons that originate in the brainstem reticular formation (RF) are organized into two reticulospinal tracts (medial and dorsal). Together, the **reticulospinal tracts** control muscles involved in posture and gait. In addition, the dorsal reticulospinal tract modifies muscle tone. Damage to the dorsal reticulospinal tract can result in hypertonic, spastic muscles.

The brainstem vestibular nuclei give rise to the medial and lateral **vestibulospinal (VS) tracts.** They innervate neck, trunk, and proximal limb extensor muscles necessary for maintaining balance. Vestibulospinal neurons also control cranial nerves that innervate the extraocular muscles. These connections help maintain focus on an object while the head is moving.

Upper motor neurons from the superior colliculus (tectum) in the midbrain form the **tectospinal tract.** This tract controls muscles responsible for reflex movements of the neck. Because the superior colliculus receives input from the optic nerves, this pathway links the visual system with neck muscles to allow visual tracking. The final group of upper motor neurons originates in the midbrain red nucleus and forms the small rubrospinal tract. This pathway has a minor role in humans.

Motor Neuron Lesions

Several diseases, such as polio and amyotrophic lateral sclerosis (ALS), target motor neurons specifically. In addition, brain injury, stroke, spinal cord injury, and other conditions can affect motor neurons. Regardless of the cause, lower motor neuron injuries result in hypotonia, hyporeflexia, skeletal muscle atrophy, and muscle weakness or paralysis. Upper motor neuron lesions can also cause paralysis or paresis, but usually result in hypertonia and hyperreflexia due to reticulospinal tract damage.

Because the impulse to move begins in the primary motor cortex, intact cortical upper motor neurons are necessary for voluntary, purposeful movement to take place. Damage to these upper motor neurons will result in loss of voluntary movement (paralysis). However, reflex muscle contraction is still possible if lower motor neurons are intact. This can occur because lower motor neurons are influenced by several other sources within the spinal

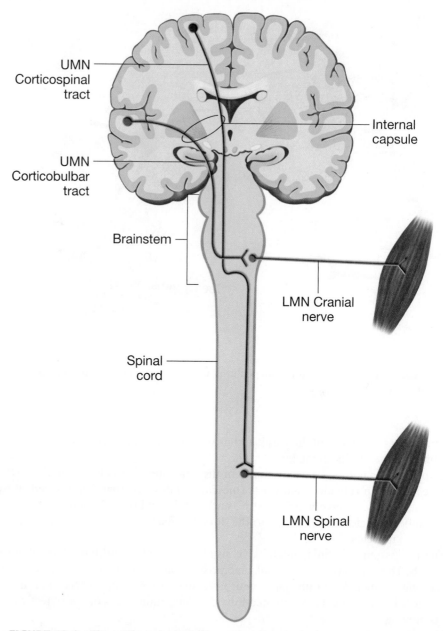

FIGURE 13-6 The corticospinal tracts contain upper motor neurons that control spinal nerves, and the corticobulbar tracts contain upper motor neurons (UMN) that control cranial nerves.

Clinical Box 13-1: Polio

Polio, a disease that specifically destroys lower motor neurons, is caused by a virus that infects lower motor neuron cell bodies. In cases where a small number of cells are damaged, the remaining lower motor neurons often produce collateral sprouts and re-innervate skeletal muscle. These patients appear to recover normal or nearly normal motor function. However, late in life the remaining lower motor neurons sometimes "wear out," leading to an increase in motor symptoms including fatigue, weakness, and muscle atrophy.

Challenge question: Would a person with polio have hypertonic muscles or hypotonic muscles?

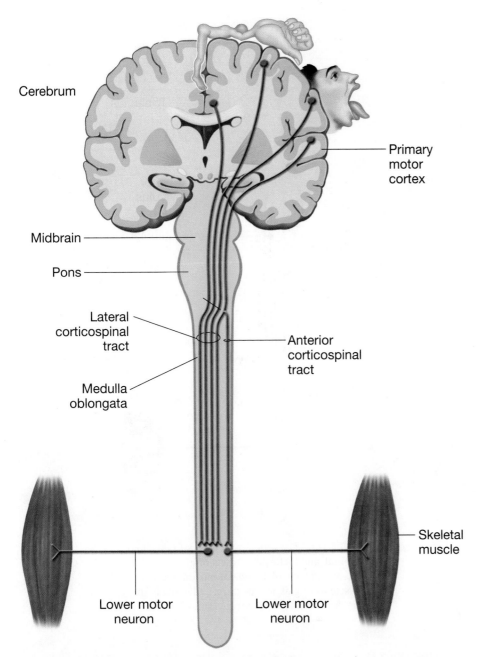

FIGURE 13-7 The lateral and anterior corticospinal tracts contain upper motor neurons that originate in primary motor cortex and that control lower motor neurons in the spinal cord.

cord: Somatosensory neurons and interneurons synapse onto lower motor neuron cell bodies and can produce activity.

Muscle Tone

Muscle tone is defined as the amount of resistance a muscle has to passive stretching. Even when relaxed, all normally innervated skeletal muscles have tone. Muscle tone has two components: a mechanical component and a neural component. The mechanical component of tone results from the physical properties of the muscle cells as well as from the muscle's connective tissue coverings. These tissues have stiffness and elasticity that cannot be altered. The neural component of tone is produced by the motor neurons that innervate each muscle fiber (see **Figure 13-9**). In every normally innervated skeletal muscle, a small number of lower motor neurons, and therefore motor units, are always "on," or firing. This means that a few muscle fibers are contracting at all times, producing a little tension in the muscle (but not causing any actual movement).

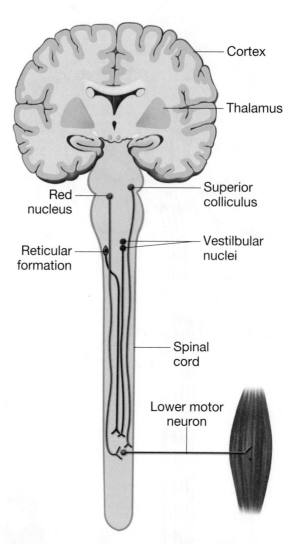

Cortex

Thalamus

Red nucleus

Superior colliculus

Reticular formation

Vestilbular nuclei

Spinal cord

Lower motor neuron

FIGURE 13-8 The reticulospinal, vestibulospinal rubrospinal, and tectospinal tracts originate in the brainstem and control aspects of movement including muscle tone, gait, and posture. Collectively they are sometimes called the extrapyramidal tracts.

Clinical Box 13-2: ALS

Amyotrophic lateral sclerosis (ALS; Lou Gehrig's disease) is a disease that affects both upper and lower motor neurons. Its cause has not yet been determined. Scientists have identified a gene (called SOD1) that is linked to about 10% of ALS cases, and have found that the motor neuron death begins at the axon terminal and moves backward toward the cell body. Patients with ALS have a mixture of flaccid and spastic paralysis, and do not have any changes in their emotional, cognitive, or sensory functions. ALS is a progressive disease that eventually paralyzes respiratory muscles, and will be fatal unless patients choose to use mechanical ventilation for breathing. In mice with a form of ALS, exercise on treadmills slowed the progress of the disease, suggesting that physical activity may be helpful in treatment. In addition, when the SOD-1 gene was partially shut down in some of the glial cells in the central nervous system, the course of the disease slowed down considerably (Boillee et al., 2006). This suggests that glial cells may play a role in the pathology of ALS.

Challenge question: Why will patients with ALS have normal sensory function?

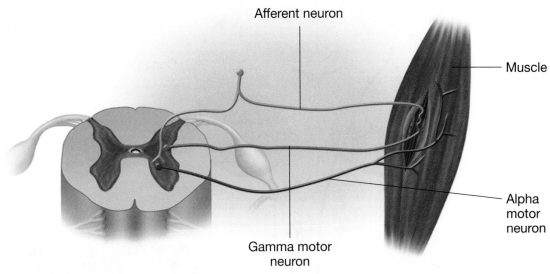

FIGURE 13-9 Muscle tone is controlled and adjusted by a reflex referred to as the gamma loop. Gamma motor neurons adjust the stiffness of muscle spindles and stimulate action potentials in the afferent neuron, which in turn stimulates activity of alpha motor neurons and contraction of motor units within the muscle.

The neural component of tone can be modified by factors such as the environment and emotions. For example, cold temperatures, anxiety, and fear can all increase tone, and warmth, massage, and relaxation can decrease it. The gamma loop reflex (see chapter 9) is responsible for adjusting muscle tone to meet short-term environmental demands. The gamma loop is controlled by the brain, via descending tracts in the spinal cord (especially by the dorsal reticulospinal tract). If the brain increases stimulation of the gamma loop, tone will increase, whereas decreased stimulation will reduce tone.

Any disruption of the gamma loop will impair the nervous system's ability to produce the muscle activity necessary for creating tone. Thus, damage to lower motor neurons will result in a skeletal muscle without tone. This would be called a hypotonic muscle (see **Table 13.1**). Typically, injury to a peripheral nerve or to lower motor neuron cell bodies in the spinal cord causes hypotonicity (see **Figure 13-10**). Hypotonic muscles feel soft and flabby, with little or no resistance to stretch or palpation. Deep tendon reflex tests yield no response, and the muscle cannot be contracted either voluntarily or via reflex stimulation.

Because the gamma loop is controlled by upper motor neurons in spinal cord descending tracts, damage to upper motor neurons also affects muscle tone. Immediately following an upper motor neuron injury, muscle tone is lost but it gradually returns and becomes excessive. This results in muscles that are hypertonic or spastic. Hypertonicity is caused by overactivity of gamma motor neurons, which increases the sensitivity of muscle spindles to stretch. In addition, alpha motor neurons become hypersensitive and depolarize at higher rates, which results in excessive muscle contraction and therefore increased tone (see **Figure 13-11**). It is probably caused by changes in receptors in the lower motor neuron cell membrane. In addition, collateral sprouting by interneurons and sensory neurons within the spinal cord after upper motor neuron injuries can result in increased lower motor neuron stimulation. Hypertonic muscles feel rigid, stiff, and tight, and are difficult to stretch

Table 13.1 Upper motor neuron injury and lower motor neuron injury

	Upper Motor Neurons	Lower Motor Neurons
Voluntary movement	Paralysis	Paralysis
Muscle tone	Hypertonia	Hypotonia
Deep tendon reflexes	Exaggerated	Lost

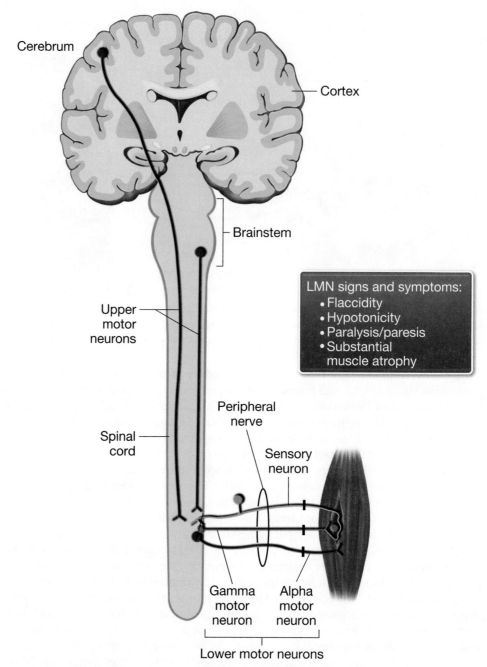

FIGURE 13-10 Injury to lower motor neurons (the gamma loop) results in a paralyzed, hypotonic muscle.

both actively and passively. Thus, a "typical" upper motor neuron injury results in muscles that are both paralyzed and hypertonic (increased resting tone) or spastic (increased resistance to passive movement; Sheean, 2002).

Control of Movement

Lower motor neurons directly innervate skeletal muscles, and upper motor neurons innervate the lower motor neurons. Damage to either type of motor neuron can cause paralysis (loss of voluntary movement). However, volitional control is not the only important component of movement. Normal motion must also be coordinated, initiated, and inhibited correctly, and movement patterns must be learned, stored, and activated at the appropriate time. The brain regions that perform these functions all act by stimulating or inhibiting upper motor neurons. Damage to any of these regions will not result in paralysis, but will cause movement to be abnormal.

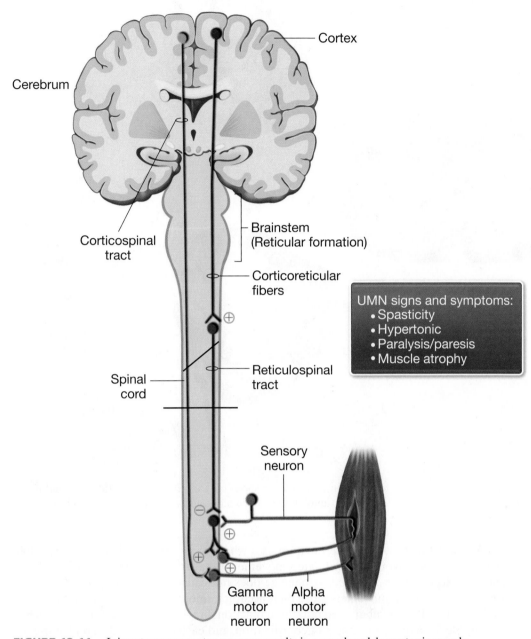

FIGURE 13-11   Injury to upper motor neurons results in a paralyzed, hypertonic muscle.

Cerebellum

The **cerebellum** is located in the posterior cranial fossa, just below the occipital lobe of the cerebral cortex (see **Figure 13-12**). The cerebellum consists of two hemispheres (right and left) that are connected by a midline structure called the vermis. The cerebellum develops as an outgrowth of the hindbrain, and is connected to the brainstem by three large nerve fiber (axon) bundles called cerebellar peduncles. All axons pass to and from the cerebellum via these three bundles.

The outer part of the cerebellum is the cerebellar cortex, composed mainly of small neurons called granule cells and large neurons called Purkinje cells. Purkinje cell dendrites are covered with numerous spines, providing an enormous surface area for synaptic contacts (about 200,000 synapses per neuron). Inside each cerebellar hemisphere are several large cerebellar nuclei. The largest is the dentate nucleus, named for its resemblance to a tooth. The others are called the fastigial nucleus, the globose nucleus, and the emboliform nucleus.

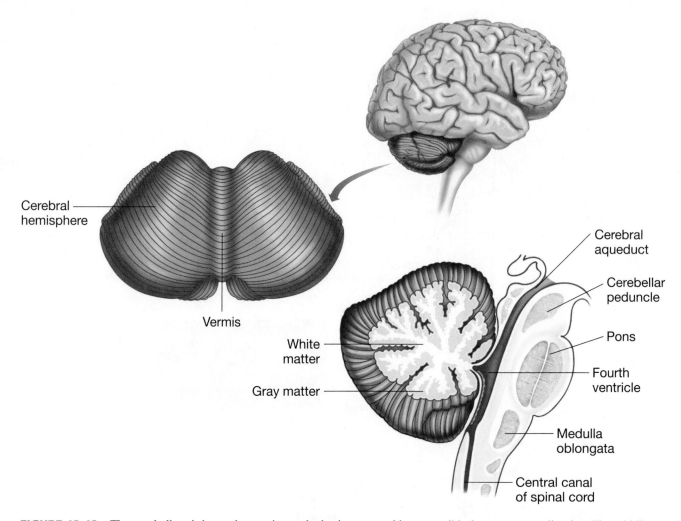

Cerebral hemisphere

Vermis

White matter

Gray matter

Cerebral aqueduct

Cerebellar peduncle

Pons

Fourth ventricle

Medulla oblongata

Central canal of spinal cord

FIGURE 13-12   The cerebellum is located posterior to the brainstem, and is responsible for motor coordination. The middle figure shows a superior view of the entire cerebellum, and the bottom figure shows a mid-sagittal section through the brainstem and cerebellum.

A major function of the cerebellum as a whole is motor coordination. Cerebellar lesions result in **ataxia** (uncoordinated movement) that is seen on the side of the body ipsilateral to the injury. Cerebellar damage does not cause paralysis or paresis (muscle weakness). However, movements lose their accuracy, smoothness, and coordination.

The cerebellum is subdivided into three functional regions (see **Figure 13-13**). Each is responsible for a different aspect of coordination, and each controls a different subset of skeletal muscles. The functional areas are the vestibulocerebellum, the spinocerebellum, and the cerebrocerebellum.

The vestibulocerebellum coordinates balance. It receives input from the vestibular apparatus in the inner ear about the position of the head in space (static information) and about changes in head position (dynamic information). This input is used to affect muscle tone in the limbs, trunk, neck, and extraocular muscles, and to coordinate muscles that maintain a normal upright posture and horizontal head position. The vestibulocerebellum sends output to the vestibular nuclei, which controls the muscles via the vestibulospinal tracts.

Damage to the vestibulocerebellum results in **disequilibrium** (difficulty maintaining and correcting balance). This is because the damaged vestibulocerebellum cannot properly coordinate the actions of numerous muscles responsible for balance. Symptoms include postural (static) tremor and truncal ataxia. Patients with postural tremor display high frequency, back-and-forth body movements while standing. In truncal ataxia, patients make large-amplitude trunk movements to maintain balance (as if they are standing on a moving train or bus).

The spinocerebellum is formed by the vermis and the adjacent parts of both cerebellar hemispheres. The function of the spinocerebellum is coordination of posture and gait. Input

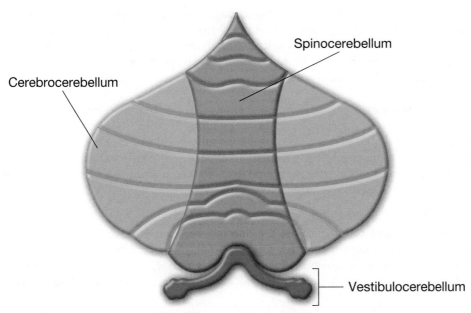

FIGURE 13-13 Schematic diagram of the cerebellum showing the three functional regions: the vestibulocerebellum is responsible for coordinating balance, the spinocerebellum is responsible for coordinating posture and gait, and the cerebrocerecellum is responsible for coordinating fine, detailed movements.

to the spinocerebellum comes from proprioceptors (muscle spindles and Golgi tendon organs) via the spinocerebellar tracts, and from the vestibular nuclei. The spinocerebellum coordinates proximal limb muscles, especially muscles of the lower extremities. There are no direct connections between the cerebellum and the lower motor neurons. Instead, the spinocerebellum projects to the vestibular nuclei and reticular formation in the brainstem, and also has connections to the primary motor cortex. The spinocerebellum acts via the vestibulospinal, reticulospinal, and corticospinal tracts. By affecting upper motor neurons located in these tracts, the spinocerebellum can coordinate muscle activity.

Lesions to the spinocerebellum result in gait ataxia. A patient with this condition displays an unsteady, wide-based, staggering gait with the legs spread far apart in an attempt to maintain postural stability. Gait ataxia can result from chronic alcoholism which damages the spinocerebellum.

The cerebrocerebellum (also called the corticocerebellum or the neocerebellum) is located in the lateral two-thirds of each cerebellar hemisphere. The cerebrocerebellum coordinates distal limb movements, as well as movements of the small muscles used for speech. Specifically, the cerebrocerebellum regulates the force, timing, and direction of movement, allowing motion to be smooth, rapid, and precise. The cerebrocerebellum is also involved in both detecting and correcting movement errors. Thus, the cerebrocerebellum is essential for movement accuracy and adaptability, and in coordinating complex voluntary movement. It also plays a role in motor learning, nonverbal communication, and the ability to shift the focus of attention.

The cerebrocerebellum gets input from the primary motor cortex, as well as from the cortical association areas of all four cortical lobes. The cerebrocerebellum integrates these signals and projects back to the cerebral cortex, forming a circuit. Because the cerebrocerebellar circuit is activated prior to firing the upper motor neurons, the motor cortex can send action potentials to the muscles with the proper timing, velocity, and sequence to permit smooth, accurate, and coordinated motion. In addition, the cerebrocerebellum is part of a complex feedback loop thought to be involved in motor learning and cognition.

Injury to the cerebrocerebellum results in ataxic (uncoordinated) movement, especially of vocal and distal limb muscles. Lesions always affect muscles ipsilateral to the lesion site. Symptoms include asynergia (a lack of cooperation between muscles that usually work together), **dysdiadochokinesis** (difficulty doing rapid, alternating movements such as pronation and supination), and ataxia (inability to coordinate muscles when performing a voluntary movement). Cerebrocerebellar damage causes disturbances in the timing, force, and direction of movement. A movement may stop before the target is attained, or the limb may overshoot the target; this is known as dysmetria or past-pointing. Patients may also display intention tremor (side to side movements when trying to reach a target) and have slurred speech (ataxic dysarthria) as a result of incoordination of muscles used in speech production.

There is some evidence that the cerebellum also has cognitive, nonmotor functions. It has connections to language, association, and limbic regions of the cerebral cortex. The cerebellum is activated during tests of language function, memory, and cognition. In addition, cerebellar damage results in deficits in executive function (planning, goal setting, abstract reasoning, working memory), and disinhibited, inappropriate behavior similar to that seen after frontal lobe injury.

Basal Ganglia

The **basal ganglia** (basal nuclei) are a group of interconnected structures located deep inside each cerebral hemisphere (see Figure 13-14). These structures are involved in initiation and inhibition of movement, as well as in initiation of thought and emotion. The basal ganglia system directs the action of all motor tracts, and thus all voluntary skeletal muscles in the body.

The basal ganglia consist of the caudate nucleus, the putamen, and the globus pallidus. Together, the caudate nucleus and putamen are referred to as the striatum or striate cortex because of their striped appearance in the sectioned brain. The putamen and globus pallidus are also known as the lentiform or lenticular (lens-shaped) nucleus. This

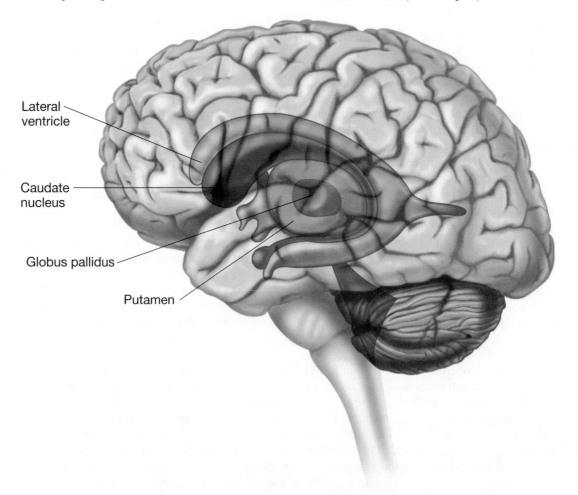

Lateral ventricle

Caudate nucleus

Globus pallidus

Putamen

FIGURE 13-14   The basal ganglia are a group of interconnected nuclei located deep inside the cerebrum, and consist of the caudate nucleus, the putamen, and the globus pallidus. Here the basal ganglia are depicted in relation to the brain's ventricles which are shown in red.

Clinical Box 13-3: Parkinson Disease

People with Parkinson disease walk with small steps and a shuffling gait, show little or no facial expression, and have difficulty shifting from one movement sequence to another. Postural instability is common because patients are unable to quickly generate a muscle contraction response that would prevent falling (for example, if pushed in a posterior direction). Falling backwards is a common sign of Parkinson Disease. In addition, spontaneous movements, such as swinging the arms while walking, or readjusting one's position while sitting, are reduced or absent. The small, slow movements seen in Parkinson disease are called bradykinesia. There is also increased resistance to passive stretch throughout joint range of motion that has a ratchet-like feel and is described as "cog-wheel rigidity." Because flexors are more affected than extensors, patients develop a flexed or stooped posture.

Some people with Parkinson Disease also have a resting tremor that is rhythmic and usually most obvious in the hands; it is sometimes called "pill-rolling" tremor. Parkinson Disease tremor is most apparent when the patient is still, and usually diminishes or disappears during purposeful movement and sleep.

People with Parkinson Disease gradually lose more substantia nigra neurons, and symptoms typically worsen. In its later stages, Parkinson Disease may be characterized by disorders of thought and mood, including depression and slowness of thinking as the cognitive and limbic basal ganglia circuits are affected. In addition, many people with Parkinson Disease lose their sense of smell (anosmia).

Treatment of Parkinson Disease is primarily pharmacological. Drugs that increase the amount of dopamine (e.g., L-dopa) or that are dopamine agonists are often prescribed. Recent evidence suggests that aerobic exercise slows the progression of Parkinson Disease, improves function, and may facilitate neuroplasticity in the basal ganglia. Thus, exercise programs may be beneficial for people with this condition (Muhlack, Welnic, Woitalla, & Mueller, 2007; Yoon et al., 2007).

Challenge question: If people with Parkinson Disease take too much of a dopamine agonist, what signs and symptoms might be expected?

entire circuit is sometimes called the kinetic system because of its role in generating and regulating movement. Four small nuclei are functionally associated with the basal ganglia. These are the substantia nigra (found in the midbrain), the subthalamic nucleus, the pedunculopontine nucleus, and the ventral tegmental area (VTA). The VTA is known to be involved in addiction and pleasure-seeking behavior (D'Ardenne, McClure, Nystrom, & Cohen, 2008).

At least four separate basal ganglia circuits have been described. These include a motor circuit (involved in movement initiation), a cognitive circuit (with extensive connections to the prefrontal cortex and cortical association areas), a limbic circuit that has many connections with emotional centers, and an oculomotor circuit that regulates eye movements. The precise functioning of each of these circuits is not completely understood, but all basal ganglia circuits affect cortical function by either increasing or decreasing the activity of cortical neurons. In this way, many important cortical functions such as thought, emotion, and movement are significantly affected by the basal ganglia.

The basal ganglia motor circuit consists of two pathways that operate in parallel (see **Figure 13-15**). The first is known as the "direct pathway." The direct pathway increases stimulation of the motor cortex and initiates movement. The other basal ganglia circuit is known as the "indirect pathway"; this circuit decreases stimulation of the motor cortex, resulting in decreased movement initiation. The direct and indirect pathways have opposite effects on body muscles: The direct pathway stimulates distal muscles and inhibits proximal ones, whereas the indirect pathway inhibits distal muscles and stimulates proximal ones. These two pathways must be balanced for normal movement to take place.

The substantia nigra (located in the midbrain) produces the neurotransmitter dopamine, which affects both basal ganglia pathways and increases the initiation of movement. Because dopamine is critical for regulating motor activity, too much or too little dopamine can have

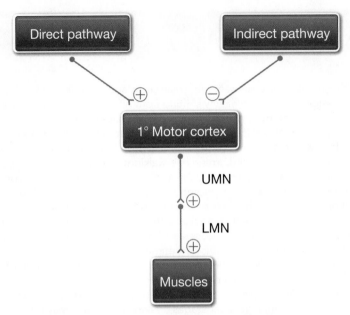

FIGURE 13-15 The direct and indirect basal ganglia pathways have opposite effects on generation of movement, and act via the upper motor neurons and lower motor neurons.

serious consequences. In general, an excess of dopamine results in unwanted and unnecessary movements **(dyskinesia),** while dopamine deficiency results in slowness of movement **(bradykinesia).** The most common disease associated with underproduction of dopamine is Parkinson Disease (PD), which results from death of neurons in the substantia nigra.

In contrast to the symptoms of dopamine deficiency, excess dopamine can cause abnormal involuntary movements **(dyskinesias).** Dyskinetic movements include dystonia (recurrent muscle spasms), akathesia (severe body restlessness and a strong compulsion to move), hemiballism (rapid, ballistic flinging movements of the limbs), and athetoid (slow, writhing) movements. Dyskinetic movements develop when there is excess dopamine, or when dopamine receptors become hypersensitive. Basal ganglia conditions that produce dyskinetic movements include Huntington disease (HD) and Tourette syndrome (TS).

The cognitive and limbic (emotional) basal ganglia circuits are less well understood than the motor circuit. These circuits modify activity of the prefrontal cortex and cortical association areas, and are important for emotion, memory, focus, and attention. Patients with basal ganglia disorders may experience problems with memory and concentration, as well as slowness of thought or dementia. Dementia typically appears relatively late in the course of Parkinson Disease, and it is a symptom of Huntington disease. In addition, several

Neuroscience Notes Box 13-1:
Huntington Disease

Huntington disease is a genetic (autosomal dominant) disorder that usually appears in late middle age. The gene responsible for Huntington disease is located on chromosome 4. It produces an abnormal form of a protein called huntingtin that damages basal ganglia neurons and causes overstimulation of the motor cortex. People with Huntington disease have involuntary (dyskinetic) movements, including chorea (rapid, jerky, arrhythmic movements), hemiballism, and athetosis. In addition to the motor symptoms, Huntington disease affects cognitive and limbic basal ganglia circuits, causing dementia and emotional disturbances. Huntington disease is a progressive, fatal disease.

Clinical Box 13-4: Tourette Syndrome

Tourette syndrome is a genetic condition characterized by hypersensitive dopamine receptors. People with Tourette syndrome exhibit brief, uncontrolled movements called tics, and report a compulsion or urgency to move that is difficult to repress. In some cases, the tics are vocal or verbal, such as the urge to repeat a particular word or phrase, grunt, or cough.

Challenge question: Since Tourette syndrome can be treated with medications that block dopamine receptors (dopamine antagonists), what signs and symptoms might result if a patient took too much of such a medication?

diseases affect the emotional and cognitive basal ganglia circuits, including schizophrenia and obsessive-compulsive disorder.

Motor Planning

The **supplementary motor area** (SMA; Brodmann's area 8) is a motor planning region. This region stores motor memories (learned movement patterns) (see **Figure 13-16**). The supplementary motor area directs the activity of primary motor cortex. A lesion to the supplementary motor area can result in **apraxia,** a motor planning deficit. Apraxia is defined as the inability to perform purposeful voluntary movement, in the absence of any sensory or motor impairment. Thus, patients with apraxia have normal sensation and are not paralyzed. However, they are unable to carry out normal movement sequences (Zadicoff & Lang, 2005), and may forget how to perform everyday routine tasks (such as brushing teeth, riding a bicycle, etc.).

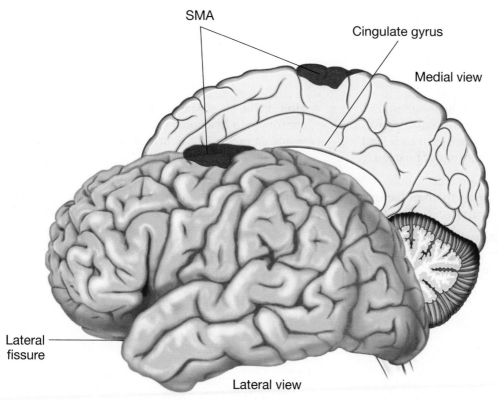

FIGURE 13-16 The supplementary motor area (SMA) stores motor memories and directs the function of the primary motor cortex.

PATIENT SCENARIOS

Patient Case 13-1 (Lucille)

Lucille is a 63-year-old woman who suffered a stroke that affected her cerebellum. She walks with a wide-based gait, and displays additional symptoms, including an intention tremor, slurred speech, and ataxia. These symptoms are evident on the right side of her body. Testing also reveals some deficits in memory and executive function, and dysdiadochokinesis.

Questions

a) Since the symptoms are on the right side of Lucille's body, on which side of the cerebellum did the stroke occur?
b) Why doesn't a lesion to the cerebellum cause paralysis?

Patient Case 13-2 (Howard)

Howard is a 75-year-old retired dentist. He presents in your clinic with a diagnosis of Parkinson Disease. Howard walks slowly and takes small steps. He is bent forward in a stooped position, and displays little facial expression. His left hand shakes when he is at rest but the tremor disappears when he reaches for a glass. He sits very still with little spontaneous movement, and his muscles feel rigid, but are not spastic.

Questions

a) In Parkinson Disease, which neurotransmitter is deficient? Where is this neurotransmitter produced in the brain?
b) What type (classification) of drug might be prescribed to treat this disease? What side effects of drug treatment might occur?
c) Would you have concerns about Howard falling? Why or why not?

Patient Case 13-3 (Stephen)

Stephen, 41 years old, has been diagnosed with amyotrophic lateral sclerosis (ALS, or Lou Gehrig's disease). This disease affects both upper and lower motor neurons. Stephen can still speak but his speech sounds garbled. He uses a wheelchair for mobility and can still move his arms but cannot perform movements with his hands. Swallowing is becoming more difficult for him, posing a risk of choking.

Questions

a) Would you expect Stephen's muscles to show spasticity, flaccidity, or a mixture of both? Why?
b) Given that ALS is a motor neuron disease, will Stephen have any sensory loss? Will his cognitive abilities be affected?

Review Questions

1. Explain how upper motor neurons and lower motor neurons work together to produce voluntary control of skeletal muscle. What effect will damage to each kind of motor neuron have on voluntary motor function?

2. Explain how normal muscle tone is created and controlled, and describe how injury to lower motor neurons and to upper motor neurons can affect tone.

3. What is the role of each functional region of the cerebellum? What are the symptoms of an injury or other pathology to each region?

4. How do the basal ganglia and substantia nigra contribute to functional movement? What effect would an excess, or a deficit, of the neurotransmitter dopamine have on movement?

5. How does the supplementary motor area (SMA) contribute to functional movement? What symptoms would be seen due to a lesion affecting the SMA?

References

1. Boillee, S., et al. (2006). Onset and progression in inherited ALS determined by motor neurons and microglia. *Science, 312,* 1389–1392.

2. D'Ardenne, K. D., McClure, S. M., Nystrom, L. E., & Cohen, J. D. (2008). BOLD responses reflecting dopaminergic signals in the human ventral tegmental area. *Science, 319,* 1264–1267.

3. Muhlack, S., Welnic, J., Woitalla, D., &Mueller T. (2007). Exercise improves efficacy of levodopa in patients with Parkinson's disease. *Movement Disorders, 22,* 427–430.

4. Sheean, G. (2002). The pathophysiology of spasticity. *European Journal of Neurology, 9,* (Suppl.1), 3–9.

5. Yoon, M. C., et al. (2007). Treadmill exercise suppresses nigrostriatal dopaminergic neuronal loss in 6-hydroxydopamine-induced Parkinson's rats. *Neuroscience Letters, 423*(1), 12–17.

6. Zadikoff, C., & Lang, A. E. (2005). Apraxia in movement disorders. *Brain, 128,* 1480–1497.

Further Reading

1. Aebischer, P., & Kato, A. C. (2007). Playing defense against Lou Gehrig's disease. *Scientific American, 297*(5), 86–93.

2. Atwood, H. L. (2006). Gatekeeper at the synapse. *Science, 312,* 1008–1009.

3. Falvo, M. J., Schilling, B. K., & Earhart, G. M. (2008). Parkinson's disease and resistive exercise: rationale, review, and recommendations. *Movement Disorders, 23*(1), 1–11.

4. Kittel R. J., et al. (2006). Bruchpilot promotes active zone assembly, Ca^{2+} channel clustering, and vesicle release. *Science, 312,* 1050–1054.

PEARSON
myhealthprofessionskit™

Use this address to access the Companion Website created for this textbook. Simply select "Physical Therapy" from the choice of disciplines. Find this book and log in using your username and password to access self-assessment questions, a glossary and more.

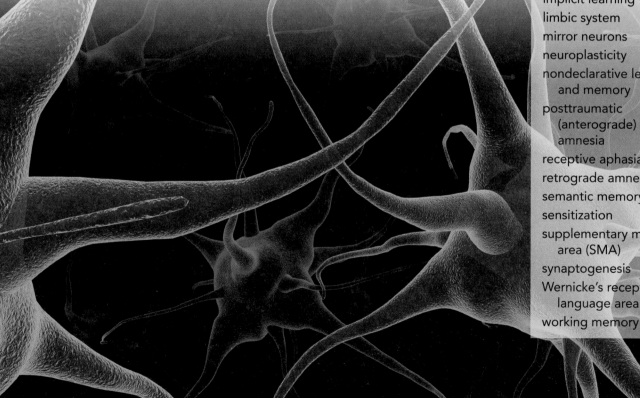

(14) Cognition, Emotion, Memory, and Language

CHAPTER OBJECTIVES

After completing this chapter, the reader will be able to:

1 Identify regions of the cerebral cortex responsible for thought (cognition) and explain the effects of lesions to those areas.

2 Describe the areas of the brain involved in emotion and explain the effects of lesions to those areas.

3 Define declarative and nondeclarative learning, identify brain regions relevant for each type of learning, and predict the functional deficits that would result from lesions to those areas.

4 Discuss the neurobiology of short-term and long-term learning.

5 Identify brain regions responsible for both receptive and expressive language, and name the types of aphasia that would result from lesions to those areas.

KEY TERMS

apraxia
Broca's expressive language area
cognition
consolidation
declarative learning and memory
dementia
emotion
episodic memory
explicit learning and memory
expressive aphasia
global aphasia
implicit learning
limbic system
mirror neurons
neuroplasticity
nondeclarative learning and memory
posttraumatic (anterograde) amnesia
receptive aphasia
retrograde amnesia
semantic memory
sensitization
supplementary motor area (SMA)
synaptogenesis
Wernicke's receptive language area
working memory

Essential Facts ···

▶ Cognition and emotion are both functions of the cerebral cortex, and they involve many brain regions acting together.

▶ Learning and memory are closely connected; learning is the process of acquiring memory.

▶ Learning and memory require changes in the brain's pattern of synapses.

▶ Language and communication have separate receptive (incoming) and expressive (outgoing) components, centered in brain regions with many interconnections.

This chapter describes the brain regions and circuits responsible for thought, emotion, learning, memory, and language. These are often described as "higher order functions" of the brain. They are centered in the cerebral cortex, and are carried out by complex, interconnected networks of neurons. Injury to these brain regions can cause striking changes in personality, emotion, behavior, and rational thought, as well as the ability to communicate and to interact socially.

Cognition and Emotion

Cognition and emotion are closely related. **Cognition** is defined as the ability to think, plan, and solve problems. It requires focus, concentration, attention, and working memory—the ability to hold a thought in the "front" of your mind. **Emotion** is harder to define, but might be thought of as the feelings and reactions that occur in response to thoughts, beliefs, or experiences. Both emotion and cognition take place internally; other people cannot access your thoughts or feelings unless you display them externally. Interestingly, the emotional centers of the brain are very closely linked to the cranial nerves that control facial muscles. These neural connections allow our faces to reflect internal emotions.

Cognition and emotion are centered in the association areas of the cerebral hemispheres. Details about the precise role of these cortical regions are incomplete, mostly because it is difficult to study them in living people. Much of what is known about cortical function comes from brain imaging studies, and from studying patients with cortical lesions. People who have had neurological injuries such as traumatic brain injury, a brain tumor, or a stroke may display cognitive or emotional deficits if the cerebral cortex is damaged.

Cognition

Cognition is centered in association areas located on the lateral and anterior parts of both cerebral hemispheres. On Brodmann's map, cognitive regions are found in areas 8–11 and 44–47 and are referred to as the *cognitive cortex* (see **Figure 14-1**). The cognitive cortex specializes in intellectual functions that include planning ahead, anticipating consequences, exercising judgment, displaying reasoning and analytical thinking, and solving problems. Proper functioning of this region allows us to delay gratification and to possess cognitive flexibility (the ability to modify or adjust based on new information, and to shift thoughts and behaviors from one topic to another). The cognitive cortex permits us to focus our minds on a problem, consider various solutions, and choose the most appropriate course of action. In particular, the prefrontal cortex is responsible for inhibition of inappropriate or potentially dangerous impulses. The prefrontal cortex is one of the last parts of the brain to mature; myelination is not complete until after age 20.

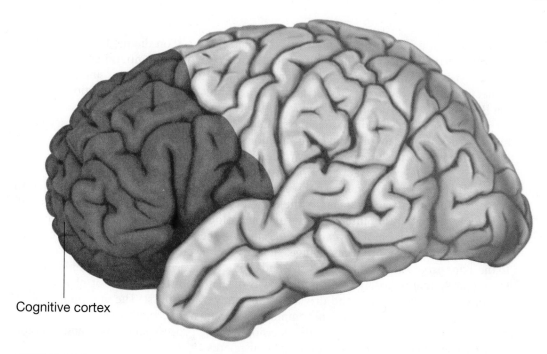

Cognitive cortex

FIGURE 14-1 Cognitive areas of the cerebral cortex are centered in the frontal lobe, and are responsible for intelligence, judgement, and behavior.

The cognitive cortex receives information from many areas of the brain, including somatosensory association cortex, auditory association cortex, visual association cortex, and the thalamus. The cognitive cortex integrates the input from these diverse sources and formulates appropriate responses.

Lesions to the cognitive cortex produce a variety of deficits in intellectual functioning. For example, a patient may have great difficulty focusing and concentrating, or (conversely) may be unable to shift attention to new topics; this is known as *perseveration*. This kind of lesion is common in patients who have suffered a traumatic brain injury, and is often characterized by an inability to plan or follow through with a task or goal. Patients may also become confused and disoriented, and have trouble following directions.

Neuroscience Notes Box 14-1:
Prefrontal Syndrome

Patients who have suffered a traumatic brain injury may display a range of behaviors, including excessive agitation, lack of self-control, and socially inappropriate behaviors. This is due to a damaged prefrontal cortex. Patients with this condition are impulsive and uninhibited, and have difficulty concentrating. Clinicians who treat people with prefrontal syndrome must structure treatment in order to manage these challenges. This might include:

- Minimizing distraction
- Setting short-term, attainable goals
- Providing easily understandable directions
- Maintaining a calm demeanor (a quiet voice and nonthreatening body language)
- Providing frequent reassurance and reorientation

Emotion

The emotional part of the human brain is located primarily on the medial aspect of the cerebral cortex. It includes the orbitofrontal cortex, the inferotemporal cortex, the cingulate gyrus, and parts of the medial temporal lobe (the hippocampus and amygdala). Collectively, these regions are referred to as the limbic system, or the emotional cortex. On Brodmann's map, this region is approximately located in areas 8–14, 23–25, and 31–33 (see **Figure 14-2**). The **limbic system** plays a major role in both emotion and memory; some limbic structures are involved in both functions, whereas others specialize in one or the other. Memory circuits and pathways are described later in this chapter.

The emotional cortex plays a critical role in cognition and behavior. It is responsible for social behavior, emotional responses, and preferences. Also, it is closely connected to sensory association areas, especially the olfactory and gustatory (taste) regions, as well as areas of the brain that interpret internal, physiological information (nausea, sweating, rapid heart rate, etc). Emotions can alter the status of the body by activating the autonomic nervous system, which produces changes in heart and respiration rates, affects blood flow to the skin (producing pallor or a blush), and causes sweating and muscle trembling. Thus, the limbic system is closely connected to parts of the brain responsible for physiological responses to danger, stress, and drives such as hunger and thirst. The emotional cortex integrates these diverse signals, and communicates them to the cognitive cortex. Cognitive areas then integrate emotions into the decision-making process, so thought and emotion are closely connected within the cerebral hemispheres

Emotion is a subjective, internal experience. It can be agreeable (good, pleasant) or disagreeable (bad, unpleasant), and can vary in intensity from mild to overwhelming. Because emotions are internal, the existence of emotion in someone else must be inferred based on that person's behavior. This means that emotions have both a private and a social, external aspect. Most people can recognize emotional states in others based on facial expressions, tones of voice, gestures, and other physical behaviors. This ability is decreased or absent in people with autism and Asperger's syndrome, who often have difficulty "reading" emotions (Shamay-Tsoory, Tomer, Yaniv, & Ahron-Peretz, 2002). In addition, observing others' emotions can produce similar feelings within us; this is the basis of empathy. A group of

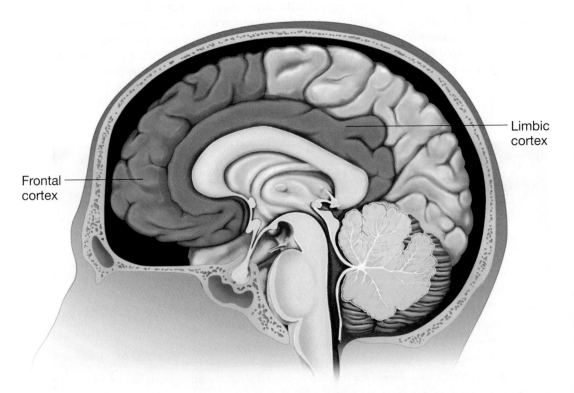

Frontal cortex

Limbic cortex

FIGURE 14-2 Emotional areas of the cerebral cortex. Most emotional regions of the cortex are located in the frontal lobes and in the limbic areas located on the medial aspect of the cerebrum.

Neuroscience Notes Box 14-2:
Prefrontal Lobotomy

The prefrontal lobotomy was a type of surgery known as "psychosurgery" and was first performed in the United States in the 1930s. The procedure involved cutting neurons that connect the prefrontal cortex with the thalamus. In some cases, this involved placing a thin metal instrument just above the upper eyelid, breaking through the bone at the top of the eye socket, and cutting axons located in the inferior part of the prefrontal cortex; this was referred to as a *trans-orbital lobotomy*. Lobotomy was performed in order to "pacify" patients with mental illnesses who displayed agitation or violent behaviors. However, it was difficult for physicians to know precisely which axons they were destroying; some patients suffered serious brain damage from lobotomy. Apathy as well as a "blunted personality" were the common side effects. When antipsychotic medications were introduced in the 1950s, fewer lobotomies were performed, and the last ones in the United States were performed in the 1970s.

mirror neurons located in the cortex are active when we observe someone else expressing emotions, and allow us to understand what other people are thinking or feeling. Mirror neurons have been found in other primates, suggesting that humans are not the only animals who can feel empathy.

Connections between the emotional cortex and the cognitive cortex run in both directions, permitting emotions to inform decision making and thinking, and also allowing the rational, thinking brain to monitor and modify emotional responses. In addition, connections between emotional regions and the hypothalamus create an internal, physiological reaction to a decision or potential course of action. This is likely the basis of the "gut" feeling, when people report that something "just feels right" or "just seems wrong." These gut feelings are signals from our emotional brain that guide our behaviors, choices, and preferences.

Lesions affecting the emotional cortex can sometimes produce a flattened affect, in which patients may display few preferences. Lesions can also have the opposite effect: Patients may have exaggerated emotional responses to less important events. Some people with injury to emotional centers lack empathy and engage in thoughtless behavior with little regard for the consequences of their actions. Damage to the emotional cortex may also affect cognitive functions, because of the many anatomical links between emotional and cognitive parts of the brain.

Learning and Memory

Learning and memory are closely connected: Learning is the process of acquiring memory, whereas memory is the result of the learning process. Almost everything that human beings know and can do is learned. The ability to learn is an essential component of rehabilitation.

Learning is based on structural changes that occur within individual neurons, along with changes in the connections between them (the synapses). The term used to describe these biological changes is **neuroplasticity.** Neuroplasticity describes the flexibility or adaptability available to the brain. Within certain limits, the brain can reorganize its neural connections and change its physical structure based on experience.

Learning and memory can be subdivided into two distinct types: declarative and nondeclarative. **Declarative learning and memory** (also called **explicit learning and memory**) refers to memories that can be described in words. Knowing your telephone number, memorizing the Gettysburg Address, and remembering your high school graduation ceremony are all examples of declarative memory. Declarative memory can be subdivided into **semantic memory** (facts and figures) and **episodic memory** (a kind of "inner diary" of your life events and experiences). Episodic memory is strongly enhanced by emotional significance: We tend to remember events that are strongly positive or strongly negative. (For example, people usually remember their wedding day, or the events of September 11, 2001, but may not be able to recall many specifics about a more ordinary day in their lives.)

In contrast, **nondeclarative learning and memory** (also called **implicit learning and memory**) cannot usually be expressed in words. Implicit memory includes both emotional responses and motor skills or habits (riding a bicycle, driving a car, using a toothbrush, etc.). Some of these skills have a cognitive component as well. For example, to be a successful driver, one must learn the rules of the road and be able to navigate around town, in addition to knowing the physical skills such as steering and braking. The motor learning component of these skills involves learning patterns of muscle activity. Once learned, these patterns can become almost automatic.

Declarative Learning and Memory

Declarative learning has four distinct stages: (1) acquisition, (2) consolidation, (3) storage, and (4) retrieval. During the acquisition stage, the brain is taking in or acquiring the new knowledge. This requires the learner to be actively engaged in the learning process: focused, attentive, and motivated to learn. The prefrontal cortex is very active during acquisition.

The second stage of declarative learning is **consolidation.** During this stage, the newly acquired knowledge is encoded into existing neural circuits. This requires activity of the hippocampus, a small region located in the medial temporal lobes that is part of the limbic system (Gardiner & Hogan, 2005). Interestingly, it appears that the two hippocampi have different functions in memory consolidation: The left hippocampus is mainly responsible for verbal learning; the right one is more important for spatial memory. Consolidation is enhanced by sleep, exercise, and repetition of the learning. (The need for repetition is the reason that students have to study for exams.) It appears that sleep may help learning because synapses are fired repeatedly during dreaming, providing a form of repetition.

After declarative learning has been acquired and consolidated, it is stored in the cerebral cortex. Different types of memory are stored in different regions—for example, visual memories are stored in the visual association cortex, and auditory memories are stored in auditory association cortex. Thus, there is no single "memory center"; memories are stored in complex networks of neurons all over the cerebral cortex (see **Figure 14-3**).

The last step in declarative learning and memory is retrieval, in which the brain accesses or remembers the learned information. This requires activation of the cortical association areas and the prefrontal cortex. Remembering stored declarative memories requires the brain to activate the storage networks across the cortex, and recombine all elements of the memory. Memories that are seldom accessed tend to fade over time, while

Clinical Box 14-1: Hippocampal Lesions

Injury to the hippocampus can cause serious difficulties with learning and memory. The hippocampus is one of the very few brain regions in which neurogenesis (growth of new nerve cells) can take place throughout life (Erikkson et al., 1998). Traumatic brain injury, Alzheimer Disease, chemotherapy (which kills rapidly dividing cells throughout the body), and chronic stress have all been shown to diminish the size of the hippocampus, thereby making learning more difficult. The hippocampus also shrinks in people with chronic depression; both psychotherapy and medication have been shown to reverse this shrinkage (Malberg, Eisch, Nestler, & Duman, 2000).

Challenge questions:

1. How would an injury to the hippocampus affect a patient's ability to learn a new exercise program?

2. Would an injury to the hippocampus affect memories that already exist?

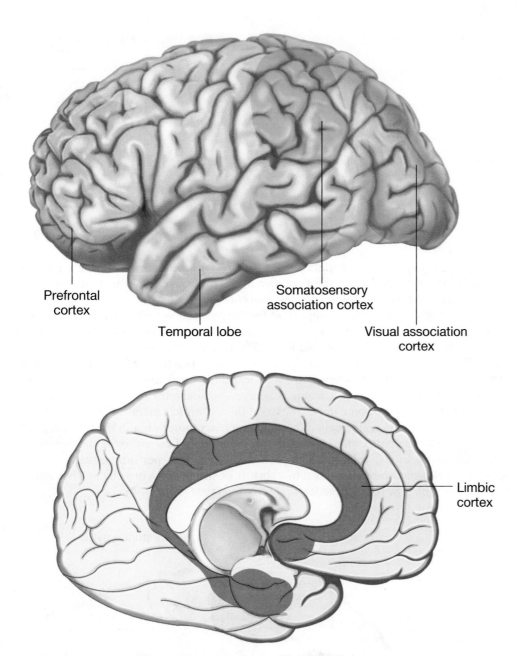

FIGURE 14-3 Cortical association areas store various aspects of memory, and are activated when the memory is retrieved. The top figure shows a lateral view of the left cerebral hemisphere, and the bottom figure depicts a mid-sagittal view of the left hemisphere.

those that are frequently accessed may become stronger. Research shows that the ability to consolidate memory (that is, to learn) is enhanced by:

- Sleep: A full night of sleep after studying improves retention of the material.
- Aerobic exercise: After studying, a walk, run, swim, or bike ride will help you remember what you studied.
- Meaningful, focused, active repetition of the material to be learned: Make your study sessions brief, focused, and active to improve your learning.

Nondeclarative Learning and Memory

Nondeclarative learning and memory includes learned emotional responses, as well as motor skill (motor) learning. Motor learning is essential for patients in physical and occupational therapy who often must learn new ways of moving following injury or disease. Motor learning uses some, but not all, of the same brain centers as declarative learning. It does not require activation of the hippocampus, but it does require activation of the brain's movement pathways and centers.

Review Concepts 14-1: Stages of Declarative Learning

- Acquisition (prefrontal cortex)
- Consolidation (hippocampus)
- Storage (cortical association areas)
- Retrieval (prefrontal cortex and cortical association areas)

Motor learning has three distinct phases. The first is *acquisition.* During the acquisition stage, all the motor areas of the brain and spinal cord are active: the primary motor cortex, the cerebellum, the basal ganglia, and the spinal cord motor tracts. In addition, the prefrontal cortex is highly active. This is important for the motivation to learn, and the ability to focus and to pay attention to one's performance. The learner must practice the new motor skill in order to acquire it. For example, learning to ride a bicycle, use a wheelchair, or play a musical instrument all require that the learner spend time practicing the new motor activity. This is why sports teams, musicians, and babies learning to walk must have regular practice.

The second stage of motor learning is *storage*—retaining the motor skills in the brain as a motor skill memory. Some people describe this as "muscle memory," but it is actually stored in a frontal lobe region called the **supplementary motor area (SMA).** In the SMA, patterns of motor activity can be stored almost indefinitely. Lesions to the supplementary motor area can cause **apraxia,** in which patients are unable to perform sequenced motor activities (making a sandwich, using a toothbrush, or sitting down in a chair). They appear to have forgotten how to do these learned activities (see Figure 14-4).

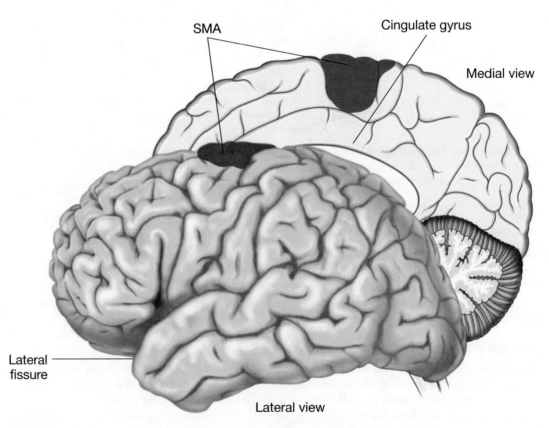

FIGURE 14-4　The supplementary motor area (SMA) stores motor or skill memory.

Finally, motor skills that have been learned and stored must be *accessed.* To use the learned motor patterns, all motor regions of the brain must be active: motor cortex, supplementary motor area, cerebellum, basal ganglia, and descending motor tracts in the spinal cord. Significantly, the prefrontal cortex is not normally active when the motor skills are being carried out. This means we can perform many activities almost automatically, while our minds are on something else. For example, most people can drive while carrying on a conversation, or looking at the passing scenery, without consciously thinking about the mechanics of braking, steering, and acceleration.

Neurobiology of Learning and Memory

Both declarative and nondeclarative (motor) learning can be short term (learned briefly, then forgotten) or long term (retained). Short-term memory includes both **working memory** (which lasts from seconds to minutes) and true short-term memory (which lasts from minutes to a few days). A good working memory is strongly correlated with intelligence: It allows us to hold a thought in "the front of the mind" and focus on it. Short-term memory lasts somewhat longer: It allows us to remember the events of the past few hours or days. These short-term memories usually fade unless they contain a strong emotional component.

Both working and short-term memory rely on biological changes in synapses that already exist within the central nervous system. When learning is taking place, synapses are fired repeatedly, and are thereby strengthened. "Strengthening" of a synapse means that presynaptic neurons put more neurotransmitters and synaptic vesicles into their axon terminals, whereas postsynaptic neurons temporarily place more receptors into the postsynaptic terminals (see Figure 14-5). This type of short-term synaptic change is called **sensitization.** It is reversible: When neural pathways are no longer being activated, the existing synapses will return to their resting states, and the memory is lost.

In contrast, long-term learning and memory involves the creation of new synapses, a process called **synaptogenesis** (see Figure 14-6). Synaptogenesis requires that synapses are fired repeatedly during the acquisition stage of learning. With enough activation, usually

Clinical Box 14-2: Amnesia

Traumatic brain injuries often cause memory loss. **Retrograde amnesia** describes memory loss of events prior to the onset of the injury. Although many of these "lost" memories return as the patient recovers, the specifics of the accident resulting in the traumatic brain injury are rarely recalled. **Posttraumatic (anterograde) amnesia** describes the inability to recall events that have occurred after the onset of a traumatic brain injury. This type of memory loss leaves patients confused and disoriented, unable to remember where they are or why they are in a hospital. Posttraumatic amnesia, like retrograde amnesia, typically fades over time, depending on the severity of the injury. Clinicians may use the duration of time that a patient displays posttraumatic amnesia to predict the severity of the traumatic brain injury (see chart below).

Duration of Posttraumatic Amnesia	Severity of TBI
5–60 minutes	Mild
1 day	Moderate
1–7 days	Severe
14 weeks	Very severe

Challenge question: What areas of the brain would be damaged in a patient with retrograde amnesia (loss of stored memories)?

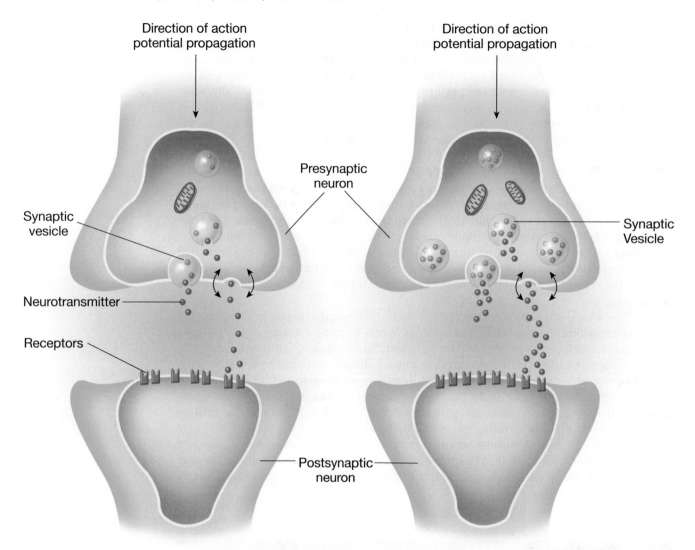

FIGURE 14-5   When a synapse is fired repeatedly, the presynaptic neuron responds by increasing the number of synaptic vesicles and neurotransmitter molecules, and the postsynaptic neuron reacts by increasing the number of neurotransmitter receptors. This is known as sensitization. The neuron on the right has been sensitized, and has more vesicles, neurotransmitters and receptors than the neuron on the left.

Neuroscience Notes Box 14-3:
Animal Geniuses

Scientists have identified a gene that appears to be important for learning. The gene codes for a receptor for the neurotransmitter glutamate. Mice that had extra copies of this gene learned twice as fast as regular mice, whereas mice that did not express the gene in a normal way were less intelligent and took longer to learn than regular mice. Similar experiments have been performed on fruit flies, creating both intelligent flies and flies that might be termed "slow learners."

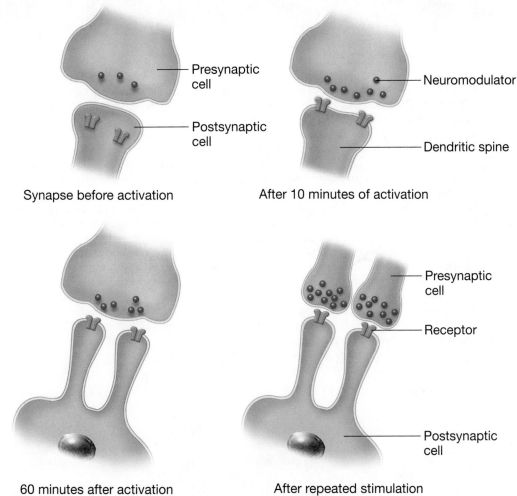

Presynaptic cell

Postsynaptic cell

Synapse before activation

Neuromodulator

Dendritic spine

After 10 minutes of activation

60 minutes after activation

Presynaptic cell

Receptor

Postsynaptic cell

After repeated stimulation

FIGURE 14-6   Repeated activation of synapses over time stimulates long-term changes in the structure of the synapse, causing the presynaptic neuron to develop more axon terminals, while the postsynaptic neuron grows additional dendrites. This development of new synapses is known as synaptogenesis.

over a period of days or weeks, genes within both the presynaptic and postsynaptic neurons will be expressed (activated). These genes code for proteins necessary to make new axon terminals, synaptic vesicles, neurotransmitters, receptors, and dendritic spines: The result is creation of a new synapse. Synaptogenesis has been studied mainly in synapses that use glutamate as the neurotransmitter. In these synapses, repeated firing causes a large, sustained flow of calcium. The high calcium levels appear to be the trigger that jump-starts activation of synaptic genes.

Long-term synaptic removal ("pruning") can also occur. When existing synapses are fired only rarely, genes that maintain these synapses are deactivated. Thus, synapses that are seldom fired will tend to decay and not be replaced. This phenomenon explains why we may forget most of a foreign language learned long ago, or the content of a course taken in the past.

Language

Language is a complex phenomenon: It involves hearing and understanding speech, as well as having the ability to formulate words and organize them into sentences, and it encompasses reading and writing. These abilities are crucial to normal communication.

Spoken language requires the ability to hear and to understand speech. These functions are located in the temporal lobe. The perception of sound takes place in the primary auditory cortex. Understanding the meaning of all sounds (not just speech) occurs in the auditory association cortex. The ability to understand the meaning of language specifically

Clinical Box 14-3: Alzheimer's Disease

Alzheimer Disease (AD) is one cause of **dementia,** defined as a loss of cognitive and memory functions. Other causes of dementia include CVA (vascular dementia), brain infections and tumors, Parkinson Disease, and many other, less common neurodegenerative diseases. People with Alzheimer Disease lose their short-term memory first, and then gradually lose long-term memory as well. Brain studies show a characteristic loss of nerve cells that begins in the temporal lobe, and gradually spreads throughout the cerebral cortex. Neurons contain "tangles" (balls of tangled fibers inside the cells) and form "plaques" (clusters of dead neurons stuck together by a mutated beta-amyloid protein). It is not clear whether the plaques and tangles are the cause of, or result from, the disease. What is known is that people with Alzheimer Disease lose cognitive and declarative memory functions, and then gradually lose the ability to function independently. Brains from people with Alzheimer Disease are smaller, lighter, and thinner than comparable healthy brains, with more space between gyri and enlarged ventricles (see **Figure 14-7**). Because the damage begins in the temporal lobe and affects the hippocampus along with regions important for facial recognition, people with Alzheimer Disease have trouble remembering names and faces, and lose their spatial memory early in the course of the disease; they may get lost easily and tend to wander. Because the amygdala is located in the temporal lobe, some people with Alzheimer Disease display hostile or aggressive behavior. Several drugs have been shown to temporarily improve cognitive function, but there are no drugs that can slow or stop the progressive and incurable course of Alzheimer Disease.

Challenge question: Why would a person with Alzheimer Disease have trouble remembering things for more than a few minutes?

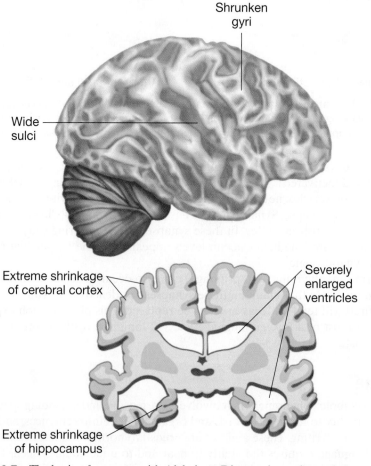

Shrunken gyri

Wide sulci

Extreme shrinkage of cerebral cortex

Severely enlarged ventricles

Extreme shrinkage of hippocampus

FIGURE 14-7 The brain of a person with Alzheimer Disease shows dramatic loss of neurons, so the cortex appears shrunken while the ventricles are greatly enlarged. The top figure is a lateral view of the right side of the brain, and the bottom figure is a transverse section through the cerebral cortex.

is centered in a region called **Wernicke's receptive language** area (see Figure 14-8). A lesion to Wernicke's area results in the inability to understand both spoken and written language, a condition called **receptive aphasia.** Patients with receptive aphasia can speak but cannot understand what others are saying to them. They also cannot understand their own speech, so they often do not make sense when talking.

The ability to formulate (create) speech is localized in **Broca's expressive (motor) language area,** in the posterior part of the frontal lobe. Broca's area stores the "programs" for speech. Broca's area permits us to organize thoughts and words in order to convey meaning. It has many connections to parts of the supplementary motor cortex where motor speech programs are stored, and to parts of the primary motor cortex that control skeletal muscles used in speech production. People with lesions to Broca's area have **expressive aphasia:** Although they can usually understand spoken language, and can think clearly, they are sometimes unable to speak at all, or may say just one word. Their speech may be described as "telegraphic" because it sometimes comes out in rapid bursts, and may contain only the essential words needed to convey meaning.

Occasionally, a stroke or brain injury will damage both Wernicke's and Broca's areas. This is known as **global aphasia.** People with this condition can neither understand nor formulate language.

In most people, both the receptive and expressive language areas are located in the left hemisphere. The corresponding regions in the right hemisphere do not have names, and are involved in nonverbal communication. For example, the region in the right temporal lobe that corresponds to Wernicke's receptive language area is active when we receive nonverbal signals (gestures, facial expressions, tone of voice, and body language). Similarly, the part of the right frontal lobe that corresponds to Broca's expressive (motor) language area is involved in producing nonverbal communication (gestures, facial expressions, etc). A few people have bilateral language areas, with smaller Wernicke's and Broca's areas on both sides of their brains, along with bilateral nonverbal communication regions.

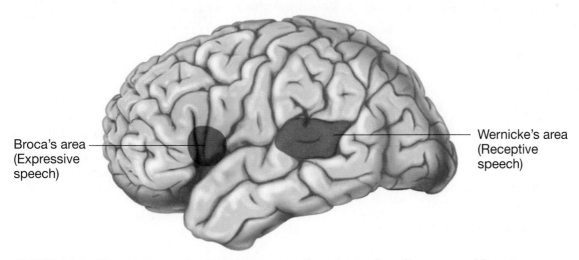

Broca's area
(Expressive
speech)

Wernicke's area
(Receptive
speech)

FIGURE 14-8   Wernicke's receptive language area permits understanding of language, and Broca's expressive language area is responsible for language production. In most people, both areas are located in the left hemisphere.

PATIENT SCENARIOS

Patient Case 14-1 (Claudia)

Claudia is an 82-year-old woman who has been diagnosed with dementia caused by Alzheimer Disease. She lives in a nursing home designed for people with severe memory impairments. Claudia often forgets the names of her caregivers, and sometimes does not recognize her children and grandchildren when they visit her. She gets lost in the dementia unit and needs help getting back to her room. However, she can remember specific events from her childhood and often speaks Polish, which was her first language (she moved to the United States from Poland as a young girl.) Claudia also remembers how to knit, a hobby she has had for many years.

Questions

a) What kind of memory does Claudia retain? What kind does she have trouble with?
b) Which brain regions are affected early in the course of Alzheimer Disease?
c) What would you expect to find if you could do an autopsy of Claudia's brain cells?

Patient Case 14-2 (John)

John is a 37-year-old man who suffered a traumatic brain injury seven weeks ago in a motorcycle accident. He is currently able to walk 100 feet with a small-based quad cane with minimal assistance from his physical therapist. His right hip displays weakness and decreased range of motion in all directions. He is often impulsive and aggressive, and is easily agitated.

Questions

a) Based on John's impulsive and aggressive behavior, what brain region do you suspect was injured in his accident?
b) How would you plan your treatment session to best limit the agitation and aggressive behaviors of this patient?

Patient Case 14-3 (Allan)

Allan, age 77, suffered a CVA (stroke) two weeks ago. He has right-side hemiplegia that is slowly improving with therapy. He is able to understand most of what is said to him, and appears oriented and alert. Allan can speak only a few words—specifically, "no," "chair," and "darn it." However, he is able to make his needs and preferences known using nonverbal communication (pointing, gesturing, facial expressions).

Questions

a) Where do you think Allan's stroke caused the most damage? What is the term that describes his language deficit?
b) How can you best communicate with Allan? How will you know what he wants or needs?

Review Questions

1. Where is cognitive function centered in the brain? Define *cognition* and provide some examples from everyday life.

2. Where is emotion centered in the brain? What are some disorders that affect emotion?

3. How are declarative and nondeclarative memory and learning different?

4. How do short-term and long-term learning occur?

5. Where are the major language centers of the brain located? Distinguish between receptive and expressive language, and define *receptive* and *expressive* aphasias.

References

1. Eriksson, P. S., Perfilieva, E., Bjork-Eriksson, T., Alborn, A-M., Nordborg, C., Peterson., D.A. & Gage, F. H. (1998). Neurogenesis in the adult human hippocampus. *Nature Medicine, 4*(11), 1313–1317.

2. Gardiner, R., & Hogan, R. E. (2005). Three-dimensional deformation-based hippocampal surface anatomy, projected on MRI images. *Clinical Anatomy, 18*, 481–487.

3. Malberg, J. E., Eisch, A. J., Nestler, E. J., & Duman, R. S. (2000). Chronic antidepressant treatment increases neurogenesis in adult rat hippocampus. *J. of Neurosci., 20*(24), 9104–9110.

4. Shamay-Tsoory, S. G., Tomer, R., Yaniv, S., & Ahron-Peretz, J. (2002). Empathy deficits in Asperger syndrome: A cognitive profile. *Neurocase, 8*(3), 245–252.

Further Reading

1. Aggleton, J. P. (1993). The contribution of the amygdala to normal and abnormal emotional states. *Trend in Neurosci, 16,* 328–333.

2. Kandel, E. R. (2006). *In Search of Memory: The Emergence of a New Science of Mind.* New York: W. W. Norton.

3. Levine, A. (2008, June/July). Unmasking memory genes. *Scientific American Mind,* 49–51.

4. Miller, G. (2004). Learning to forget. *Science* (News focus), *304,* 34–36.

5. Morgane, P. J., Galler, J. R., & Mokler, D. J. (2005). A review of systems and networks of the limbic forebrain/limbic midbrain. *Progress in Neurobiology, 75,* 143–160.

6. Rempel-Clower, N.L., Zola, S.M., Squire, L.R., and Amaral, D.G. (1996). Three cases of enduring memory impairment after bilateral damage limited to the hippocampal formation. Journal of Neuroscience, *16,* 5233–5255,

7. Scheff, S. W., Price, D. A., Hicks, R. R., Baldwin, S. A., Robinson, S., & Brackney, C. (2005). Synaptogenesis in the hippocampal CA1 field following traumatic brain injury. *J. of Neurotrauma, 22*(7), 719–732.

8. Scoville, W. B., & Milner, B. (1957). Loss of recent memory after bilateral hippocampal lesions. *J. Neurol Neurosurg Psychiatry, 20,* 11–21.

PEARSON
myhealthprofessionskit™

Use this address to access the Companion Website created for this textbook. Simply select "Physical Therapy" from the choice of disciplines. Find this book and log in using your username and password to access self-assessment questions, a glossary and more.

Development and Aging

CHAPTER OBJECTIVES

After completing this chapter, the reader will be able to:

1. Describe how the nervous system develops, both before and after birth.

2. Explain the changes that take place in the brain due to environmental influences and experiences during infancy and childhood.

3. Discuss the neurobiology of common developmental disorders, including spina bifida, Down syndrome, autism, cerebral palsy, epilepsy, hydrocephalus, and Arnold-Chiari malformation.

4. List changes that occur in the nervous system due to aging.

KEY TERMS

anencephaly
Arnold-Chiari malformation
ataxic cerebral palsy
athetoid cerebral palsy
autism
cerebral palsy (CP)
critical periods (sensitive periods)
differentiation
Down syndrome
epilepsy
hydrocephalus
hypoxia
myelination
neural crest
neural groove
neural plate
neural tube
Schwann cells
spastic hemiplegia
spina bifida
status epilepticus
synaptogenesis

Essential Facts··

▶ The nervous system begins developing at 18 days of gestation, and has established its basic pattern by the end of the first trimester.

▶ Development of the nervous system requires cells to divide, migrate, specialize, form synapses, and lay down myelin.

▶ Normal sensory and movement experiences are necessary for normal development.

▶ Many developmental disorders result from genetic or environmental disruptions in nervous system development.

▶ In healthy people, age-related changes in brain function are small, and involve some decline in sensation and in processing speed.

This chapter describes how the nervous system develops before and after birth, and how the system changes during childhood and adolescence. As people age, the nervous system experiences a number of alterations that affect its function. These include thinning of the myelin sheath, loss of some motor neurons, and decreased sensitivity of sensory receptors. As a result, older people have slower transmission of action potentials, less muscle strength, decreased control of movement, and a decline in sensory function. These changes are often compounded by other complications of aging such as arteriosclerosis, loss of mobility, and diseases like diabetes, Alzheimer Disease, and Parkinson Disease that affect neuron function.

Nervous System Development

The human nervous system begins its development a few weeks after the sperm and egg unite, and continues into early adulthood. During development, cells divide, rearrange, specialize, and form many connections with one another as well as with other body organs, including muscles and glands. Many developmental disabilities result from disruptions of these basic developmental processes.

Before Birth: Prenatal Development

Development of the human nervous system begins 18 days after the egg is fertilized. A sheet of cells called the **neural plate** forms on the dorsal side of the embryo (see **Figure 15-1**). Over the next several days, the neural plate enlarges, and then begins to buckle or fold in the center. This creates a **neural groove**. Gradually, the neural groove deepens until its two edges touch. As the edges come into contact, they fuse together to create a hollow tube of cells (the **neural tube**) that is evident by gestational day 21. Some cells from the edges of the neural plate are pinched off to form the **neural crest.** The embryonic neural tube and neural crest form the basic structure of the nervous system.

The neural tube develops first in the lower cervical region, and then closes or "zips up": first in a cranial direction, and then toward the sacrum (caudally). By 24 days of gestation, the neural tube is almost completely closed. Failure of the tube to close completely results in serious neurological deficits, including **anencephaly** (lack of brain development) and **spina bifida** (incomplete closure of the spinal cord).

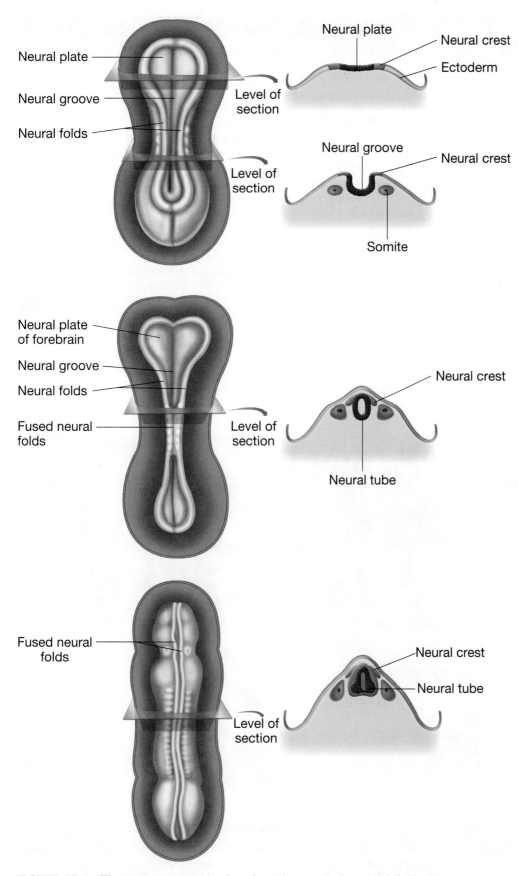

FIGURE 15-1 The nervous system develops from the neural plate, which folds up to create a hollow neural tube and the adjacent neural crest. The neural tube forms the brain and spinal cord, whereas the neural crest forms the autonomic and sensory ganglia as well as the adrenal medulla.

Clinical Box 15-1: Neural Tube Defects

Anencephaly results from incomplete closure of the cranial end of the neural tube. In most cases, the forebrain fails to develop along with the overlying skull bones so the baby is born with an exposed brainstem and dies before or shortly after birth.

Spina bifida is caused by incomplete closure of the sacral end of the neural tube (see **Figure 15-2**). In spina bifida occulta, the spinal cord and cauda equina develop normally and are covered by skin, but the vertebral arches are incomplete. This usually occurs in the lower lumbar part of the spine. In spina bifida cystica, the vertebral arches fail to develop and a large sac of meninges protrudes from the back. Sometimes the spinal cord is in place within the vertebral column (meningeocele), or the cord may be located within the sac of meninges (myelomeningeoceole). Spina bifida can cause paralysis and sensory loss in the lower extremities, as well as loss of bladder and bowel control. Spina bifida is associated with folic acid deficiency; other contributing factors are not known.

Challenge question: Why might spina bifida cause lack of bladder and bowel control? (*Hint:* Which spinal cord levels contain nerves to the bladder and bowel?)

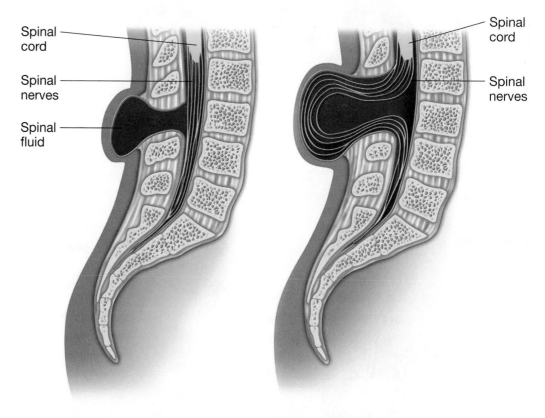

Spinal cord

Spinal nerves

Spinal fluid

Spinal cord

Spinal nerves

Meningocele   Myelomeningocele

FIGURE 15-2   Types of spina bifida include meningocele, in which the vertebral arch is incomplete but the spinal cord is in place, as well as myelomeningocele, where a sac of meninges protrudes from the dorsal aspect of the spinal column, sometimes containing the spinal cord and spinal nerves. Spina bifida results from incomplete closure of the neural tube.

Review Concepts 15-1: Summary of Nervous System Subdivisions

- Forebrain (prosencephalon)
  1. Cerebrum (cerebral cortex and subcortical nuclei) (telencephalon)
  2. Thalamus and hypothalamus (diencephalon)

- Midbrain (mesencephalon)

- Hindbrain (rhombencephalon)
  1. Pons (metencephalon)
     Cerebellum
  2. Medulla oblongata (myelencephalon)

- Spinal cord

The brain and spinal cord both develop from the neural tube. Beginning on gestational day 28, the superior (cranial) end of the tube begins to form three subdivisions: the forebrain, midbrain, and hindbrain (see **Figure 15-3**). The forebrain then separates into the two cerebral hemispheres, the thalamus and the hypothalamus. The midbrain changes relatively little, whereas the hindbrain gives rise to the pons, cerebellum, and medulla oblongata. The inferior part of the neural tube becomes the spinal cord.

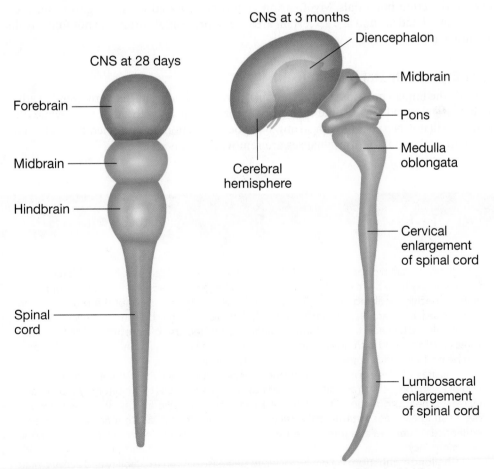

FIGURE 15-3 The nervous system is divided into the forebrain, midbrain, hindbrain, and spinal cord. The forebrain undergoes tremendous growth, while the midbrain and hindbrain remain relatively small.

While the neural tube is growing and subdividing, the neural crest cells are migrating throughout the body. They form the autonomic nervous system (the sympathetic and parasympathetic nerves), somatosensory neurons and receptors, and part of the adrenal gland (the adrenal medulla). In addition, the **Schwann cells** that form the myelin sheath in the peripheral nervous system develop from the neural crest (see **Figure 15-4**).

By the end of the first trimester of pregnancy (12 weeks), the basic organizational structure of the nervous system is in place. After that, developing neurons and their supporting glial cells divide to form about 100 billion neurons and 5 trillion glial cells. After birth, the glial cells continue to multiply, but neurons in most parts of the nervous system lose that ability. Only the hippocampus and olfactory epithelium continue to form new neurons throughout life.

In addition to cell division (mitosis), three other important cellular processes take place before birth. The first of these is migration, in which neurons move to their proper locations. They are attracted or repelled by chemical cues that guide them to their correct place in the CNS. Failure of nerve cells to migrate properly can create ectopic ("out of place") neuron cell bodies, and can cause abnormal generation of action potentials (seizures).

Once neurons have reached their correct locations, they must differentiate (specialize). This means that the cells acquire a specific structure and function. **Differentiation** is controlled by chemical cues and by the location of the neurons. For example, nerve cells located on the dorsal aspect of the neural tube will become sensory neurons, whereas those located ventrally become motor neurons. Failure to differentiate properly is associated with several nervous system abnormalities, including **Down syndrome** and fetal alcohol syndrome.

The last step in prenatal nervous system development is **myelination** of axons. Myelin is formed by glial cells: oligodendroglial cells in the central nervous system, and Schwann cells in the peripheral nervous system. The myelin sheath insulates axons and speeds transmission of action potentials. Myelination begins at about 20 weeks of gestation, and is mostly completed around age 2. Certain areas (e.g., prefrontal cortex) do not fully myelinate until early adulthood.

After Birth: Postnatal Development

At birth, the human nervous system contains many more neurons than are found in adults. As babies grow and learn, some neurons will form synapses with other cells, while other neurons will not. Nerve cells with strong synaptic connections are retained throughout life, but neurons that fail to form synapses are removed ("pruned").

Clinical Box 15-2: Epilepsy (Seizure Disorder)

Epilepsy is a brain disorder that is characterized by repeated seizures. Many different kinds of epilepsy have been described. Seizures may be generalized (of diffuse origin) or partial (with a specific, localized origin). Seizures occur when specific areas of the brain become overexcited, firing action potentials randomly. The disorder may be caused by genetic brain abnormalities, by head trauma, tumors, or strokes, or because of **cerebral palsy.** Many seizures can be treated with drugs that decrease nerve cell excitability. In some cases, surgery can be performed to remove the sites where the seizures begin.

Seizures can be harmful because the excessive nerve activity can cause overproduction of excitatory neurotransmitters, excess calcium release, loss of inhibitory synapses, and increased heat production. If seizures last too long, the toxic effects of overactivity and overheating can cause **status epilepticus,** which may result in death if not halted. Status epilepticus is defined as a generalized seizure that lasts 30 minutes or more, and is a medical emergency.

Challenge question: If a drug is given to decrease neuron excitability and activity, what might some side effects of the drug be?

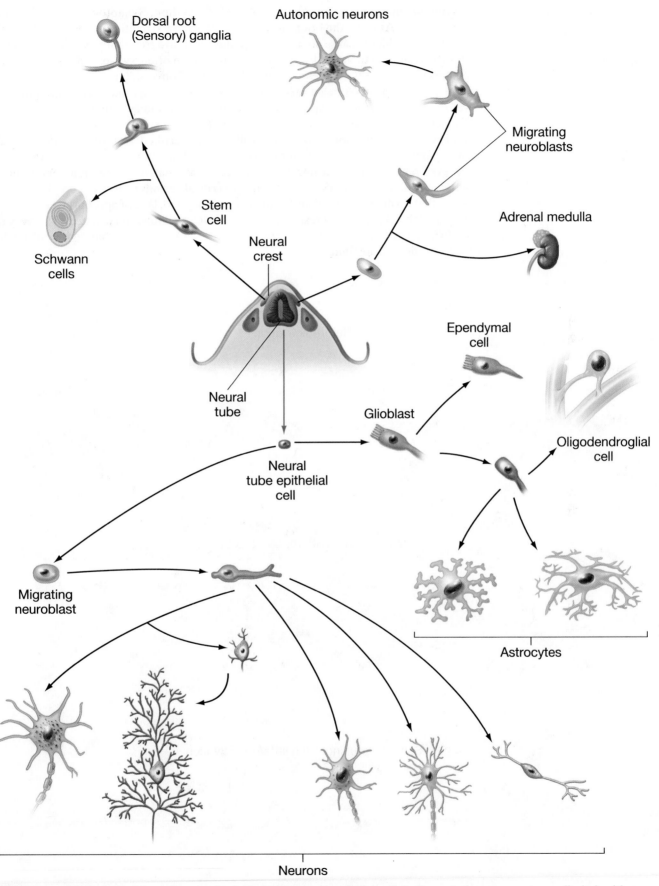

FIGURE 15-4 Cells derived from the neural tube include neurons and glial cells in the central nervous system; cells derived from the neural crest include autonomic and sensory neurons, as well as the adrenal medulla.

Synaptogenesis is the process of synapse formation. Synaptogenesis takes place throughout life. At birth, the brain contains relatively few synaptic connections. As a child grows, life experiences cause some neural pathways to fire frequently, whereas others are seldom activated. In those pathways that are stimulated often, synapses are strengthened, and many new synapses are created (synaptogenesis). Conversely, pathways that are rarely fired will not form synaptic connections (see Figure 15-5). Synaptogenesis requires the developing brain to receive appropriate sensory stimulation as well as opportunities for movement and exploration of the environment. If these experiences are lacking, the pattern of synaptic connections established will be impoverished. Neurons that do not make strong synaptic connections to other nerve cells are eliminated.

Developmental stages during which synapses are created in large numbers in certain functional regions of the CNS are referred to as **critical periods (sensitive periods)**. Because neurons that do not make enough synapses are eliminated, lack of appropriate stimulation during the critical period will result in a poorly developed functional system. This very difficult to make up later, as the brain's ability to establish synapses in that region will decline after the critical period ends.

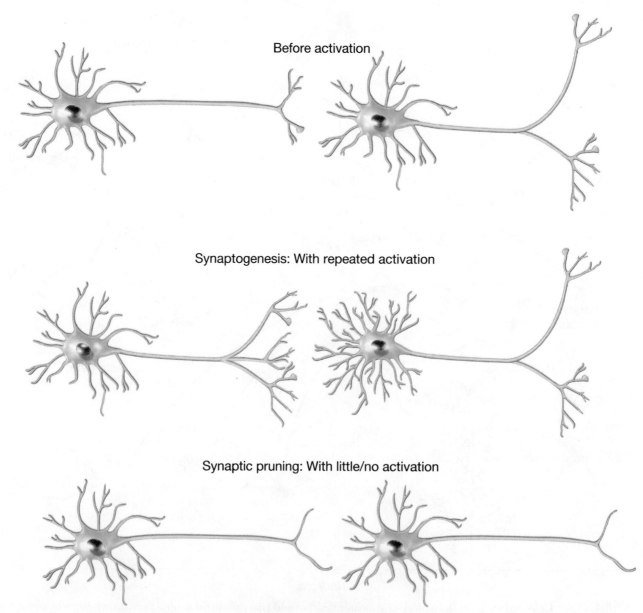

Before activation

Synaptogenesis: With repeated activation

Synaptic pruning: With little/no activation

FIGURE 15-5   Frequent activation of synapses stimulates synaptogenesis (growth of new synapses), whereas little or no synaptic activation results in synaptic pruning (removal of synapses).

Neuroscience Notes Box 15-1:
Critical Periods

Critical periods have been described for the brain's visual system and language centers. For example, if a newborn animal's eyelids are sewn shut at birth, the visual cortex fails to organize properly. When the eyelids are opened later, the animal is unable to see normally. In humans, a critical period for learning language is thought to exist during the first several years of life; the ability to learn new languages decreases with increasing age. Compare the accent of a person who learned a new language as an adult with the accent of a native speaker. Even if they have been speaking English for the same amount of time, the two accents will probably sound quite different.

At birth, some parts of the nervous system have well-developed myelin sheaths that allow rapid transmission of nerve signals. In the peripheral nervous system, sensory neurons are well-myelinated, so newborn babies can feel touch, pain, and pressure. Cranial nerves necessary for smell and taste are fully myelinated, but the optic nerves are not; newborns can see clearly for only a short distance. Motor pathways are not completely myelinated at birth except for the cranial nerves needed to suck and swallow. Thus, healthy newborn babies are well-prepared to nurse. However, babies born too early (premature babies or "preemies") may not be ready for life outside the mother, and may have difficulty with the motor skills necessary for nursing.

During the first few years of life, a baby's brain grows and matures. It will double in size during the first year, and will use over 50% of the energy the baby consumes. The primary postnatal cellular processes are myelination, synaptogenesis, and apoptosis (programmed cell death). Most neurons (except in the hippocampus and olfactory epithelium) do not divide after birth.

Myelination of axons is due to growth of glial cells that thicken the myelin sheath and speed the transmission of action potentials. The primary motor and primary sensory cortex are myelinated by about 16 months of age. The last part of the brain to be fully mature is the prefrontal cortex; myelination is not complete there until early adulthood.

Clinical Box 15-3: Deficits Caused by Premature Birth

The last several weeks of pregnancy are a critical period of rapid brain growth and maturation. Babies born prematurely are more susceptible to brain trauma than those born at full term. The trauma usually results from disruption of blood flow or oxygen to the brain. Brain tissue near the lateral ventricles (periventricular regions) is especially prone to injury. Two common pathologies of prematurity are periventricular leukomalacia (PVL) and interventricular hemorrhage (IVH; see **Figure 15-6**). PVL refers to damage to the white matter (axons) next to the lateral ventricles. It is caused by lack of blood flow or decreased oxygen in the blood. PVL can cause motor impairments that affect the lower extremities. IVH involves bleeding into the ventricles of the brain. It results in varying degrees of motor impairment, depending on the extent of the bleeding. The severity of IVH is related to the degree of prematurity. Infants born before 30 weeks of gestation are at highest risk of IVH (Dubowitz, Dubowitz, & Mercuri, 1999).

Challenge question: If the cerebral cortex is injured by premature birth, what kind of functional deficits (other than motor impairments) might be expected?

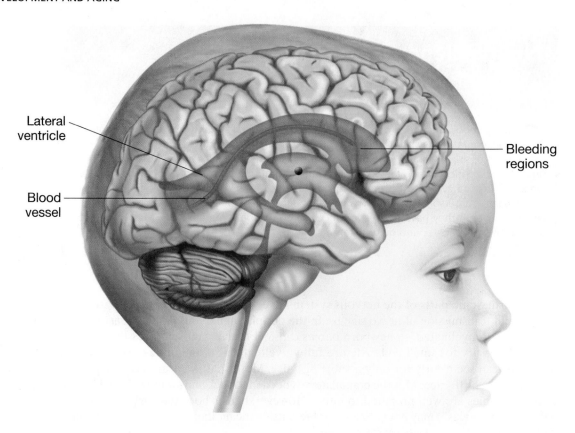

Lateral ventricle

Blood vessel

Bleeding regions

FIGURE 15-6 Bleeding into the ventricles (interventricular hemorrhage) is one cause of cerebral palsy that can occur when babies are born before 30 weeks of gestation.

Developmental disorders of the nervous system are caused by abnormal growth and development of the CNS. In addition, disabilities that occur as a result of the birth process, or that occur shortly after birth, are often classified as developmental disorders. Many disorders have a genetic origin, whereas others result from environmental causes, including infections, prematurity, or oxygen deprivation to the brain. Some disorders have no known cause.

Cerebral palsy (CP) is a nonprogressive motor disorder that occurs prenatally, during the birth process, or shortly after birth. This disorder has a variety of causes, including infection, lack of oxygen to the brain, intraventricular hemorrhage, premature birth, and brain injury. It is always classified by the type of motor dysfunction present, even if there are other kinds of problems with sensation, language, or cognition.

There are four major types of cerebral palsy. Spastic cerebral palsy results from damage to upper motor neurons, often to the corticospinal tracts on one side of the brain. A common form of spastic CP is **spastic hemiplegia** (spastic paralysis on one side of the body). **Athetoid cerebral palsy** is characterized by slow, writhing movements of the limbs and is caused by damage to the basal ganglia. **Ataxic cerebral palsy** results from cerebellar injury; patients display uncoordinated movements. Finally, some people have mixed CP, with two or more movement dysfunctions at the same time. Speech disorders, sensory impairments, hearing and visual problems, seizures, and cognitive dysfunction may accompany the motor system injuries. Musculoskeletal impairments are also common as a result of the neurological deficits.

The motor and sensory deficits caused by cerebral palsy vary. Most clinicians who treat people with cerebral palsy attempt to improve functional ability by reducing the number and degree of impairments that the child exhibits. For example, someone with spastic cerebral palsy may have very tight plantar flexor and hip adductor muscles that can prevent ambulation. The clinician will focus treatment on stretching, preventing contractures, and weight-bearing activities to help prevent this impairment from leading to a decrease in potential function.

Clinical Box 15-4: Arnold-Chiari Malformation

Arnold-Chiari malformation is characterized by a malformed hindbrain (see **Figure 15-7**). In Type I malformations, the pons and medulla oblongata are small and abnormally formed; the inferior medulla and part of the cerebellum protrude down through the foramen magnum into the spinal canal. Symptoms include severe headache, ataxia due to compression of the cerebellum, and weakness of muscles of the face and tongue. Dizziness and hearing loss can result from compression of cranial nerves in the pons and medulla. Type II Arnold-Chiari malformation is similar to Type I, with the addition of hydrocephalus due to blockage of cerebrospinal fluid (see below). Type II frequently accompanies spina bifida.

Challenge questions: Which cranial nerve could cause weakness of tongue muscles? Which cranial nerve could cause hearing loss and dizziness?

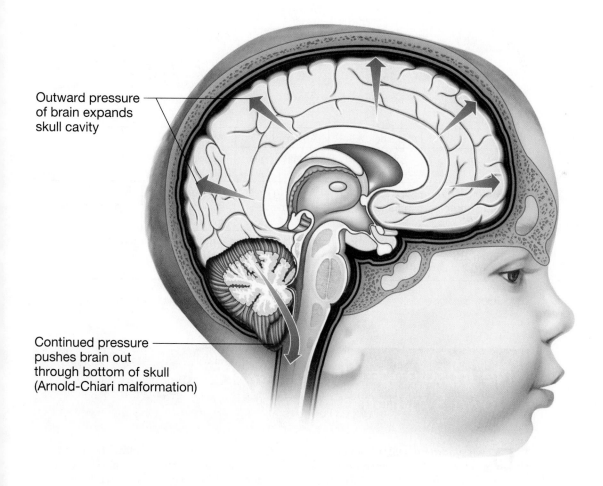

Outward pressure
of brain expands
skull cavity

Continued pressure
pushes brain out
through bottom of skull
(Arnold-Chiari malformation)

FIGURE 15-7 In Arnold-Chiari malformation, the brainstem and cerebellum protrude down into the spinal canal, and enlargement of the ventricles may occur causing hydrocephalus.

Clinical Box 15-5: Hydrocephalus

Hydrocephalus results from blockage of CSF flow through the ventricles and subarachnoid space (see **Figure 15-8**). It may accompany spina bifida or Arnold-Chiari malformation, or it may occur as a result of head injury, tumor, or scar tissue within the brain. Because CSF drainage is blocked, the brain's ventricles will begin to swell. In young children whose skull bones have not yet fused, expansion of the ventricles causes enlargement of the cerebral cortex and skull, resulting in formation of a huge head with paper-thin cerebral cortex and cranial bones. In adults, brain injuries and tumors that block CSF flow also cause increased CSF pressure that compresses the brain against the skull and results in **hypoxia** (lack of oxygen to nerve cells) and brain damage. If diagnosed early enough, doctors can implant a shunt with a one-way valve to drain the excess fluid and prevent damage to the brain.

Challenge question: If CSF flow were blocked in the cerebral aqueduct, which ventricles would become distended?

Review Concept 5-2: Types of Cerebral Palsy

	Spastic	Athetoid	Ataxic	Mixed
Lesion	Upper motor neurons	Basal ganglia	Cerebellum	Mixture of motor areas
Motor signs and symptoms	Spastic paralysis	Writhing movements	Ataxia (unco-ordinated movements)	Mixture of motor deficits
Possible nonmotor problems	Sensory impairments, vision and hearing deficits, language problems, cognitive impairments, musculoskeletal impairments			

Neuroscience Notes Box 15-2: Down Syndrome

Down syndrome (DS) is a genetic disorder that occurs in about 1/800 births. The disorder results from the presence of an extra (third) copy of chromosome 21; it is also known as trisomy 21. People with Down syndrome have a variety of brain abnormalities in addition to other physical characteristics. Cognitive disability and hypotonia are common. The brains of people with Down syndrome are smaller than normal, with fewer cortical neurons and abnormally formed dendrites. The cerebellum contains many undifferentiated (unspecialized) cells. The ability to form synapses is decreased in people with this disorder; this may be why they learn more slowly. Microscopically, nerve cells in people with Down syndrome resemble those of people with Alzheimer disease.

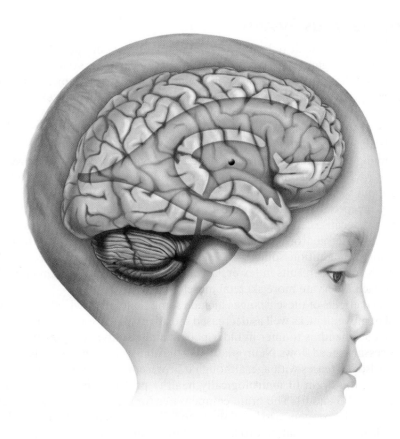

FIGURE 15-8 When cerebrospinal fluid drainage is blocked, the brain's ventricles enlarge; in babies this can result in enlargement of the skull. This is referred to as hydrocephalus.

Clinical Box 15-6: Autism (Pervasive Developmental Disorder)

Autism (pervasive developmental disorder) is a neurodevelopmental genetic disorder characterized by impaired social interaction and communication. Some people with autism display stereotypical, repetitive behavior patterns and some have cognitive impairments. The cerebral cortices of some people with autism have more neurons than normal, but the cerebellum has fewer. In addition, brains of people with autism produce less serotonin than normal, and treatment with serotonin reuptake inhibitors (SSRIs) seems to improve social functioning. This condition is often described as a "spectrum disorder," spanning from people with severe impairments all the way to people who are very intelligent and highly functional.

Challenge question: Since the cerebellum is abnormal in people with autism, would you expect any type of movement dysfunction?

The Aging Nervous System

The effects of age on the healthy brain are not completely understood. It is important to separate the normal aging process from development of nervous system diseases, and from the effects of other systemic diseases on brain function. For example, both diabetes and heart disease can harm the nervous system. Healthy people can have excellent brain function throughout life, and retain the ability to learn via neuroplasticity.

The healthy aging brain shows a small loss of neurons (less than 10% of the total). However, the brain shrinks with age (about 0.8% per year after age 30) and weighs a bit less due to thinning of myelin. Older brains have fewer synapses, postsynaptic receptors, and dendrites, as well as smaller amounts of neurotransmitters. For example, the substantia nigra secretes about 50% less dopamine at age 60 than at age 20. In the peripheral nervous system, sensory receptors become less sensitive because the action potential threshold increases with age. Because cell membranes in older people contain more cholesterol than in younger people, older neurons are stiffer and less fluid, and respond less effectively to sensory stimulation. In addition, some lower motor neurons in the spinal cord and brainstem are lost with age. This results in fewer, larger motor units, since the remaining lower motor neurons each innervate more skeletal muscle fibers.

The functional effects of these changes include some skeletal muscle atrophy and less precise control of movement, as well as decreased sensitivity of the somatosensory system. Because the myelin sheath is thinner in older people and because synapses function less effectively, processing speed slows. Neuroplasticity (the ability to form new synapses based on experience) also decreases with age, although it is present throughout life.

Blood flow to the brain of neurologically healthy people declines by about 23% between the ages of 33 and 61. The brain compensates for this decrease by extracting a larger proportion of the oxygen carried by the blood. The factors responsible for the flow decline are unclear but the small neurons controlling dilation and contraction of brain arterioles may be responsible. These small nerve cells decrease in number with normal aging.

PATIENT SCENARIOS

Patient Case 15-1 (Brittany)

Brittany is 7 years old. She was born with cerebral palsy that affects the left side of her body. She was born early because her mother contracted an infection during pregnancy. Brittany has spasticity and paresis of the left upper and lower extremities, and also has some vision loss as well as a mild cognitive deficit.

Questions

a) Why might premature birth affect the brain and cause cerebral palsy?
b) Which side of Brittany's brain was probably affected to cause her left-sided paresis?
c) Which type of CP does Brittany have?

Patient Case 15-2 (Jack)

Jack is a 21-year-old man who was born with spina bifida. He has flaccid paralysis of both lower extremities, and lacks control of his bladder and bowel function. He also lacks sensation below the T10 dermatome. When Jack was born, he was diagnosed with mild hydrocephalus, but an implanted shunt has successfully prevented any further skull enlargement. Jack is a college student majoring in business who hopes to work in the financial industry when he graduates.

Questions

a) At which spinal cord level did Jack's neural tube fail to fuse correctly?
b) Why are Jack's bladder and bowel functions affected?
c) Where is Jack's shunt probably implanted? What is its purpose?

Review Questions

1. Describe the formation of the neural tube. What are the four primary divisions of the tube? What structures does each division form in the fully developed brain? What structures form from the neural crest?

2. Describe the major cellular processes that occur during neurogenesis. When does myelination begin in the developing nervous system? When is it completed? What purpose does myelination serve?

3. Describe the nervous system at birth. What effect will appropriate stimulation have on the nervous system? What structural changes in the brain are correlated with learning?

4. Describe the cause (if known), and signs/symptoms associated with each of the following developmental disorders:
   • Arnold-Chiari malformation
   • Autism (pervasive developmental disorder)
   • Cerebral palsy
   • Down syndrome
   • Epilepsy
   • Hydrocephalus
   • Spina bifida

5. Explain the process of normal aging in healthy individuals. What functional effects do aging-related changes have?

References

1. Dubowitz, L. M., Dubowitz, V., & Mercuri, E. (1999). *The neurological assessment of the preterm and full-term newborn infant.* London: Cambridge University Press.

2. Ozonoff, S., Rogers, S. J., & Pennington, B. F. (2006). Asperger's syndrome: Evidence of an empirical distinction from high-functioning autism. *J. of Child Psychology and Psychiatry, 32*(7): 1107–1122.

PEARSON
myhealthprofessionskit™

Use this address to access the Companion Website created for this textbook. Simply select "Physical Therapy" from the choice of disciplines. Find this book and log in using your username and password to access self-assessment questions, a glossary and more.

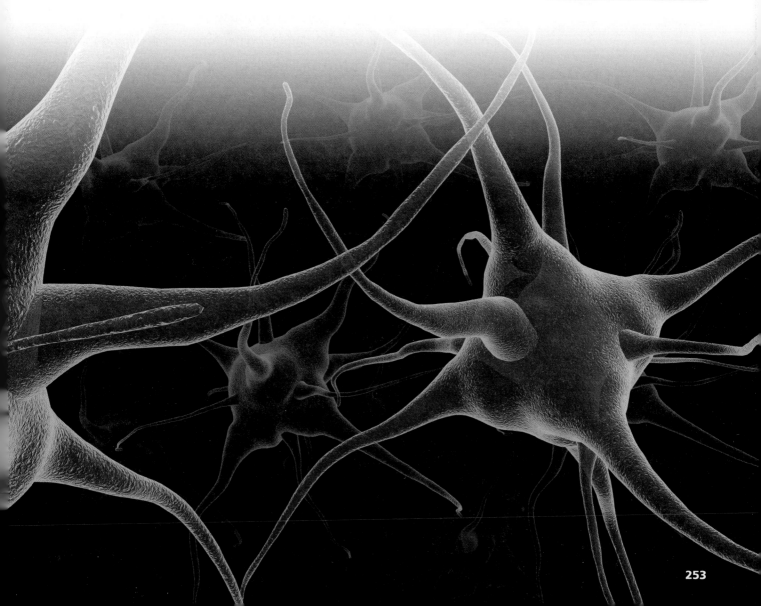

16

Brain Injury and Neuroplasticity

CHAPTER OBJECTIVES

After completing this chapter, the reader will be able to:

1. Discuss mechanisms of CNS injury, including trauma, ischemia, infection, and hemorrhage, and their effects on neuron function.

2. Describe the major mechanisms behind neural plasticity.

3. Explain how exercise and mental stimulation affect neural plasticity and functional recovery.

KEY TERMS

anoxia
contre-coup injury
coupe injury
diffuse axonal injury
encephalopathy
hypoxia
neurogenesis
neuroplasticity
traumatic brain injury
(TBI)

Essential Facts··

▶ Nervous system injury is caused by trauma, disease, or anoxia, and it results in the death of neurons.

▶ Neurons in the central nervous system do not regenerate, but neurons in the peripheral nervous system can regenerate.

▶ Recovery following brain injury occurs by several methods, including synaptogenesis, axon sprouting, functional reorganization, and neurogenesis.

▶ Functional recovery is enhanced by physical activity.

The central nervous system can be damaged by disease, trauma, or vascular problems such as strokes (CVAs). Diseases such as Parkinson Disease or Alzheimer Disease harm cells directly, whereas trauma, strokes, and lack of blood flow to the brain or spinal cord can produce swelling and inflammation that compress the nervous system, damaging neurons and depriving them of blood and oxygen. This chapter will focus on the mechanisms of brain injury, the brain's response to damage, and the process of healing and recovery.

Brain Injury

Traumatic brain injury (TBI) describes mechanical trauma to the brain that occurs when the head strongly impacts an object (for instance, during a car accident) or when an object strikes the head. Brain injury can also occur if a strong force shakes the brain without direct impact on the skull; this can happen after a bomb blast creates intense shock waves. If the head meets something solid, the brain is often injured at the site of the impact; this is called a **coupe injury** (see Figure 16-1). If the force of the initial impact is large enough, it may cause the brain to bounce against the opposite side of the skull; this is referred to as a **contre-coup injury.** In many cases, the contre-coup injury is more severe than the coupe lesion. Both are considered focal lesions, in which a specific region of brain tissue (neurons, glial cells, and blood vessels) is injured by the force of impact.

Focal lesions are localized to specific parts of the brain, so the symptoms that result are relatively predictable. For example, if someone hits her or his forehead on a solid object (e.g., car steering wheel), that person might have a coupe injury at the front of the brain (affecting the prefrontal cortex) and a contre-coupe lesion at the back of the brain (affecting the primary visual cortex). Knowing this, one could predict that this person might have prefrontal syndrome and cortical blindness or other visual dysfunctions from the accident.

Another type of brain damage can occur from rotational forces that result in the brain twisting within the skull. This type of injury can be very devastating as the soft tissues of the brain are dragged across the jagged bony structures located at the base of the skull (see Figure 16-2). This causes widespread shearing of CNS axons, and is called **diffuse axonal injury.** A sad example of both coupe/contre-coup and diffuse axonal injuries is

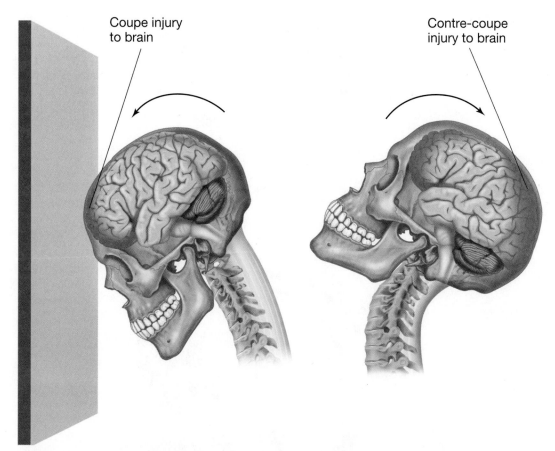

Coupe injury
to brain

Contre-coupe
injury to brain

FIGURE 16-1   Focal lesions are injuries to specific regions of the brain. In coupe/contre-coupe injuries, the brain is affected at the side of impact and on the opposite side as the brain moves within the skull.

that of shaken baby syndrome. When young children are shaken with great force, their brains vibrate back and forth within their skulls. This type of injury can cause multiple focal lesions, and also shears numerous axons, causing wide-ranging damage that cannot be localized to any specific area.

Neurons can also be damaged by events that deprive the brain of blood and oxygen. Such events include prolonged immersion in water (as in near drowning), heart attacks that cause the heart to stop pumping blood for a period of time, and surgical mishaps in which blood flow to the brain is compromised. These events produce **hypoxia** (decreased oxygen) or **anoxia** (lack of oxygen). Neurons have a very high metabolic rate; they can survive without oxygen for only about 3 minutes. After that, they are unable to synthesize ATP and begin to die. This is especially true of neurons in the cerebral cortex. Anything that causes prolonged lack of blood flow to the brain will cause widespread neuronal loss and therefore brain damage.

When neurons are injured, they respond with a series of biological and biochemical events. If neurons are damaged badly enough to die, or are killed because they are deprived of oxygen, they react by swelling. Eventually the neuron cell body ruptures, spilling the cell's contents into the intercellular space. Enzymes, calcium ions, and neurotransmitters are released from the dying cells, and can damage nearby neurons and glial cells. Thus, a kind of chain reaction of cell death can be created, spreading the damage beyond the initial site (see **Figure 16-3**).

At the same time, injury to capillaries and other small blood vessels (arterioles and venules) causes blood to pool in the damaged areas. Blood loss deprives nearby tissue of blood, and the pooled blood compresses adjacent neurons. This also increases the area of cell death. In addition, the pooled blood attracts immune system cells, which arrive to

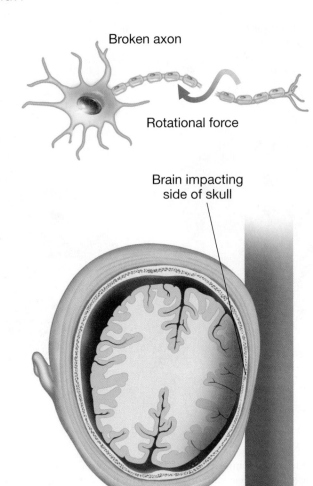

Broken axon

Rotational force

Brain impacting
side of skull

FIGURE 16-2 When rotational forces affect the head, the brain can rotate
inside the skull resulting in twisting and shearing that can tear axons within
their myelin sheaths. This type of damage can be widespread and is known
as diffuse axonal injury.

secrete chemicals that can intensify the swelling. Because there is little space within the
skull, the swelling further compresses brain tissue. A similar reaction occurs when there
is an infection within the skull or spinal column (e.g., bacterial meningitis). Swelling
and inflammation caused by the infection will damage cells, producing **encephalopathy.**
All of these factors increase the size and scope of the damaged area beyond the initial
infarct.

In some injuries, axons are damaged (as in axonal shearing) and the cell bodies are
initially left intact. In the central nervous system, axon injury causes the distal segment of
the axon to swell and die. Within a few days, the proximal segment of the axon also dies,
and is removed by microglial cells (see **Figure 16-4**). Next, the cell body begins to grow
another axon, putting out a small sprout or growth cone. However, the growth cone cannot
elongate, and eventually the entire central nervous system neuron dies. This is different
from the peripheral nervous system, where growth cones do elongate to form new axons. It
appears that the peripheral nervous system contains specific growth factors to assist regeneration, whereas the central nervous system contains factors that impair axon outgrowth
(Liu, Fournier, GrandPre, & Strittmatter, 2002).

Severe brain injury causes a long list of problems for patients. Generally, brain injury
results in unconsciousness. Neurologists typically describe three levels of consciousness
caused by brain damage:

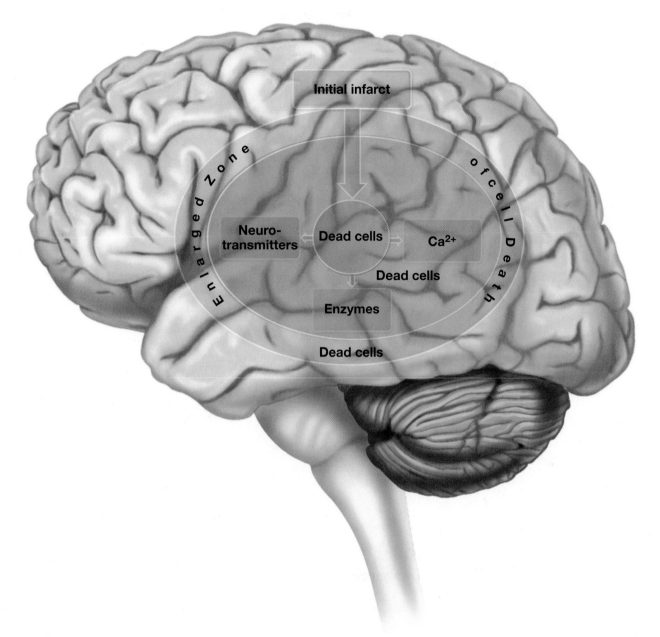

FIGURE 16-3 After brain injury, dead and dying neurons release chemicals that can damage adjacent neurons and magnify the initial infarct.

1. Coma: Eyes are closed, patient is unaware of anything; this stage lasts up to 4 weeks
2. Vegetative state: Eyes are open, patient can sleep and wake but is unaware of environment
3. Minimally conscious state: Patient has some awareness of the environment and may be able to respond to simple questions or commands

The longer a person is in a coma or vegetative state, the worse the prognosis. (See chapter 7 for more information on states of unconsciousness and the Glasgow Coma Scale.)

In addition to disorders of consciousness, severe brain injury can also result in seizures, language deficits, paralysis and sensory loss, ataxia, and long-term cognitive problems. The specific deficits depend on which brain regions have been affected by the injury. If a patient is immobilized due to the injury, problems resulting from immobility can also arise—these include pressure sores, heterotopic ossifications, and contractures (Zasler, 2007).

1)

Axon degeneration

Injury

2)

degeneration

degeneration

CNS   PNS

3)

Neuron removed

Neuron retained

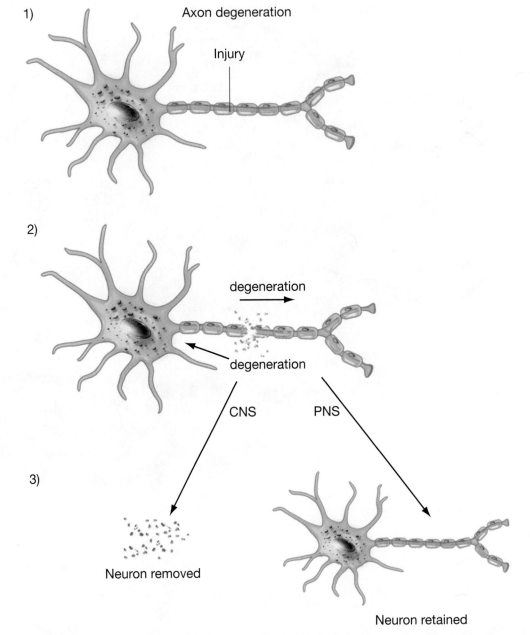

FIGURE 16-4 When axons are injured, they degenerate back to the neuron cell body. Neurons in the CNS die and are not replaced, but neurons in the PNS can usually regenerate their axons.

Mechanisms of Recovery

Although most parts of the CNS do not regenerate after injury, some functional recovery may be possible. This is because many surviving neurons are able to form new connections (synapses), essentially rewiring the brain and spinal cord. Rewiring explains why some people are able to achieve a degree of functional recovery even from serious traumatic, infectious, or anoxic events.

Several mechanisms that contribute to this recovery have been described. They include axonal sprouting, activation of parallel pathways, and neurogenesis (growth of new neurons). *Axonal sprouting* has been demonstrated in the spinal cord (Kraft, 2005). In incomplete spinal cord injury, some axons in motor and/or sensory spinal cord tracts are not damaged. These healthy, intact axons can produce new branches that travel through the injured area of the cord and form synapses with target cells on the other side of the damaged zone (see **Figure 16-5**). This allows some recovery of motor or sensory function.

A   Before injury

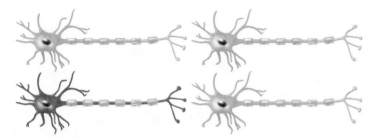

Collateral sprouting following the death of one
presynaptic neuron

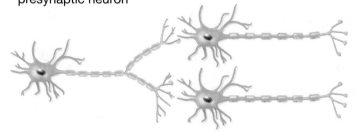

B   Before injury

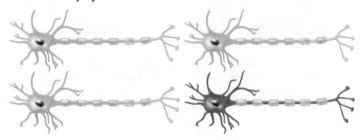

Rewiring after the death of one postsynaptic neuron

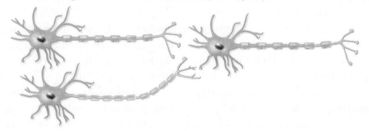

FIGURE 16-5   When a neuron dies, the remaining neurons can often create
new connections (synapses) to rewire the nervous system in order to restore
function. Existing neurons can develop new axon terminals (shown in A), or
can form new connections (shown in B).

Activation of parallel pathways (rewiring) is another method of potential recovery. In
this recovery mechanism, intact neurons can take on new functions and create new synaptic
connections that allow the central nervous system to carry out its essential functions. For
example, if the primary motor cortex in one cerebral hemisphere is injured by a stroke
(CVA), the opposite side (contralateral) cortex can assume some control of skeletal muscle
movements. With enough time and enough practice (rehabilitation), more synaptic connections are formed along the new pathways, allowing improved function.

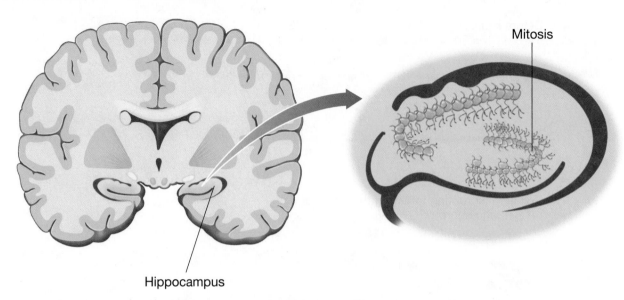

FIGURE 16-6 Neurogenesis takes place throughout life in the hippocampus, a region involved in creating new long-term memories and in learning.

Table 16.1 Factors Affecting Neurogenesis in the Hippocampus

Stimulated by	Inhibited by
Aerobic exercise	Stress, Depression
Mental stimulation	Chemotherapy

Neurogenesis (growth of new neurons) has been shown to occur in two distinct areas of the brain: the hippocampus and the olfactory epithelium (see **Figure 16-6**). In the hippocampus, new neurons are generated throughout life (Erikkson et al., 1998). These new cells must establish synaptic connections with other neurons, or they will be removed (pruned away). Neurons in the hippocampus form more connections in people who are physically active and mentally stimulated. This is consistent with evidence that people who walk daily show improved performance on cognitive function tests, including an improved ability to concentrate and to handle multiple complex tasks. In animals, exposure to physically and mentally stimulating environments helps to retain new nerve cells, whereas stress and drugs that decrease cell division result in fewer new neurons (see **Table 16.1**). For example, chemotherapy drugs (which are designed to prevent cell division in order to kill cancer cells) can also decrease the size of the hippocampus; some people taking chemotherapy report having trouble with memory and concentration that is consistent with an effect on the hippocampus. In addition, people with clinical depression have a smaller hippocampus that increases in size when the depression is treated effectively.

Effects of Exercise and Therapy on Functional Recovery

Scientists have studied the effects of physical activity and exercise on the brain for a number of years. Among the many benefits of aerobic exercise are (1) an improved blood supply to the brain (as shown by new growth of capillaries), (2) an increased number of cells in the hippocampus and parts of the frontal and temporal lobes involved in memory and concentration, and (3) more synapses among neurons. In addition, exercise has been shown to improve the return of function in the brains and spinal cords of people with conditions such as ALS, Parkinson Disease, CVA, and TBI (DiFillipo et al, 2008; King & Horak, 2009; Moore, Roth, Killian, & Hornby, 2010). This indicates that patients who exercise even at moderate levels have a better chance of regaining function.

The brain's ability to reorganize itself based on experience is referred to as **neuroplasticity.** It means "adaptability" or "flexibility" and it has been observed in the central nervous system at all ages. Neuroplasticity is responsible for learning and for the ability to recover (fully or partially) from nervous system injury, infection, and disease. The biological mechanisms involved in neuroplasticity include synaptogenesis (formation of new synapses; Briones, Suh, Jozsa, & Woods, 2006) and neurogenesis (formation of new neurons; Scheff et al., 2005). Neurons that are frequently activated form many more synapses than those that are activated less often ("neurons that fire together wire together"). For clinicians, this means patients recovering from a central nervous system injury should be encouraged to activate neurons and pathways to promote functional recovery. An area of therapy known as "forced use" utilizes this by preventing patients from using an uninvolved (unaffected) limb and forcing them to use an involved (affected) one; there is evidence that this can promote clinically significant functional improvement (van der Lee et al., 1999).

In addition to exercise, exposure to mentally and socially enriched environments has been shown to improve learning, memory, and function in animals with healthy nervous systems and in those with nervous system diseases or injuries. Although not all of the mechanisms underlying neuroplasticity have been identified, it appears that physical exercise and mental and social stimulation can increase levels of chemicals called neurotrophic factors in the brain, and can activate genes that code for synapse formation. This evidence indicates that neuroplasticity is enhanced by both physical and mental stimulation.

Clinical Box 16-1: Neglect and Neuroplasticity

Some patients who suffer from strokes or traumatic brain injuries that largely affect the right side of the brain display "neglect." For example, patients with a cerebrovascular accident (CVA) in the right side of the brain will ignore the left side of the body. In severe cases, a person may dress only the right half of the body, and literally not notice that he or she is wearing only one pant-leg and one shirt-sleeve. In order to capitalize on the mechanisms of neural recovery, clinicians can focus their treatments on weight bearing through the affected extremities, reaching activities toward the neglected side, and improving awareness of the neglected side by positioning themselves toward that visual field and encouraging active and passive control of the affected side.

Challenge question: How would focusing on the neglected side of the body affect the opposite side of the brain? Would it stimulate neuroplasticity?

PATIENT SCENARIOS

Patient Case 16-1 (Ned)
Unilateral Neglect
Ned is a 73-year-old man who suffered a CVA during hip replacement surgery. The stroke affected the right side of his brain. Ned displays left-side neglect: He shaves only the right side of his face, combs the hair on the right side of his head, and eats food only from the right side of his plate. He seems to be unaware of the left side of his body, even when other people remind him about it.

a) Using the principles of neural plasticity and recovery, how can a clinician help Ned improve awareness of his left side?

b) What precautions would a clinician need to be aware of when working with Ned?

Patient Case 16-2: (Xang)
Traumatic Brain Injury
Xang, a 23-year-old man, sustained a traumatic brain injury due to a motorcycle accident. He is experiencing frontal lobe syndrome (impulsive, uninhibited behavior) and cortical blindness.

a) Which specific areas of the cerebral cortex have probably been injured? What is the term used to describe this type of lesion?

b) If Xang experienced axon shearing due to his accident, could you pin-point the damaged areas(s)? Explain what happens in the brain to cause this type of injury.

Patient Case 16-3 (Betty Ann)
Healthy Aging Brain
Betty Ann is a 58-year-old woman who is worried about her brain health. She has seen several older relatives struggle with memory problems as they aged. She works at a sedentary job and does not enjoy exercise. Her sister Ellie Mae is two years older; Ellie Mae bikes for fun on weekends and swims at the "Y" twice a week.

a) What advice would you give Betty Ann to keep her brain as healthy as possible? Is there anything she can do now to minimize her chances of having memory problems?

b) If Betty Ann and Ellie Mae both had a stroke or suffered a brain injury, which sister might have a better chance of functional recovery? Why?

Review Questions

1. Describe the effects of coupe/contre-coupe, axonal shearing and anoxia/hypoxia injuries on brain function.

2. Explain the major biological mechanisms of neuroplasticity.

3. Describe how exercise and mental/social stimulation affect neuroplasticity.

References

1. Briones, T. L., Suh, E., Jozsa, L., & Woods, J. (2006). Behaviorally induced synaptogenesis and dendritic growth in the hippocampal region following transient global cerebral ischemia are accompanied by improvement in spatial learning. *Experimental Neurology, 198,* 530–538.

2. DiFilippo, M., Tozzi, A., Costa, C., Belcastro, V., Tantucci, M., Picconi, B., & Calabresi, P. (2008). Plasticity and repair in the post-ischemic brain. *Neuropharmacology, 55,* 353–362.

3. Erikkson, P. S., Perfilieva, E., Bjork-Erikkson, T., Alborn, A-M., Nordborg, C., Peterson, D. A., & Gage, F. H. (1998). Neurogenesis in the adult human hippocampus. *Nature Medicine, 4*(11), 1313–1317.

4. King, L. A., & Horak, F. B. (2009). Delaying mobility disability in people with Parkinson disease using a sensorimotor agility exercise program. *Physical Therapy, 89,* 384–393.

5. Kraft, U. (2005, November 21). Mending the spinal cord. *Scientific American Mind.*

6. Moore, J. L, Roth, E. J., Killian, C., & Hornby, T. G. (2010). Locomotor training improves daily stepping activity and gait efficiency in individuals poststroke who have reached a "plateau" in recovery. *Stroke, 41,* 129–135.

7. Scheff, S. W., Price, D. A., Hicks, R. R., Baldwin, S. A., Robinson, S., & Brackney, C. (2005). Synaptogenesis in the hippocampal CA1 field following traumatic brain injury. *Journal of Neurotrauma, 22*(7), 719–732.

8. van der Lee, J. H., Wagenaar, R. C., Lankhorst, G. J., Vogelaar, T. W., Devillé, W. L., & Bouter, L. M. (1999). Forced use of the upper extremity in chronic stroke patients: Results from a single-blind randomized clinical trial. *Stroke, 30*(11), 2369–2375.

9. Zasler, N. D. (2007). A physician talks about brain injury: The basics. Brain Injury Association of America.

Further Reading

1. Chen, R., Cohen, L. G., & Hallet, M. (2002). Nervous system reorganization following injury. *Neuroscience, 111*(4), 761–773.

2. Conceptualizing Brain Injury as a Chronic Disease. (2009). Brain Injury Association of America.

3. Cotman, C. W., & Berchtold, N. C. (2002). Exercise: A behavioral intervention to enhance brain health and plasticity. *Trends in Neuroscience, 25*(6), 295–301.

4. Dunlop, S. A. (2008). Activity-dependent plasticity: Implications for recovery after spinal cord injury. *Cell, 31*(8), 410–418.

5. Gould, E., Reeves, A. J., Graziano, M. S. A., & Gross, C. G. (1999). Neurogenesis in the neocortex of adult primates. *Science, 286,* 548–552.

6. Li, Y., Field, P. M., & Raisman, G. (1998). Regeneration of adult corticospinal axons induced by transplanted olfactory ensheathing cells. *J. of Neuroscience, 18(4),* 10514–10524.

7. Lowenstein, D. H., & Parent, J. M. (1999). Brain, heal thyself. *Science, 283,* 1126–1127.

8. Rakic, P. (2006). No more cortical neurons for you. *Science, 313,* 928–929.

9. Scherer, M. R., & Schubert, M. C. (2009). Traumatic brain injury and vestibular pathology as a comorbidity after blast exposure. *Physical Therapy, 89,* 980–992.

10. Wernig, A., Nanassy, A., & Muller, S. (1998). Maintenance of locomotor abilities following Laufband (treadmill) therapy in para- and tetraplegic persons: Follow-up studies. *Spinal Cord, 36,* 744–749.

PEARSON

myhealthprofessionskit™

Use this address to access the Companion Website created for this textbook. Simply select "Physical Therapy" from the choice of disciplines. Find this book and log in using your username and password to access self-assessment questions, a glossary, and more.

abducens nerve: cranial nerve VI; innervates lateral rectus (extraocular) muscle

acetylcholine (Ach): neurotransmitter found in the parasympathetic nervous system and in parts of the sympathetic nervous system

action potential (nerve impulse): signal transmitted along neurons by inward flow of Na^+ ions; voltage = +35 mV

acute pain: short-term pain that results from injury or disease and serves a protective function

alpha motor neurons: large-diameter lower motor neurons found in peripheral nerves that innervate skeletal muscle to produce muscle contraction

amnesia: loss of memory

amygdala: almond-shaped nucleus in the temporal lobe; responsible for strong visceral emotions (fear, anger, rage)

anencephaly: lack of brain development caused by failure of superior end of neural tube to close

anosmia: loss of sense of smell

anoxia: lack of oxygen, usually due to interruption of blood supply

anterior cord syndrome: spinal cord injury in which the anterior portion of the cord is damaged leaving posterior regions intact; dorsal columns are usually unaffected

anterior corticospinal tract: descending tract found in anterior spinal cord white matter; controls muscles of neck and shoulder

anterior spinothalamic tract: ascending tract located in anterior spinal cord white matter; conveys light touch and pressure sensations to the brain

aphasia: language deficit caused by damage to language-specific regions of the brain

apraxia: motor planning disorder; patients are unable to plan, sequence, and carry out learned movement patterns; a result from damage to supplementary motor area (SMA)

Arnold-Chiari malformation: brain abnormality in which the brainstem and cerebellum are small and protrude down into the spinal canal

ascending (somatosensory) tract: group of sensory axons in the spinal cord that convey sensation to the brain

ascending reticular activating system (ARAS): part of reticular formation that maintains conscious awareness; damage can cause coma

ascending tracts: bundles of axons located in spinal cord white matter that carry sensory action potentials to the brain

association nuclei: small nuclei in the thalamus that connect sensation to emotion

astrocyte: glial cell found in central nervous system that regulates the environment surrounding neurons and stimulates formation of the blood-brain barrier

ataxia: uncoordinated voluntary movement

ataxic cerebral palsy: lack of coordinated movement caused by injury to the cerebellum around the time of birth

athetoid cerebral palsy: uninhibited writhing movements of the limbs caused by injury to the basal ganglia around the time of birth

auditory cortex: region of temporal lobe responsible for perception of sound

auditory ossicles: small bones in middle ear that transmit vibration through the middle ear cavity to the oval window

autism: developmental disorder characterized by impaired social communication

autonomic neuron: nerve cell in peripheral nerve that affects function of internal organs

axon: long nerve fiber that is part of a neuron and transmits action potentials

axon terminal (synaptic terminal, synaptic knob): structure found at the end of an axon that releases neurotransmitters for communication with other cells at synapses

Babinski sign: extension and abduction of the toes when the sole of the foot is stroked; normal in children under age 2 and evidence of upper motor neuron damage in adults

basal ganglia (nuclei): group of nuclei (grey matter) located deep in the brain that work together to initiate movement, thought, and emotion; composed of caudate nucleus, putamen, and globus pallidus. Also called *striatum* or *kinetic system*

blood-brain barrier: formed by tight connections between cells in capillary walls; protects nerve tissue from substances in the blood

bradykinesia: slowness of movement; may result from underactive basal ganglia circuits, decreased dopamine, or dopamine antagonists

brainstem: brain region composed of midbrain, pons, and medulla oblongata; controls breathing, heart rate, and cranial nerves

Broca's expressive language area: region in frontal lobe that controls speech/language production

Brodmann's map: numbered regional map of cerebral cortex

Brown-Sequard syndrome: spinal cord injury in which one side of the cord is damaged

calvaria: skull bones that protect brain

cauda equina: motor and sensory nerve roots from lumbar and sacral spinal cord found inside sacral portion of vertebral column

central autonomic fibers: neurons from the hypothalamus that control the autonomic nervous system

central cord syndrome: spinal cord injury in which the central portion of the cord is damaged leaving peripheral regions intact; typically affects upper extremities more than lower extremities

central nervous system (CNS): brain and spinal cord

cerebellum: brain region located posterior to brainstem and inferior to occipital lobe; major function is motor coordination

cerebral cortex: outer layer of cerebrum; composed of neuron cell bodies and dendrites and divided into frontal, parietal, temporal, and occipital lobes

cerebral hemisphere: one side of cerebrum

cerebral palsy (CP): developmental disorder caused by damage to motor and other areas of the brain before, during, or shortly after birth

cerebrospinal fluid: watery fluid produced inside ventricles of brain; fluid supports and nourishes CNS

cerebrum: largest part of the brain; composed of cerebral cortex and subcortical nuclei, including basal ganglia, thalamus, and hypothalamus

cervical plexus: peripheral nerves from cervical spinal cord that innervate skin and muscles of neck and the thoracoabdominal diaphragm

chronic pain: long-term pain that persists when injury or disease has ended

clonus: a series of rapid, rhythmic alternating movements seen after spinal cord injury

cochlea: part of inner ear containing receptors for hearing

cognition: ability to think, plan, reflect, and solve problems

colliculi: small structures in midbrain that are part of pathways for vision and hearing

coma: state of prolonged and profound loss of consciousness

complete spinal cord injury: damage to spinal cord that produces loss of anal sensation and loss of anal sphincter contraction

cones: sensory receptors for color vision

consolidation: stage of learning during which memory is solidified and transferred to cortical association areas for long-term storage

contre-coupe injury: brain damage on the side of the brain opposite to a blow or injury; caused by motion of the brain within the skull

corpus callosum: large bundle of commissural axons connecting right and left cerebral hemispheres

cortical blindness: loss of vision caused by damage to primary visual cortex

corticobulbar tract: descending (motor) tract containing upper motor neurons from cerebral cortex that will synapse onto interneurons and lower motor neurons in the brainstem to innervate cranial nerves

corticospinal tract: descending (motor) tract containing upper motor neurons from cerebral cortex that will synapse onto interneurons and lower motor neurons in spinal cord to innervate spinal nerves

coupe injury: brain damage on the side of the brain where an injury occurred

cranial base: bones inside skull that support the brain; contains many holes (foraminae) for blood vessels and cranial nerves that run to and from the brain

critical periods (sensitive periods): times during nervous system development during which many synapses are formed in specific CNS circuits (vision, hearing, etc)

declarative learning and memory: memory that can be described in words (e.g., facts and figures, life events)

dementia: cognitive and memory deficit caused by injury or disease that damages the cerebral cortex

dendrite: extensions of neuron cell body that form receptive site for synapses

denervation: loss of nerve connection to a muscle cell or another neuron

depolarization: inward flow of sodium ions sufficient to generate nerve impulse (action potential) in neuron

dermatome: region of the body innervated by sensory nerves arising from one spinal cord segment

descending tracts: bundles of axons located in spinal cord white matter that carry motor action potentials from the brain to control muscle function

diencephalon: part of the forebrain that contains the thalamus and hypothalamus

differentiation: specialization of nerve cells based on structure and function

diffuse axonal injury: brain damage that is widespread and cannot be localized; caused by shearing and rotation of the brain within the skull

diplopia: double vision; may result from injury to cranial nerves serving extraocular muscles

disequilibrium: difficulty maintaining and correcting balance

dorsal columns: ascending tract found in anterior spinal cord white matter; conveys conscious proprioception, vibration, and two-point discriminative touch to the brain

dorsal (posterior) horn: portion of spinal cord grey matter that receives sensory axons from peripheral nerves

dorsal (posterior) ramus: portion of spinal nerve that innervates skin and muscles of the back; contains sensory, motor, and sympathetic autonomic nerve fibers

dorsal respiratory nucleus: small area in medulla oblongata that controls phrenic nerve to diaphragm; allows breathing to take place automatically

Down syndrome (DS): genetic disorder that affects cortical function and ability to learn

dysarthria: difficulty speaking caused by injury to vocal muscles or the nerves that control them

dysdiadochokinesis: loss of the ability to perform rapid, alternating movements

dyskinesia: excessive, unnecessary movements; may result from overactive basal ganglia circuitry, excessive dopamine or dopamine agonists, or overexpression of dopamine receptors

dysphagia: difficulty swallowing caused by injury to muscles of the pharynx or the cranial nerves that control them

emotion: feelings associated with internal and external stimuli that are centered in the brain's limbic system and medial emotional cortex

encephalopathy: swelling of the brain

endoneurium: connective tissue covering of individual axons

ependymal cells: glial cells that secrete cerebrospinal fluid

epilepsy: disorder characterized by repeated seizures

epineurium: connective tissue covering of an entire peripheral nerve

episodic learning and memory: memory of one's life events that is a subset of declarative memory

epithalamus: small region of diencephalon that contains pineal gland

excitatory postsynaptic potential (EPSP): change in membrane potential caused by neurotransmitter binding that causes inside of cell to become more positively charged

exocytosis: process of releasing a substance from a cell using small vesicles

explicit learning and memory: memory that can be described in words (also known as *declarative learning/memory*)

expressive aphasia: loss of the ability to form sentences and communicate expressively using language; results from damage to Broca's expressive language area in frontal lobe

extraocular muscles: muscles that move the eyeball

facial nerve: cranial nerve VII; innervates muscles of facial expression as well as taste buds, salivary glands, and lacrimal (tear) glands

frontal lobe: cortical lobe located beneath frontal bone; contains motor areas and regions involved in thinking, problem solving, and emotion

gamma motor neurons: small-diameter lower motor neurons that form part of peripheral nerves; innervate muscle spindles to maintain and adjust tone

glial cell (neuroglial cell): cell in the nervous system that supports neurons

global aphasia: loss of both receptive and expressive language; results from injury to the Wernicke's and Broca's areas

glossopharyngeal nerve: cranial nerve IX; innervates pharynx and palate as well as the parotid salivary gland

Golgi tendon organ (GTO): sensory receptor located in tendons; detects muscle tension/contraction

grey matter: region in center of spinal cord that contains neuron cell bodies and dendrites

growth cone: process that emerges from a regenerating axon and grows toward target in periphery; guided by connective tissue, Schwann cells, and growth factors

hair follicle receptors: sensory receptor located in hair follicles; detects movement of hairs (light touch)

hemianopsia: loss of vision in one visual field

hemiplegia: paralysis of one side of the body

hippocampus: small nucleus located in medial temporal lobe; responsible for creating new long-term memories

homeostasis: a state of internal physiological balance within the body

hydrocephalus: "water on the brain"; a condition resulting from blockage of cerebrospinal fluid drainage that causes swelling of the ventricles and enlargement or compression of the cerebrum

hypertonicity: excessive tone in skeletal muscle; evidence of spinal cord injury

hypoglossal nerve: cranial nerve XII; innervates muscles of the tongue

hypophysis (pituitary gland): pea-sized gland located inferior to brain; controls endocrine system under direction of hypothalamus

hypothalamus: part of diencephalon that controls appetite, water balance, hunger and thirst, as well as the autonomic nervous system and the endocrine system

hypoxia: lack of oxygen to a tissue or organ

implicit learning and memory: memory that cannot be easily described in words; includes motor skill (procedural) learning/memory

incomplete spinal cord injury: damage to spinal cord where either anal sensation or anal sphincter contraction are retained

infarct: region of dead cells in brain or spinal cord; results from lack of oxygen to nerve cells

inhibitory postsynaptic potential (IPSP): change in membrane potential caused by neurotransmitter binding that causes inside of cell to become more negatively charged

internal capsule: region of cerebrum containing upper motor neurons from the entire motor cortex as well as sensory neurons traveling to the entire sensory cortex

intralaminar nuclei: small structures in the thalamus that maintain consciousness

ion: small charged molecule

ion channel: protein located in neuron cell membrane that allows one or more kinds of ions to enter or exit cell

lateral corticospinal tract: descending bundle of axons conveying motor signals from primary motor cortex to spinal cord; contains upper motor neurons that control voluntary movement

lateral horn: regions in center of spinal cord that contains neuron cell bodies for autonomic motor neurons; found at spinal cord levels T_1–L_2 and S_2–S_4

lateral spinothalamic tract: ascending tract in lateral spinal cord white matter that conveys pain and temperature sensations to the brain

limbic system: portions of cortex responsible for memory and emotion

local potential: small ion flow into or out of nerve cell

locked-in syndrome: bilateral paralysis of all cranial nerves except those that move the eyes, along with bilateral paralysis of the entire body; results from stroke or injury to the pons

lower motor neuron: a nerve cell that forms a synapse with skeletal muscle and is part of a peripheral nerve (cranial nerve or spinal nerve)

lumbar plexus: peripheral nerves emerging from lumbar portion of spinal cord that innervate muscles of the hip and thigh regions

macula: part of retina with highest concentration of cones; site of sharpest visual acuity

medulla oblongata: part of brainstem that is adjacent to cervical spinal cord

Meissner's corpuscle: sensory receptor located in subcutaneous tissue and dermis; detects two-point discriminative touch ("fine touch")

melatonin: hormone produced by pineal gland (epithalamus) that induces sleep

membrane pump: protein found in cell membrane that allows molecules to enter or exit cell against their concentration gradient

Meniere's disease: vertigo caused by excess fluid in inner ear

meninges: connective tissue surrounding and protecting brain and spinal cord; consists of dura mater, arachnoid, and pia mater

Merkel's disc: sensory receptor located in subcutaneous tissue and dermis; detects pressure/texture

microglia cells: glial cells found in central nervous system that remove debris

mirror neurons: neurons in parietal lobe that are activated when we empathize with the emotions or experiences of another

monoplegia: paralysis of one limb

motor cortex: region of frontal lobe responsible for controlling skeletal muscles

motor end plate: cell membrane of a skeletal muscle fiber that forms the postsynaptic side of a neuromuscular junction

motor homunculus: specific, regional (somatotopic) organization of upper motor neurons on the primary motor cortex

motor neuron: a nerve cell that innervates muscle

motor point: place on the surface of a skeletal muscle where a peripheral nerve penetrates the muscle

motor unit: one lower motor neuron and all skeletal muscle fibers innervated by that motor neuron

muscle fiber (myofiber): a muscle cell

muscle spindle: small capsule located in many skeletal muscles that contains intrafusal muscle fibers, sensory nerve endings, and gamma motor neurons; detects muscle stretch

muscle tone: amount of resistance to passive stretching found in skeletal muscles

myelin: fatty material that wraps around axons to provide insulation and increase speed of action potentials; formed by glial cells

myelination: insulation of axons; produced by neuroglial cells

myotome: a muscle or group of muscles innervated by motor neurons arising from a single spinal cord segment

necrosis: cell death due to disease or injury

neural crest: cells that arise from the developing neural plate and are pinched off when the neural tube closes

neural groove: fold in the neural plate that forms as the plate grows and begins to develop into the neural tube

neural plasticity: flexibility of synapses/connections among neurons, based on experience

neural plate: sheet of cells located on the dorsal side of the developing embryo that becomes the entire nervous system

neural tube: cylinder of cells formed by the neural plate that gives rise to the brain and spinal cord

neurogenesis: development of new neurons; in humans, neurogenesis occurs in the hippocampus throughout life

neuromuscular junction: synapse between a motor neuron and a skeletal muscle fiber

neuron: cell in the nervous system that can generate and transmit information

neuropathic pain: pain caused by damage to peripheral nerve axons

neuropathy: pain, tingling, and numbness in a peripheral nerve caused by disease or injury

neuroplasticity: flexibility or adaptability of the brain; the brain's ability to rewire itself based on experience

neurotransmitter: chemical released from axon terminal that binds to receptors at synapses

nociceptive pain: pain caused by disease or injury to tissue that stimulates pain receptors

nociceptor: pain receptor

nondeclarative learning and memory: memory that cannot be easily described in words; includes motor (procedural) learning/memory

norepinephrine (NE): neurotransmitter found in the sympathetic nervous system that is chemically related to adrenaline

occipital lobe: smallest cortical lobe located below occipital bone; contains regions responsible for visual perception and interpretation

oculomotor nerve: cranial nerve III; innervates extraocular muscles as well as smooth muscle located in the eye

olfactory cortex: region of temporal lobe responsible for perception of odor

olfactory nerve (tract): cranial nerve I; neurons that convey sense of smell to brain

olfactory receptors: receptors for smell located in top of nose

oligodendrocyte: glial cell found in central nervous system that forms myelin sheath around axons

optic chiasm: place where optic nerves cross

optic nerve: cranial nerve II; innervates visual receptors in the eye

optic tract: neurons connecting the optic chiasm to the thalamus; transmits action potentials from the contralateral visual field

organ of Corti: site of sensory receptors for hearing; located inside cochlea of inner ear

otolithic organs: utricle and saccule; contain sensory receptors for head movement

oxytocin: hormone produced in posterior pituitary gland that stimulates uterine contractions and milk flow from mammary glands

Pacinian corpuscle: sensory receptor found in dermis, subcutaneous tissue, and periosteum; detects vibration and deep pressure

paralysis: loss of voluntary motor function

paraplegia: paralysis of both lower extremities

parasympathetic system: subdivision of the autonomic nervous system responsible for maintaining body homeostasis (physiological balance and energy conservation)

paresis: weakness or partial paralysis of a skeletal muscle

paresthesia: pain and numbness caused by peripheral neuropathy; pain is described as burning, aching, "pins and needles" feeling

parietal lobe: cortical lobe located beneath parietal bone; contains regions responsible for somatosensory perception and interpretation

perineurium: connective tissue that wraps around bundles of axons in a peripheral nerve to form fascicles

peripheral nerve: nerve fibers in the body that connect muscles, skin, and other structures with the spinal cord and brain

peripheral nervous system (PNS): cranial nerves and spinal nerves

photoreceptors: rods and cones; sensory receptors for vision located on retina

pineal gland: region of epithalamus that produces the hormone melatonin

pituitary gland: gland located just below brain; produces hormones under the influence of the hypothalamus

plexus: network of nerve fibers

pons: part of brainstem between midbrain and medulla oblongata

postsynaptic neuron: nerve cell with receptors on cell membrane that receives binding of a neurotransmitter at a synapse

posttraumatic (anterograde) amnesia: memory loss extending from a traumatic event forward in time; often caused by traumatic brain injury

prefrontal cortex: part of frontal lobe responsible for problem solving, impulse control, and connecting emotion with thought

prefrontal syndrome: loss of impulse control due to lesions of the prefrontal cortex

presynaptic neuron: nerve cell that releases a neurotransmitter at a synapse

primary auditory cortex: region in temporal lobe for perception of hearing

primary motor cortex: region of frontal lobe located on precentral gyrus that contains cell bodies of cortical upper motor neurons; beginning of the lateral corticospinal, anterior corticospinal, and corticobulbar tracts

primary olfactory cortex: region in temporal lobe for perception of smell

primary somatosensory cortex: region of cerebral cortex located in parietal lobe; site of perception (conscious awareness) of sensation

primary visual cortex: site of visual perception; located in occipital lobe

proprioception: movement and position sense

proprioceptors: sensory receptors located in muscle, tendon and joint capsules that detect body position and movement

quadriplegia: paralysis of all or part of four limbs; also called tetraplegia

receptive aphasia: loss of the ability to understand language; caused by damage to Wernicke's receptive language area in temporal lobe

receptor: peripheral end of a sensory neuron that converts a stimulus into an action potential

reflex: nerve connection in the spinal cord that allows for rapid, nonvoluntary movement in response to a stimulus

refractory period: time period after generation of action potential when another action potential cannot occur

relay nuclei: nuclei in the thalamus that send action potentials to cerebral cortex

resting membrane potential: charge difference across neuron cell membrane when neuron is at rest; averages –70 mV

reticular formation (RF): network of neurons located in brainstem that extends into diencephalon; controls sleeping and waking and conscious awareness

reticular nucleus of the thalamus: small nucleus in the thalamus that controls relay nuclei and decides which information is sent to cerebral cortex

reticulospinal tract: descending (motor) tract containing upper motor neurons from brainstem reticular formation that control posture, gait, and muscle tone

retina: region at the back of the eyeball that contains photoreceptors (rods and cones)

retrograde amnesia: memory loss preceding a traumatic event; often caused by injury to cortical association areas where memory is stored

rods: photoreceptors located in retina that provide black and white vision

Ruffini corpuscle: sensory receptor that detects stretching of the skin

sacral plexus: network of nerve fibers formed by sacral spinal nerves; innervates lower extremity and pelvic floor

sacral sparing: the ability to perceive anal sensation or contract the anal sphincter voluntarily; evidence of an incomplete spinal cord injury

safety factor: ratio of current that is available to stimulate an action potential to the current that is needed to stimulate an action potential; should be 5 or 6 in a healthy neuron

saltatory conduction: method of propagating action potentials rapidly in myelinated axons; current flows only at gaps in myelin sheaths

Schwann cells: supporting (glial) cells found in the peripheral nervous system that provides the myelin sheath surrounding many axons

semantic learning and memory: memory for facts and figures; a subset of declarative learning/ memory

semicircular canals: three small regions of inner ear that detect rotational head movement

sensitization: physiological change in sensory receptors that causes them to be more easily stimulated

somatosensory cortex: region of parietal lobe responsible for perception of somatosensation

somatosensory system: neurons that detect, transmit, and interpret sensations from the skin, subcutaneous tissue, muscles, tendons, and joints

spastic hemiplegia: paralysis and hypertonia on one side of the body resulting from injury to the motor cortex or upper motor neurons around the time of birth

spasticity: exaggerated skeletal muscle contractions in response to muscle stretch or other sensory stimuli

special sensory system: neurons that detect, transmit, and interpret sensations for vision, hearing, balance, taste, and smell

spina bifida: condition caused by incomplete closure of the neural tube in which part of the spinal cord is exposed

spinal accessory nerve: cranial nerve XI; controls trapezius and sternocleidomastoid muscles

spinal cord segments: thirty regions of the spinal cord that correspond to vertebrae of the spinal column; each segment gives rise to paired spinal nerves

spinal cord: structure connecting brain with peripheral nerves; located inside spinal column

spinal meninges: three layers of connective tissues that surround and protect the spinal cord (dura mater, arachnoid, pia mater)

spinal nerves: peripheral nerves that arise from the spinal cord and provide sensory, voluntary motor, and autonomic innervation to the body

spinal shock: two- to four-week period following traumatic spinal cord injury during which all sensory and motor function below the area of injury ceases

spinocerebellar tracts: axons in the spinal cord that convey unconscious proprioception (muscle length and tension) to the cerebellum

splanchnic nerves: autonomic nerves that innervate structures in the abdomen and pelvis

spondylosis: chronic compression of spinal cord caused by bony growths inside the vertebral column

status epilepticus: condition caused by seizures lasting as long as 30 minutes that produce brain damage or death; it is a medical emergency

stereognosis: the ability to identify objects by touch

substantia nigra: region in medulla oblongata that produces dopamine and has many connections to basal ganglia in the cerebrum; named for its dark appearance in a sectioned brain

subthalamic nucleus: small nucleus in diencephalon that has many connections to basal ganglia

supplementary motor area (SMA): region of frontal lobe located anterior to primary motor cortex; stores movement patterns and sequences (motor memories)

sympathetic system: portion of the autonomic nervous system responsible for responding to stress, danger, and exercise

sympathetic trunk: chain of sympathetic ganglia found along posterior body wall in neck, thorax, abdomen, and pelvis

synapse: point of connection between neurons, or between neurons and other cell types, where information is transmitted (often in the form of a chemical signal)

synaptic cleft: space between two neurons at a synapse

synaptic pruning: removal of rarely used synapses

synaptic receptors: molecules found on postsynaptic neurons that bind neurotransmitters

synaptic vesicles: small hollow spheres made of phospholipid that contain chemical neurotransmitters

synaptogenesis: process of synapse formation; enhanced by repeated activation of synapses

tectospinal tract: descending (motor) tract containing upper motor neurons from brainstem superior colliculus that control neck movements and allow visual tracking

temporal lobe: region of cerebral cortex located below temporal bone; contains regions for language, hearing, olfaction, emotion, and memory

tetraplegia: paralysis of all four limbs; also called quadriplegia

thalamic syndrome: condition caused by damage to the thalamus, including sensory ataxia, contralateral sensory loss, and intense pain

thalamus: paired structures located inferior to cerebral cortex; transmits nerve impulses to cortex

thermal receptor: sensory receptor that detects changes in temperature

traumatic brain injury (TBI): damage to the brain caused by a blow to the head, hitting the head on a solid object, or trauma such as violent shaking

trigeminal nerve: cranial nerve V; innervates muscles of jaw (mastication) and provides sensory innervation to the face, tongue, teeth, and palate

trochlear nerve: cranial nerve IV; innervates superior oblique extraocular muscle

upper motor neuron (UMN): motor neuron with its cell body in the cerebral cortex or brainstem that controls activation of lower motor neurons

vagus nerve: cranial nerve X; innervates muscles of pharynx and larynx and provides parasympathetic innervation to structures in the thorax and abdomen

vasopressin: hormone produced in the hypothalamus that affects body's water balance and blood pressure; also called antidiuretic hormone (ADH)

ventral (anterior) horn: region of spinal cord grey matter that contains voluntary lower motor neuron cell bodies

ventral (anterior) ramus: portion of spinal nerve that innervates anterior body wall structures as well as all parts of the upper and lower extremities

ventricles: fluid-filled spaces located inside of brain; contain cerebrospinal fluid

vertebral column: spine; consists of vertebrae that surround and protect the spinal cord; divided into cervical, thoracic, lumbar, sacral, and coccygeal regions

vertigo: dizziness

vestibular apparatus: part of inner ear that contains sensory receptors for head position and movement; consists of three semicircular canals and two otolithic organs

vestibular nuclei: small brainstem structures that receive input from the vestibular apparatus in the inner ear and connect to the cerebellum, motor cortex, and spinal cord

vestibulocochlear nerve: cranial nerve VIII; conveys sensations of hearing and balance to the brain

vestibulospinal tract: descending (motor) tracts containing upper motor neurons from brainstem vestibular nuclei that control muscles used for balance and the extraocular muscles

visual cortex: region of occipital lobe responsible for perception of vision

Wernicke's area: region located in temporal lobe responsible for perception/understanding of language

white matter: axons covered with myelin; forms inner layer of brain and outer region of spinal cord

working memory: very short-term memory; associated with focus and attention to a problem or thought

APPENDIX B
Answers to Patient Scenarios

CHAPTER 2
2-1 (RYAN): MENINGITIS

a) Dura mater, arachnoid, subarachnoid space, pia mater. CSF is contained in the subarachnoid space.
b) The dura mater has many pain receptors, so inflammation causes intense pain.
c) Bacteria and viruses that infect the dura can be seen in the CSF, along with white blood cells. The dura mater and arachnoid would be punctured in order to perform a spinal tap.

2-2 (FLORENCE): CVA

a) The lateral part of the cerebral cortex, including areas that control movement, sensation, and language; also the basal ganglia and diencephalon.
b) Neurons usually live about 3 minutes without oxygen; the longer the brain is deprived of blood and oxygen, the more nerve cells die and the larger the infarct will be.

2-3 (MARIA): HYDROCEPHALUS

a) The brain has four ventricles. Each hemisphere contains a lateral ventricle that drains into a central third ventricle. From there, cerebrospinal fluid (CSF) drains through the cerebral aqueduct to the fourth ventricle. CSF leaves the fourth ventricle and enters the subarachnoid space that surrounds the brain and spinal cord.
b) In young children whose skull bones have not yet fused, the brain and skull will enlarge due to excess CSF within the ventricles.
c) The shunt contains a one-way valve that drains CSF out of the ventricles to prevent the fluid from building up and causing brain damage.

CHAPTER 3
3-1 (WAYNE): MS

a) In multiple sclerosis (MS), the immune system damages myelin. This slows transmission of nerve impulses.
b) MS affects the central nervous system (CNS).
c) Oligodendroglia are affected in MS.

3-2 (ALISON): GBS

a) In Guillain-Barre syndrome (GBS), the immune system damages myelin. This slows the transmission of nerve impulses.
b) GBS affects the peripheral nervous system (PNS).
c) In GBS, the immune system damages Schwann cells.

CHAPTER 4
4-1 (ANDY): SPASTICITY

a) Inhibiting neurotransmitter release prevents the synapse from functioning.
b) Botox prevents release of acetylcholine at the neuromuscular junction. This will prevent muscle cells from contracting. If Andy's adductors are too tight (contracted), the injections will relieve this.
c) Synapses can be inhibited if the neurotransmitters are destroyed in the synaptic cleft, or if they cannot detach from their receptors. You could also block or destroy the receptors so that the neurotransmitter cannot bind.

4-2 (JOHNNIE): MYASTHENIA GRAVIS

a) If acetylcholine receptors are blocked, the neurotransmitter cannot bind and the synapse cannot function.

b) Muscles will be weak or paralyzed, depending on how many neuromuscular junctions are affected.

CHAPTER 5
5-1 (HENRY): PREFRONTAL SYNDROME

a) Prefrontal syndrome; prefrontal cortex
b) Cortical blindness

5-2 (GEORGIA): CVA AND APHASIA

a) Expressive aphasia; Georgia's Broca's/expressive language area is affected.
b) Probably the left hemisphere was injured. Broca's area is located on the left side in most people.

5-3 (MARY ANNE): CVA AND NEGLECT

a) This patient has unilateral or left-sided neglect, caused by injury to her premotor cortex.
b) The left-sided paralysis is due to an infarct in the right primary motor cortex.

CHAPTER 6
6-1 (TED): THALAMIC SYNDROME

A clinician treating someone with thalamic syndrome needs to avoid causing pain if possible. The clinician can begin by asking the patient what has invoked pain previously. It is also important to let the patient direct treatment as much as feasible. People with this condition often learn methods of moving that prevent the onset of the pain. Although many studies are inconclusive, some evidence suggests that both high-frequency and low-frequency TENS (transcutaneous electrical nerve stimulation) can help decrease thalamic pain in some people.

CHAPTER 7
7-1 (WILLIAM): BRAINSTEM INFARCT

a) Cranial nerves VIII-XII arise from the medulla. Injury could impair hearing and balance (CN VIII), swallowing and speech (IX and X), movement of the neck and shoulder (XI), and movement of the tongue (XII).
b) The neurons in motor tracts on one side of the brainstem control movement on the opposite side of the body; the largest motor tract (lateral corticospinal tract) crosses in the medulla oblongata.

7-2 (ANN): BELL'S PALSY

a) Bell's palsy is caused by injury to the facial nerve (CN VII).
b) The facial nerve also contains neurons that supply salivary glands, the lacrimal gland, and taste receptors on the tongue. Ann might experience dry mouth and a dry eye, and may lose her sense of taste on part of her tongue.

7-3 (DAVID): TRIGEMINAL NERVE DAMAGE

a) Cranial nerve V (trigeminal nerve), on the right side.
b) Because the trigeminal nerve does not innervate the muscles of facial expression, David should be able to smile, close his eyes, and display other facial expressions; those muscles are innervated by the facial nerve.

CHAPTER 8
8-1 (JEREMY): TRAUMATIC SPINAL CORD INJURY

a) Physical injury level is C8 on the right and C7 on the left. Functional level is C7 on the right and C6 on the left.
b) Test for sacral sparing by assessing anal sphincter contraction and sensation using a gloved finger. If either is present, the injury is defined as incomplete.
c) The diaphragm is innervated by C4, which is intact in this patient, but intercostal and abdominal wall muscles are innervated below the lesion level and would be lost. Jeremy

will not need mechanical ventilation but will have some loss of respiratory function. He will lose voluntary control of both bladder and bowel.

8-2 (ANNETTE): SPINAL STENOSIS

a) The hypertonicity is likely due to damaged reticulospinal tracts, and the ataxia could result from damage to the spinocerebellar tracts or the vestibulospinal tracts.
b) Spinal stenosis is progressive, so symptoms will worsen over time, whereas traumatic spinal cord injury is a nonprogressive condition that does not get worse.

8-3 (KATHY): BROWN-SEQUARD SYNDROME

a) Kathy's right leg should function normally.
b) No; pain from the right lower extremity travels in the lateral spinothalamic tract, which passes through the left side of the spinal cord at T4, and would therefore be damaged by this tumor.
c) No; the upper extremities are innervated by C5-T1, above the region of the tumor.

CHAPTER 9
9-1 (CINDY): CARPAL TUNNEL SYNDROME

a) Median nerve.
b) Because the median nerve is a peripheral nerve, it will probably recover. Peripheral nerves express genes that aid regeneration.

9-2 (RUFUS): DIABETIC PERIPHERAL NEUROPATHY

a) People with diabetes often have nerve damage in their feet, so they cannot feel pain; they also have poor circulation, so healing is very slow.
b) The best way to minimize foot problems is to control blood sugar through diet, medications, and regular exercise. In addition, the feet should be checked regularly for sores.

CHAPTER 10
10-1 (JERRY): AUTONOMIC DYSREFLEXIA

a) Sympathetic overactivity causes a dramatic blood pressure elevation.
b) High-level spinal cord injury (SCI) damages the central autonomic fibers that control the autonomic nervous system (ANS).
c) If autonomic dysreflexia is not addressed rapidly, blood pressure can become so high that a stroke can occur.

10-2 (EDUARDO): COMPLEX REGIONAL PAIN SYNDROME (CPRS)

a) He probably has overactivity of sympathetic nerves causing the pain fibers to become hypersensitive.
b) The swelling is probably caused by lack of use due to the pain Eduardo is experiencing.

CHAPTER 11
11-1 (WILMA): CVA

a) The right side of the cortex has been damaged.
b) Pain is transmitted in the lateral spinothalamic tract, light touch in the anterior spinothalamic tract, and conscious proprioception in the dorsal columns.

11-2 (PAUL): PERIPHERAL DIABETIC NEUROPATHY

a) The pain is probably caused by damage to peripheral axons due to the diabetes. This is an example of neuropathic pain.
b) Small-diameter peripheral axons are damaged first, followed by larger ones. This means that pain is usually the first sensation affected, followed by axons carrying light touch, and then by those conveying proprioception.

   c) Local anesthetics affect small-diameter axons that carry pain and temperature first, followed by axons conveying light touch. The last axons affected are those conveying proprioception, which are the largest-diameter fibers in peripheral nerves.

CHAPTER 12
12-1 (JENNIE): VERTIGO

a) Otoconia (ear sand) in the utricle and saccule were dislodged.

b) Otoconia have entered the semicircular canals and are bending the hair cells, producing a sensation of dizziness.

c) Vertigo can result from Meniere's disease, tumors that affect the vestibulocochlear nerve, and infections or inflammation of the nerve.

12-2 (HAZEL): HEMIANOPSIA

a) Hemianopsia or visual field deficit.

b) The CVA (cerebrovascular accident, or stroke) damaged her right visual cortex, which perceives visual signals from the left visual field.

c) You may need to approach this patient from her good (right side), and call her attention to her left side.

CHAPTER 13
13-1 (LUCILLE): ATAXIA

a) Each side of the cerebellum affects muscles on the ipsilateral side of the body, so the CVA affected the right side of her cerebellum.

b) The cerebellum controls activity of motor cortex, so cerebellar lesions do not affect voluntary muscle contraction; instead, they affect the ability to coordinate muscles.

13-2 (HOWARD): PARKINSON DISEASE

a) Dopamine is deficient in Parkinson disease (PD); it is normally produced in the substantia nigra (in the midbrain).

b) Because PD results from a dopamine deficit, dopamine replacement medications can treat the signs and symptoms. A potential side effect is dyskinesia, which can result from excess dopamine.

c) Howard is at risk for falls because people with PD often cannot initiate muscle contraction rapidly enough to catch themselves if they stumble.

13-3 (STEPHEN): AMYOTROPHIC LATERAL SCLEROSIS

a) Because amyotrophic lateral sclerosis (ALS) affects both upper motor neurons and lower motor neurons, most people with this disease have a mixture of spastic and flaccid paralysis.

b) People with ALS usually have no sensory loss and no cognitive changes; sensation and cognition remain normal.

CHAPTER 14
14-1 (CLAUDIA): ALZHEIMER DISEASE

a) Claudia retains her motor skill memories, but has difficulty with declarative memory.

b) The medial temporal lobe is affected early in Alzheimer disease (AD), including the hippocampus, the amygdala, and regions important for recognizing faces.

c) The brain cells of someone with Alzheimer disease contain tangles and plaques.

14-2 (JOHN): TRAUMATIC BRAIN INJURY

a) Prefrontal cortex.

b) Keep the treatment session short and simple, maintain a calm demeanor, and choose goals that the patient can attain to minimize frustration.

14-3 (ALLAN): APHASIA

a) Allan has Broca's or expressive aphasia, caused by a lesion to Broca's motor language area.
b) Allan will probably understand language and nonverbal communication, but will be unable to communicate verbally with others. He will need to use gestures, body language, and facial expressions to make his needs known.

CHAPTER 15
15-1 (BRITTANY): CEREBRAL PALSY

a) Babies born too early may have leakage of blood into the brain's ventricles, or lack of blood flow to certain regions of the brain.
b) Left-sided paresis results from damage to the right side of the brain.
c) Cerebral palsy is defined by the type of motor dysfunction present, so her CP is referred to as spastic hemiplegic cerebral palsy.

15-2 (JACK): SPINA BIFIDA

a) Since Jack lacks sensation below the T10 dermatome, his neural tube failed to close at about level T11.
b) Bladder and bowel function are controlled by S2-S4, so neural tube damage above that can affect these functions.
c) Shunts to treat hydrocephalus are implanted in one lateral ventricle in order to drain excess cerebrospinal fluid (CSF) so it cannot cause the ventricles to enlarge and damage the brain.

CHAPTER 16
16-1 (NED): UNILATERAL NEGLECT

a) Keep calling his attention to the neglected side, remind him to move it as needed, use a visual cue (bright colored shoe or bracelet).
b) Remember that he won't be able to see what is on his left and is at risk for injury (e.g., by bumping into things or tripping over obstacles on the left).

16-2 (XANG): TRAUMATIC BRAIN INJURY (TBI)

a) Frontal lobe syndrome is caused by damage to the prefrontal cortex, and cortical blindness results from injury to the primary visual cortex in the occipital lobe. This is a coupe/contre-coup injury, in which there are specific focal lesions.
b) Axon shearing can affect neurons across the cortex, so it is difficult to identify specific lesions. This kind of injury results from shaking or twisting of the brain within the skull.

16-3 (BETTY ANN): HEALTHY AGING BRAIN

a) Betty Ann can improve the chances of maintaining brain health and memory by exercising regularly, performing mentally stimulating activities, and maintaining social connections and relationships.
b) Since Ellie Mae is more physically active, she might have a better chance of recovery from brain damage because evidence shows that physical activity improves neuroplasticity, the brain's recovery mechanism.

APPENDIX C
Answers to Review Questions

CHAPTER 1

1. These functions are all located in the brain.

2. The spinal cord transmits sensation to the brain from the body and sends signals from the brain to the body to control muscles. A spinal cord injury would impair both of these functions, so patients would lose the ability to feel pain and to move muscles voluntarily.

3. Peripheral nerves transmit sensation from the body to the brain and spinal cord, and transmit signals from the brain and spinal cord to the skeletal muscles, skin, bones, joints, and internal organs.

4. Neuroplasticity means that the brain is flexible and can change or adjust its connections based on experience.

CHAPTER 2

1.
- *Cerebral cortex:* movement, sensation, thought, emotion, language, problem solving
- *Diencephalon:* sensory processing (thalamus); autonomic functions (hypothalamus)
- *Brainstem:* basic life functions (heart rate, breathing) and cranial nerves
- *Cerebellum:* motor coordination and motor learning

2. Spinal cord segment is a region of the cord that contains motor, sensory, and autonomic nerves to a specific body region; there are 8 cervical, 12 thoracic, 5 lumbar, and 5 sacral segments.

3. Dura mater, arachnoid, pia mater; meninges surround and protect the brain and spinal cord. The subarachnoid space is deep to the arachnoid and contains cerebrospinal fluid; the epidural space is outside the dura and contains nerve roots.

4.
- *Anterior cerebral artery:* anterior part of frontal lobes
- *Middle cerebral artery:* lateral portion of each cerebral hemisphere; thalamus, hypothalamus
- *Posterior cerebral artery:* occipital lobes, thalamus, midbrain
- *Basilar artery:* pons and cerebellum
- *Vertebral arteries:* medulla oblongata and cerebellum
- *Anterior and posterior spinal arteries:* spinal cord

5. The barrier protects the nerve cells from potentially harmful substances contained in the blood. Oxygen, water, glucose, and amino acids can cross the barrier, as can alcohol and many drugs.

CHAPTER 3

1.
- *Cell body:* contains DNA; makes proteins for cell
- *Dendrites:* extensions of cell body; other neurons form synapses with dendrites
- *Axon:* long process that connects neuron to other cells
- *Axon terminals:* end of axons that form synapses with other cells

2. Each kind of gated ion channel opens its gate in response to a different kind of stimulus. Modality-gated channels open in response to a physical stimulus such as touch or vibration. Ligand-gated channels open when a chemical binds (attaches) to them. Voltage-gated channels open when there is a significant change in ion concentrations across the neuron cell membrane (a change in membrane voltage or potential).

3. When the neuron is at rest, the inside of the cell contains large, negatively charged molecules so the inside has an overall negative charge. The outside of the cell has many positively charged ions, primarily Na^+. The difference in charges across the cell membrane is called the resting membrane potential; its average value is about −70 mV.

4. Action potentials are generated when a stimulus causes enough gated ion channels to open so that there will be a large Na^+ influx into the neuron. The Na^+ influx constitutes the action potential.

5. Action potentials move along the neuron in the direction of the axon terminal. As each section of membrane depolarizes, some Na^+ channels in the next section open, whereas channels in the previous section close. In myelinated axons, the myelin sheath insulates the axon. Small gaps in the myelin called *nodes of Ranvier* contain many ion channels, so that the action potential can "hop" from one node to the next. This is called *saltatory conduction*. It allows the action potential to move about 100 times faster.

6. Astrocytes stimulate formation of the blood-brain barrier to protect neurons. Oligodendroglial cells form myelin in the brain and spinal cord. Microglia remove dead and dying cells, whereas ependymal cells secrete cerebrospinal fluid. These four cells are all found in the central nervous system. Schwann cells are located in the peripheral nervous system, where they form the myelin sheath covering peripheral nerve axons.

7. If a neuron's cell body is damaged, the neuron will die and not be replaced. In the CNS, damage to an axon usually causes the whole cell to die. However, in the peripheral nervous system, damage to an axon is not fatal; the axon degenerates and then regrows until it finds a target cell with which to connect. If the neuron forms a synapse, it will survive.

CHAPTER 4

1. This would be a diagram (Figure 4-1).

2. Action potentials cause an inflow of Ca^{2+} ions in axon terminals; this results in exocytosis of the neurotransmitter into the synaptic cleft. The neurotransmitter diffuses across to the postsynaptic membrane and binds to its receptor. Binding causes the postsynaptic cell to depolarize (stimulatory synapse) or be inhibited (inhibitory synapse).

3. Neuromuscular junction = acetylcholine. Parkinson disease = dopamine. Pain = substance P. Learning = glutamate. Seizures = glutamate, GABA. Spasticity = GABA.

4. Learning is correlated with synaptogenesis, the development of new synapses. A synapse could be pruned if it is seldom activated.

CHAPTER 5

1.

Region	Function	Effects of a Lesion
Primary motor	Controls contralateral muscles	Contralateral paralysis
Premotor	Body image and awareness; controls trunk and proximal limb muscles	Unilateral neglect
Supplementary motor	Motor planning, motor memory	Motor planning deficit (apraxia)
Broca's expressive language	Expressive language (speech)	Expressive aphasia
Prefrontal	Thinking, planning, emotion, impulse control	Prefrontal syndrome
Primary somatosensory	Somatosensory awareness/perception	Sensory loss, contralateral side
Somatosensory association	Interpretation of somatosensory stimuli	Astereognosis
Parietotemporal association	Reading, writing, mathematical skills, abstract thinking	Dyslexia, dysgraphia, dyscalculia
Primary visual	Visual perception	Cortical blindness
Visual association	Interpretation of visual stimuli	Visual agnosia
Primary auditory	Auditory perception	Hearing loss
Auditory association	Interpretation of auditory stimuli	Auditory agnosia

Continued

Region	Function	Effects of a Lesion
Wernicke's receptive language	Understanding of language	Wernicke's/receptive aphasia
Inferotemporal	Recognition of faces, colors	Prosopagnosia
Primary olfactory	Olfactory perception	Anosmia or olfactory hallucinations
Amygdala	Strong negative emotion: fear and anger	Loss of fear or uncontrolled rage
Hippocampus	Long-term memory formation	Anterograde amnesia

2. The left hemisphere usually controls language, and the right side controls nonverbal communication and musical abilities.

3.
- *Speech/language:* Broca's expressive and Wernicke's receptive language centers
- *Vision:* primary visual and visual association cortices
- *Thinking and problem solving:* prefrontal cortex and inferotemporal cortex
- *Movement:* primary motor, premotor, and supplementary motor areas
- *Sensory perception:* primary somatosensory cortex

4. Areas that take up the most space on the motor homunculus are body regions containing many small muscles that perform delicate, precise movements: lips, tongue, vocal cord muscles, and fingers. Areas that take up the most space on the somatosensory cortex are those with a high density of sensory receptors: lips, tongue, face, and fingertips. These areas require many nerve cells and are controlled very precisely by the brain.

CHAPTER 6

1.

Nucleus	Function
Sensory relay	Relay sensation from one side of body to opposite side sensory cortex
Special sensory relay	Relay vision and sound to visual or auditory cortex
Motor	Project to motor cortex
Association	Regulate emotion
Nonspecific	Maintain consciousness
Reticular	Regulate relay nuclei

2. The hypothalamus regulates basic body functions such as drinking and eating. It controls the autonomic nervous system that regulates blood pressure, and releases hormones that affect elimination of fluid in the kidney. The hypothalamus also controls the body's endocrine system via the pituitary gland.

3. Thalamic syndrome is characterized by severe intractable pain that does not usually go away. Patients may display extreme pain when touched or moved.

CHAPTER 7

1.

Region	Structure	Function
Midbrain	Red nucleus	Motor coordination
	Substantia nigra	Produces dopamine
	Superior colliculus	Visual relay nucleus

Continued

Region	Structure	Function
	Inferior colliculus	Auditory relay nucleus
Pons	Connections to cerebellum	Ataxia and balance disorders
Medulla Oblongata	Dorsal respiratory nucleus	Controls breathing by contracting diaphragm
	Inferior olive	Motor error detector

2. The reticular formation is responsible for mood, modification of pain, sleep/wake cycles, and motivation. The ascending reticular activating system (ARAS) is part of the reticular formation, and it is responsible for maintaining consciousness. A lesion to the ARAS can result in coma or a vegetative state.

3. This question is answered by Summary Box 7-1 (Cranial Nerves).

SUMMARY BOX 7-1: CRANIAL NERVES

Number	Name	Function	Effect of a Lesion	Test
1	Olfactory	Smell (olfactory perception)	Anosmia (loss of sense of smell)	Wave peppermint oil or vanilla under patient's nose
2	Optic	Visual perception	Blindness (loss of visual perception)	Ask if patient can see object on far wall and close up
3	Oculomotor	Eye movement	Diplopia (double vision)	Ask patient to track object by moving the eyes
		Pupil constriction, lens accommodation (for far/near vision)	Dilated pupil, loss of accommodation	Shine light into eyes; see if pupils constrict
4	Trochlear	Eye movement	Diplopia (double vision)	Ask patient to track object by moving the eyes
5	Trigeminal	Sensation to face (includes teeth, tongue, dura mater)	Loss of sensation on face and inside mouth	Touch patient's forehead, cheek, and chin with wisp of cotton or paper
		Movement of jaw (mastication or chewing)	Paralysis of jaw muscles	Ask patient to move jaw and make chewing motions; watch for symmetry
6	Abducens	Eye movement	Diplopia (double vision)	Ask patient to track object by moving the eyes laterally

Continued

Number	Name	Function	Effect of a Lesion	Test
7	Facial	Muscles of facial expression; move face to convey emotion	Facial paralysis	Ask patient to smile, raise eyebrows, close eyes
		Taste to anterior tongue	Loss of taste (aguesia)	Place a drop of juice or soda on tongue with dropper
		Production of tears and saliva	Dry eye, dry mouth	Ask patient if there are problems with dry eye or mouth
		Sensation to palate and pharynx (part)	Loss of sensation on palate	None
8	Vestibulo-cochlear (acoustic)	Balance and hearing	Vertigo, unilateral hearing loss	Test hearing by holding watch a few inches from one ear (do this in a quiet room)
9	Glosso-pharyngeal	Sensation to pharynx, palate, posterior tongue, carotid sinus, and carotid body	Loss of blood pressure control, loss of gag reflex (can cause choking)	Ask patient about difficulty swallowing; observe for gagging when eating and/or drinking
		Taste to posterior tongue	Loss of taste (aguesia)	None
		Stylopharyngeus muscle (swallowing)	Difficulty swallowing	None
		Saliva production	Dry mouth	Ask patient about problems with dry mouth
10	Vagus	Sensation to larynx, dura mater, ear, and thoracic and abdominal viscera	Loss of sensation from viscera	None
		Swallowing movements, voice production (controls laryngeal muscles)	Difficulty swallowing, hoarse voice	Ask patient about difficulty swallowing; listen for hoarse voice

Continued

Number	Name	Function	Effect of a Lesion	Test
		Controls viscera of thorax and abdomen	Rapid heart rate, decreased digestive functions	None
		Taste to back of throat	Loss of taste, back of throat	None
11	Spinal accessory	Contraction of sternocleidomastoid and trapezius muscles	Weakness in neck and shoulder movements	Ask patient to shrug shoulders and rotate neck
12	Hypoglossal	Tongue movements	Paralysis and atrophy of tongue	Ask patient to stick out tongue; watch for symmetry

CHAPTER 8

1. Central grey matter is divided into three horns: anterior/ventral, lateral, and posterior/dorsal. Peripheral white matter is divided into regions: anterior/ventral, lateral, and posterior/dorsal. White matter contains ascending and descending tracts; grey matter contains neuron cell bodies. Cord contains 30 segments: 8 cervical, 12 thoracic, 5 lumbar, and 5 sacral. Cord is covered by three layers of meninges: pia mater, arachnoid, and dura mater. Cerebrospinal fluid is located deep to arachnoid.

2.

Pathway	Type of Sensation	Location
Anterior spinothalamic	Light touch, pressure	Anterior white matter
Lateral spinothalamic	Pain, temperature	Lateral white matter
Dorsal columns	Conscious proprioception, vibration, two-point discriminative touch	Posterior white matter
Spinocerebellar	Unconscious proprioception	Lateral white matter

3.

Pathway	Function	Location
Lateral corticospinal	Voluntary movement, all body muscles	Lateral white matter
Anterior corticospinal	Voluntary movement, upper extremity	Anterior white matter
Reticulospinal	Muscle tone	Lateral white matter
Vestibulospinal	Posture and balance	Lateral white matter

4. Anterior spinal artery supplies anterior two-thirds; posterior spinal arteries supply posterior one-third; segmental arteries supply lateral portion.

5. Classified by lesion level, by lowest functional level, by number of limbs affected, by whether they are complete or incomplete.

6. Sensory loss in dermatomes at and below the physical lesion level; flaccid paralysis in myotomes at the lesion level and spastic paralysis below. A deep tendon reflex test can distinguish a flaccid muscle (no detectable contraction) from a spastic/hypertonic muscle (a hyperactive response).

7. Diaphragm is innervated by C4, intercostal muscles by thoracic nerves, and abdominal wall muscles by lower thoracic and lumbar nerves. Injury at or above C4 paralyzes diaphragm; injury above thoracic/lumbar levels paralyzes intercostals and abdominal muscles that assist with respiration. Bladder, bowel, and genitals innervated by S2–S4; injury at or above sacral levels causes loss of voluntary control and sensation from these organs.

CHAPTER 9

1. Spinal nerves all contain somatosensory, voluntary motor, and sympathetic neurons. Each axon is wrapped in endoneurium; each group of axons (fascicle) is wrapped by perineurium, and each peripheral nerve is covered by epineurium.

2. A plexus is a network of axons (nerve fibers). The cervical plexus innervates the neck and diaphragm; the brachial plexus innervates the upper extremity; the lumbar plexus innervates the lower extremity; and the sacral plexus innervates the lower extremity and pelvic floor.

3. Following injury, axons degenerate. After that, new axons sprout from the cell body and form a growth cone that elongates until it reaches a target and creates a new synapse. Scar tissue can impair regeneration. Connective tissue and Schwann cells can assist regeneration and guide the growth cone toward its target.

CHAPTER 10

1.

Organ	Sympathetic Effect	Parasympathetic Effect
Heart	Faster and stronger beat	Slower beat, less forceful
Bronchi	Dilation, more airflow	Constriction, less airflow
Adrenal gland	Stimulation; adrenalin released into blood	None
Skeletal muscle	Increased blood flow	None
Digestive tract	Decreased function	Increased function
Skin	Decreased blood flow	None
Sweat glands	Stimulation	None
Salivary glands	Less saliva	More saliva
Bladder	Urinary retention	Urine release
Penis/clitoris	Emission/ejaculation	Erection/lubrication
Pancreas	Increased blood sugar	Decreased blood sugar
Pupil	Dilation	Constriction

2.
- *Alpha receptors:* sweat glands, arterioles to skeletal muscle
- *Beta-1 receptors:* heart, blood vessels, GI tract
- *Beta-2 receptors:* bronchi
- Beta blockers slow the heart; asthma medications stimulate beta-2 receptors to increase airflow to the lungs. Cocaine and amphetamines increase norepinephrine levels and mimic a sympathetic response, including increased heart rate and blood pressure.

3. Central autonomic fibers connect the hypothalamus in the brain to the autonomic nerves. This allows the brain to control function of the autonomics.

4. Autonomic dysreflexia is caused by overactivity of the sympathetic neurons and usually follows a traumatic injury. Signs and symptoms include red, shiny skin, swelling, and excruciating pain. It is thought that this is caused by hypersensitivity of pain receptors due to overactive sympathetic nerve cells.

CHAPTER 11

1.

Sensation(s)	Receptor(s)	Ascending (sensory) Tract
Pressure, texture, light touch, stretching of the skin	Merkel's discs, Ruffini endings, hair follicle receptors	Anterior spinothalamic
Pain, temperature	Nociceptors, thermal receptors	Lateral spinothalamic
Vibration, two-point discriminative touch, conscious proprioception	Pacinian corpuscles, Meissner's corpuscles, joint receptors	Dorsal columns
Unconscious proprioception	Muscle spindles, Golgi tendon organs	Spinocerebellar

2. All ascending tracts that reach somatosensory cortex contain axons that cross over from one side of the spinal cord or brainstem to the other side on their way to the cortex. Thus, damage to the cortex causes loss of sensation on the opposite side of the body.

   Acute pain results from direct injury to tissue and the resulting inflammation. It directs attention to the injured area and encourages behaviors that promote healing. Acute pain is usually of short duration, ending once the injury heals. *Nociceptive pain* is pain caused by long-term stimulation of pain receptors, usually resulting from chronic diseases or conditions. *Neuropathic pain* is caused by direct injury to neurons.

CHAPTER 12

1. Light enters the eye through the cornea, passes through the lens, and strikes photoreceptors on the retina. Light activates chemical reactions in the rods and cones, generating action potentials that travel in the optic nerve to the brain.

2. The optic nerve connects to the brainstem for visual reflexes, to the hypothalamus for sleep/wake cycles, and to the primary visual cortex for visual perception. From the primary visual cortex, the "what" pathway connects to the temporal lobe for identification of people and objects by sight, and the "where" pathway connects to the parietal lobe for spatial location.

3.

Region	Effect of Lesion
Eye	Loss of vision in the ipsilateral eye
Retina	Loss of vision in the ipsilateral eye
Optic nerve	Loss of vision in the ipsilateral eye
Optic tract	Loss of vision in contralateral visual field
Primary visual cortex (unilateral)	Loss of vision in contralateral visual field
Primary visual cortex (bilateral)	Cortical blindness

4. Sound waves are transmitted through the middle ear via movement of the auditory ossicles. This causes movement of the oval window, and movement of endolymph within the cochlea. Endolymph movement causes motion of the hair cells in the cochlea, which generates action potentials that are transmitted to the brain via the vestibulocochlear nerve. Hearing is perceived in the auditory cortex, located in the temporal lobe.

5. The vestibular system is located in the inner ear, where vestibular receptors respond to movement of the head and generate action potentials. These travel to the brain in the vestibulocochlear nerve.

6. In Meniere's disease, excess endolymph causes vertigo and hearing loss. People with BPPV experience vertigo but not hearing loss.

7. Smell receptors are located in the olfactory epithelium inside the nose, and taste receptors are found on the tongue. Olfaction is transmitted to the brain via the olfactory nerve (CN I), and taste is transmitted via three cranial nerves (facial VII, glossopharyngeal IX, and vagus X).

CHAPTER 13

1. Upper motor neurons control lower motor neurons, which activate muscles for voluntary movement. Upper motor neuron lesions cause spasticity and paralysis or paresis, whereas lower motor neurons cause flaccid/hypotonicity and paralysis or paresis.

2. Normal tone is maintained by the gamma loop reflex, and requires sensory neurons as well as both gamma and alpha motor neurons. Tone is adjusted by the brain via descending spinal cord tracts. In particular, the reticulospinal tracts keep tone under control, so injury to this tract results in hypertonicity. Lower motor neuron injuries cause loss of tone (hypotonia).

3. As a whole, the cerebellum is responsible for motor coordination. The vestibulocerebellum controls balance, the spinocerebellum is responsible for coordinating gait and posture, and the cerebrocerebellum coordinates fine movements. Vestibulocerebellar injury causes truncal ataxia, spinocerebellar damage results in gait ataxia, and cerebrocerebellar damage causes coordination dysfunction, including past-pointing, disdiadochokinesis, and intention tremor.

4. The substantia nigra produces dopamine that acts on the basal ganglia to allow movement initiation. Excess dopamine can produce unwanted movements (dyskinesia) and a dopamine deficit can cause movement inhibition (bradykinesia).

5. The supplementary motor area (SMA) is a movement planning region that stores motor memories. Lesions to the SMA cause apraxia, a motor planning deficit.

CHAPTER 14

1. Cognition is mainly located in the lateral part of the cerebral cortex. Cognition is the ability to think, plan, and solve problems. It includes functions such as balancing a checkbook, passing an exam, and reading and writing.

2. Emotion is mainly located in the limbic system on the medial aspect of the cerebral cortex.

3. Declarative learning can be expressed in words, and includes sematic memory (facts and figures) as well as memories of life events. It requires the prefrontal cortex, hippocampus, and cortical association areas of the brain. Nondeclarative learning encompasses motor learning, which requires activity of motor circuits and pathways, but does not involve the hippocampus.

4. Short-term learning involves modifying existing synapses and is reversible. Long-term learning involves synaptogenesis, the creation of new synapses.

5. The brain's major language centers are Broca's motor speech area and Wernicke's receptive speech area. In most people, both of these regions are located in the left hemisphere. Receptive language refers to the ability to understand language, whereas expressive language is the ability to produce language. Lesions to Broca's area cause motor or expressive aphasia, whereas damage to Wernicke's area results in receptive or sensory aphasia.

CHAPTER 15

1. The neural tube forms early in development by formation of a plate of cells that rolls up to create the neural tube. The neural tube has four major subdivisions: forebrain (forms cerebrum, thalamus, and hypothalamus); midbrain; hindbrain (forms pons, cerebellum, and medulla oblongata); and spinal cord. The neural crest gives rise to sensory neurons, autonomic neurons, and the adrenal medulla.

2. There are four cellular processes that are important in nervous system development: mitosis (production of new neurons); migration (movement of neurons); differentiation (specialization); and myelination. Of these, myelination begins prenatally and continues through early adulthood; all others are completed prior to birth. Myelination increases the transmission speed of action potentials.

3. At birth, the nervous system has all neurons in place, some myelination has occurred, and there are relatively few synapses. Stimulation causes synaptogenesis, which is correlated with learning.

4. Describe the cause (if known) and the signs/symptoms associated with each of the following developmental disorders:

Disorder	Cause	Signs/Symptoms
Arnold-Chiari malformation	Unknown	Compression of cerebellum and brainstem
Autism	Genetic	Impaired communication and social interaction
Cerebral palsy	Birth injury or premature birth	Various motor, sensory, language, and cognitive disorders
Down syndrome	Genetic	Cognitive disorder
Epilepsy	Genetic or brain injury	Seizures
Hydrocephalus	Blockage of CSF	Enlargement of ventricles and brain
Spina bifida	Probably genetic; also linked to low folic acid	Sensory and motor loss below level of spinal cord involvement

5. Small loss of neurons and thinning of myelin sheath causes slower transmission of action potentials, decreased sensory sensitivity, and less synaptogenesis.

CHAPTER 16

1. A coupe/contre-coupe injury causes focal lesions, typically on opposite sides of the brain. This results from a strong force exerted on one side of the head that can cause the brain to bang into the opposite side of the skull. Axonal shearing damages axons across the brain and is more likely to affect long axons; this means that the damage cannot be located to any specific region. The same is true of anoxia/hypoxia injuries, caused by lack of blood flow and oxygen delivery to neurons.

2. The major mechanisms of neuroplasticity are axon sprouting (axons make new connections to replace damaged ones); activating parallel pathways (neurons take on new functions); and neurogenesis (new neurons are made and create synapses).

3. Evidence shows that physical exercise, mental stimulation, and social activity all improve the ability of the brain to create and retain new synaptic connections.

APPENDIX D
Answers to Clinical Boxes

CHAPTER 2

2-1   Motor coordination and motor learning.

2-2   Dura mater and arachnoid.

2-3   Sensory nerve roots.

CHAPTER 3

3-1   If Na$^+$ channels in motor axons were blocked, the brain and spinal cord would not be able to send action potentials to skeletal muscles, so there would be muscle weakness (if partially blocked) or paralysis (if completely blocked).

3-2   A medication that decreases immune function would probably improve sensation in a person with multiple sclerosis (MS) because MS is an autoimmune disease, in which the immune system attacks and damages cells that produce myelin. If myelin is healthy, transmission of action potentials will improve.

3-3   Both MS and Guillain-Barre syndrome (GBS) are demyelinating diseases. In MS, myelin is damaged in the central nervous system, whereas in GBS, there is injury to myelin in the peripheral nervous system.

CHAPTER 4

4-1   Dopamine receptors.

4-2   Denervation hypersensitivity might cause excessive muscle contraction or spasms; it could also cause patients to have a very strong response to sensory stimuli (e.g., painful sensations would feel even more painful).

4-3   Excess botulism toxin could paralyze important body muscles, including the diaphragm.

CHAPTER 5

5-1   Paralysis of contralateral upper extremity and face, loss of sensation on contralateral upper extremity and face, and aphasia (if CVA is in left hemisphere).

5-2   Middle cerebral artery (MCA).

5-3   Lateral and inferior part of motor cortex (the portion that controls lip, tongue, and vocal cord muscles).

5-4   Most people with receptive aphasia can still understand nonverbal communication, so gestures and facial expressions can be used to communicate.

CHAPTER 7

7-1   If there are no cells in the substantia nigra making dopamine, there will be no "black stuff" in the midbrain.

7-2   The oculomotor and trochlear nerves control eye movements and arise from the midbrain, so they would be spared from an infarct in the pons.

7-3   Ask the patient to open and close the eyes, or move the eyes to follow a moving target (a pencil or finger works well).

7-4   Since the trigeminal nerve (not the facial nerve) provides sensation to the face, patients with Bell's palsy will have normal facial sensation.

CHAPTER 8

8-1   A positive Babinski sign indicates damage to descending tracts.

8-2   The posterior part of the spinal cord contains the dorsal columns that transmit conscious proprioception, two-point discrimination, and vibration to the brain; these sensations would be lost.

8-3   The lateral spinothalamic tract transmits pain to the brain; this pathway is injured in patients with autonomic dysreflexia.

8-4

    1. Brown-Sequard syndrome.

    2. All of them.

8-5   No, a person with complete spinal cord injury above the sacral levels cannot feel sensation from the genitals.

8-6   Cervical spinal nerves innervate the upper extremity, so any cervical pathology can affect the arms.

CHAPTER 9

9-1   No, because the intercostal muscles assist with exhalation (internal intercostals) and external intercostals (inhalation).

9-2   The median nerve provides sensation to the lateral two-thirds of the palm and digits 1 through 4.

9-3   The piriformis is elongated in internal rotation and adduction while the hip is flexed.

9-4   C5 innervates elbow flexors (biceps brachii, brachialis); C7 innervates elbow extensors (triceps brachii); and L3 innervates knee extensors (quadriceps femoris).

9-5   Lumbosacral level dermatomes would be affected early in Guillain-Barre syndrome.

CHAPTER 10

10-1   Norepinephrine is mainly responsible for producing vasoconstriction to increase systemic blood pressure.

CHAPTER 11

11-1   Local anesthetics block Na^+ channels on small-diameter axons first; these are the axons that carry pain signals to the central nervous system. Touch and pressure are conveyed in larger diameter axons that would be affected only if a large dose of local anesthetic were given.

CHAPTER 12

12-1   Call for help; this is evidence of swelling in the skull and is an emergency situation.

12-2   A patient with tunnel vision will be able to see in the center of each visual field, but not the periphery. Someone with hemianopsia will lose vision in one entire visual field, whereas optic nerve damage causes loss of vision in one eye.

CHAPTER 13

13-1   People with polio would have hypotonia, because polio is a lower motor neuron disease that damages the motor neurons responsible for producing muscle tone.

13-2   Amyotrophic lateral sclerosis (ALS) is a motor neuron disease that does not affect sensory neurons.

13-3   Excess dopamine or a dopamine agonist could produce excessive involuntary movements (dyskinesia).

13-4   An excess of a dopamine antagonist could cause signs and symptoms of Parkinsonism, including bradykinesia, muscle rigidity, postural instability, and resting tremor.

CHAPTER 14

14-1

    1. A patient with a hippocampus injury will have difficulty remembering the parts of the exercise program, because it is required for new long-term learning.

    2. Hippocampal injuries do not usually affect pre-existing memories, since the hippocampus is not needed to access old memories.

14-2   Cortical association areas would be damaged in retrograde amnesia.

14-3   In Alzheimer disease, the hippocampus is often one of the first areas of the brain affected; this will cause problems with the patient's ability to consolidate new long-term memories.

CHAPTER 15

15-1   The bladder and bowel are controlled by spinal cord levels S2-S4, and are often affected in people with spina bifida.

15-2 Drugs used to treat epilepsy decrease neuron activity, so sedation (sleepiness) is a very common side effect.

15-3 All functions located in the cerebral cortex may be affected by prematurity. These include motor deficits, sensory deficits, language problems, and cognitive disabilities.

15-4

1. The hypoglossal nerves (CN XII) innervate muscles of the tongue and are located in the medulla oblongata, so they are vulnerable to injury in Arnold-Chiari malformation.

2. The vestibulocochlear nerves (CN VIII) innervate the inner ear cochlea (for hearing) and vestibular apparatus (for balance); injury to these nerves can cause hearing loss and dizziness.

15-5 The cerebral aqueduct drains cerebrospinal fluid from the third ventricle into the fourth ventricle, so a blockage of the aqueduct will cause fluid to build up in the lateral ventricles and the third ventricle.

15-6 The cerebellum is responsible for coordination, so people with autism may have difficulties coordinating their movements normally.

CHAPTER 16

16-1 Because sensation and movement on each side of the body map to the contralateral side of the brain, using the neglected side of the body will stimulate neuron activity in the damaged side of the brain and promote neuroplasticity.

INDEX

Note: Page numbers with *f* indicate figures; those with *t* indicate tables.

A

Abdominal aortic plexus, 153*f*
Abducens nerve, 87*f*, 92*f*, 93*t*, 96, 192*f*
Accessory nerve, 92*f*, 94*t*, 99, 130*f*, 192*f*
Accommodation, 179
Acetylcholine (ACh), 52*f*, 55–57, 55*t*, 56*f*, 150
Action potential, 40–43, 41*f*, 42*f*
Activation of parallel pathways (rewiring), 259, 260*t*
Acute inflammatory polyneuropathy, 143
Acute pain, 174, 175
Adenosine triphosphate (ATP), 36, 114
Adrenal gland, 147*t*
Adrenal medulla, 148*f*, 153*f*, 242, 243*f*
Adrenergic nerve endings, 150
Adrenergic synapses, 150
Adrenocorticotropic hormone (ACTH), 80*f*
Afferent nerve fibers, 140*t*, 162*f*, 165–67, 166*f*, 166*t*
Afferent nerves, 104, 109*f*
Afferent neurons, 163*f*, 164, 165, 174, 209*f*
After-hyperpolarization, 40
Aging nervous system, 250
Alpha motor neurons, 140, 140*t*, 209, 209*f*, 210*f*, 211*f*
Alzheimer disease (AD), 71, 232, 232*f*
American Spinal Injury Association (ASIA), 116, 118*f*, 137, 138*t*
Amnesia, 73, 229
Amygdala, 72, 72*f*, 92
Amyotrophic lateral sclerosis (ALS), 205, 208
Anencephaly, 238
Anesthetics
  local, 129
  topical, 41
Animal geniuses, 230
Anosmia, 72, 92, 191, 193
Anoxia, 255
Ansa cervicalis, 129, 130*f*
Anterior branch, 134*f*
Anterior cerebral arteries, 24*f*, 25*f*, 26
Anterior cingulate gyrus, 68

Anterior cord syndrome, 121, 122*f*
Anterior corticospinal tract (ACST), 110, 110*t*, 111*f*, 204, 207*f*
Anterior cutaneous branch, 133*f*, 134*f*
Anterior nucleus, 78*f*
Anterior pituitary, 80*f*
Anterior spinal artery, 26, 113–14, 114*f*
Anterior spinocerebellar tract, 172*t*
Anterior spinothalamic tract, 89, 108–9, 108*f*, 167–68, 168*f*
Anterograde amnesia, 4
Anterograde transport, 35, 36*f*
Anterolateral system, 108, 108*f*, 109
Antidiuretic hormone (ADH), 81, 82
Aphasia, 72, 233
Apraxia, 66, 217, 228
Arachnoid, 20, 22*f*, 29*f*
Arachnoid mater, 104*f*
Arachnoid trabeculae, 20–21
Armpit (axilla), 130, 131
Arnold-Chiari malformation, 247, 247*f*, 248
Arteries
  basilar, 23, 24*f*, 26
  brain, 23–26, 24*f*
  carotid, 23, 24*f*
  cerebral, 24*f*, 25*f*, 26
  spinal, 26
  vertebral, 23, 24*f*
Arterioles in skeletal muscle, 151*t*
Arteriosclerotic plaque, 23
Ascending reticular activating system (ARAS), 91
Ascending tracts, 106–10, 106*t*
  dorsal columns, 106–7, 107*f*
  somatosensory, 167, 167*t*
  spinocerebellar, 109–10, 109*f*
  spinothalamic, 89*f*, 108–9, 108*f*
Association areas, cortical, 226, 227*f*
Association fibers, 62, 64*f*
Association nuclei, 76